Welcome to ...

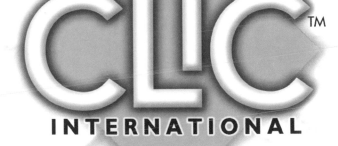

CLIC™
INTERNATIONAL

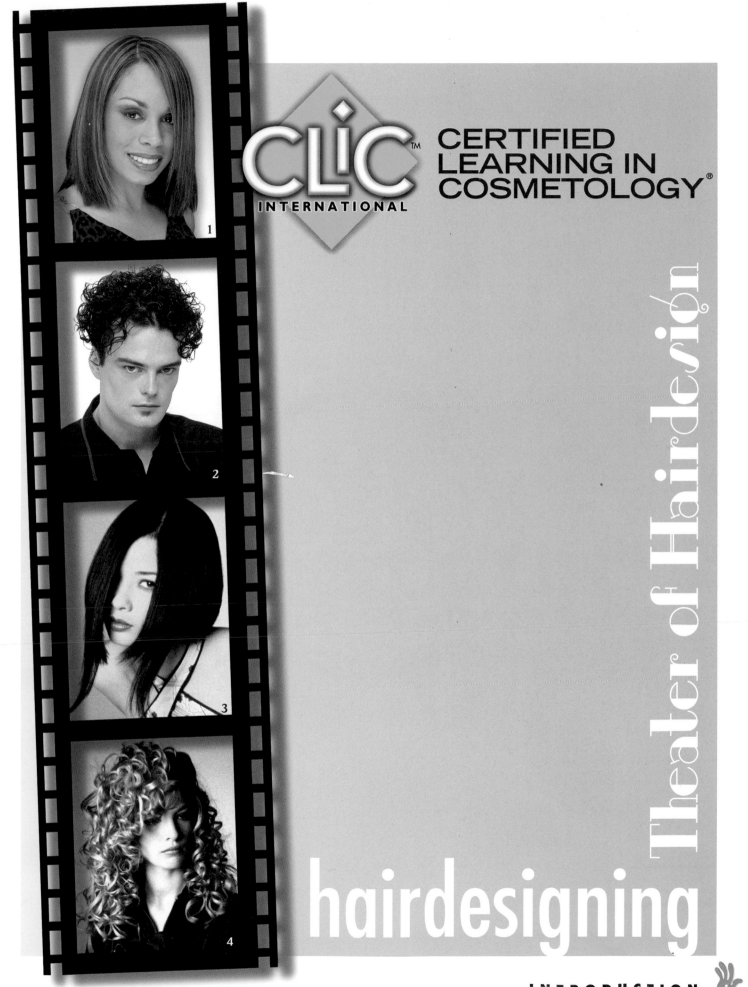

CLiC™ INTERNATIONAL

CERTIFIED LEARNING IN COSMETOLOGY®

Theater of Hairdesign

hairdesigning

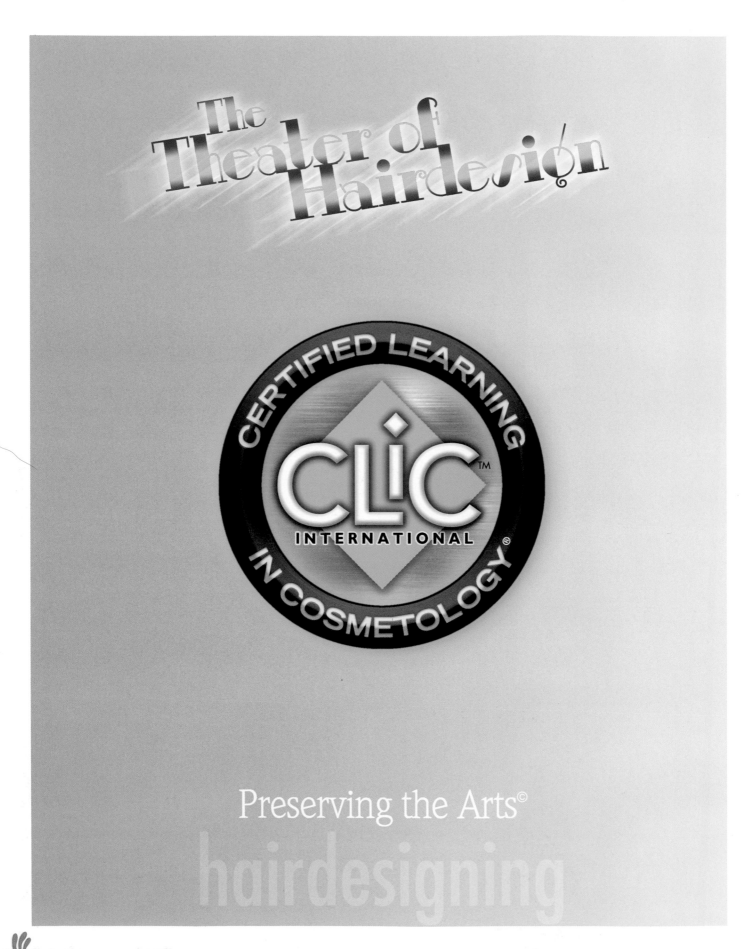

The Theater of Hairdesign

CERTIFIED LEARNING

CLiC™

INTERNATIONAL®

IN COSMETOLOGY

Preserving the Arts©

hairdesigning

Dedication...

Special thanks to all the dedicated teachers and educational support staff members who unselfishly devote their time and energy to make a difference in the lives of their students.

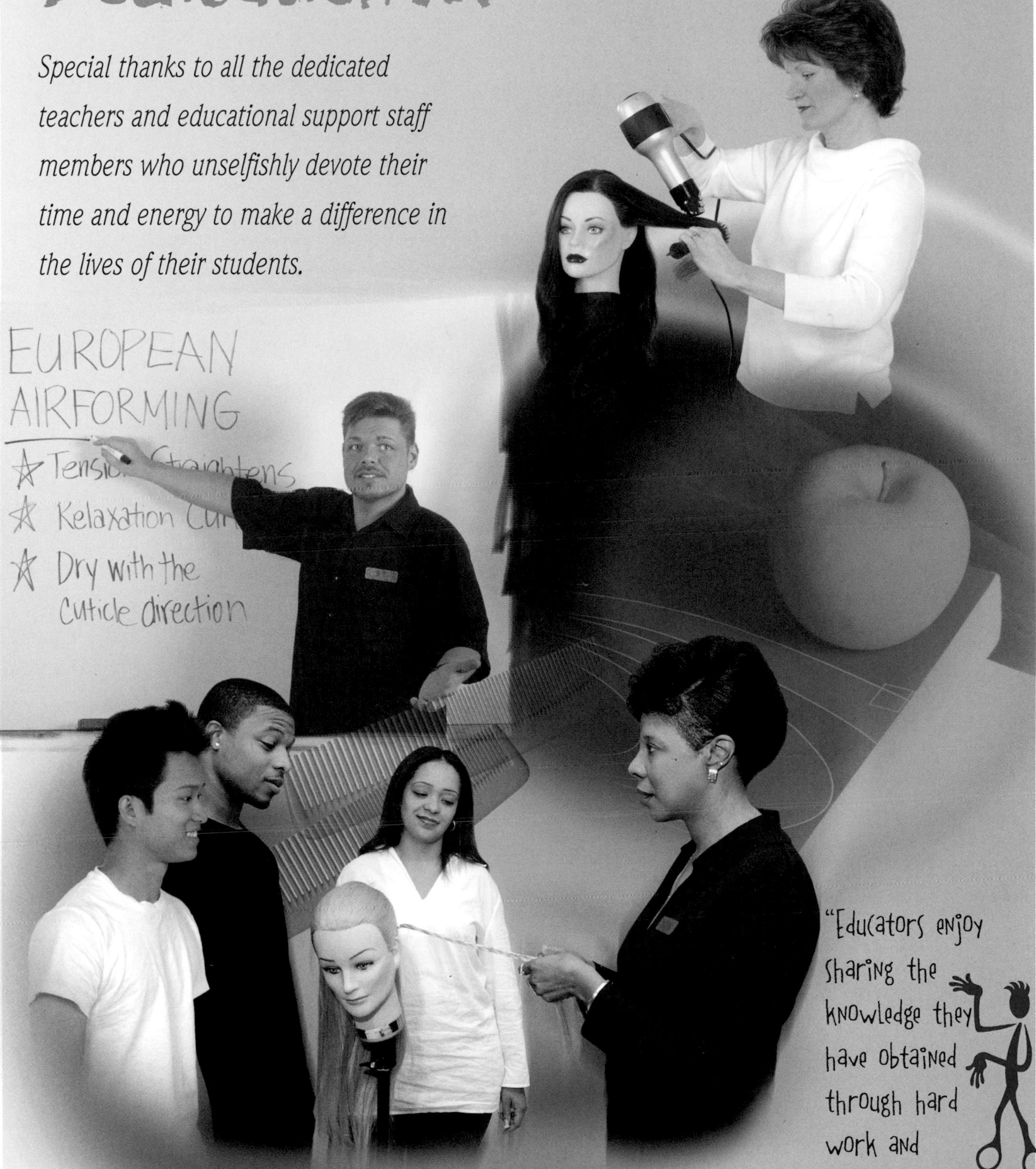

EUROPEAN
AIRFORMING
★ Tension Straightens
★ Relaxation Cur...
★ Dry with the
   cuticle direction

"Educators enjoy sharing the knowledge they have obtained through hard work and experience. They deserve admiration and respect."

SPECIAL ACKNOWLEDGEMENTS

Chapter 2 Tools Contributors:
Golden Supreme, Inc., Santa FE Springs, CA
Helen of Troy
Marianna Industries
Marilyn Brush Company

Chapter 9 Hair Extension Contributor:
Charlotte Jayne/Garland Drake International

CLiC Artists and Hair Style Contributors:
Ben DeCordova
Lyal McCaig
Maria Garcia
Randy Rick
Ron Hawkins

CLiC Photo Shoot
Contributors:
Dorothy Hayward
Ella Jarrett
Linda Kleckley
Lorrie Weinhold
Randy Rick
Theresa Kysniak

Director of Education
Margie Wagner

Curriculum Development
Manager
Theresa Ksyniak

CLiC Photographer
John Dalton

Illustration
Laura Gelsomini

Graphic Design
James Wosochlo

Graphic Design Intern
Jennifer Smoot

History Tool Artifacts
Joseph Dave Rose

Layout, Design and
Illustration
Condict and Company

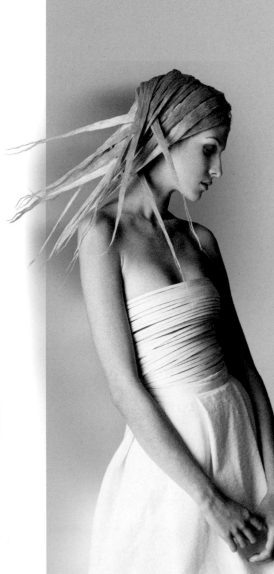

HAIR

Artist page(picture number)

CREDITS AND ACKNOWLEDGEMENTS

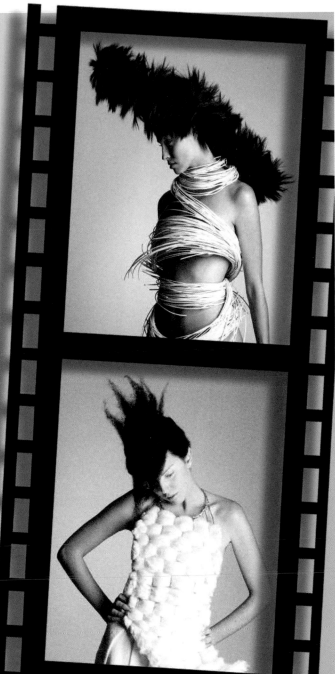

Larhonda Fields – Royal Designs 207(3)

Latonia Vasquez – Hair of Essence 207(2)

Maria Norman 24(1), 240(1)

Michael Christopher Salon 147, 160(2), 211(3)

Monica Summers – Salon Jon'z 22(8)

Morris Gargiule 159(2)

Ms. Scottie – T.B.C. Salon 251(2)

Nacole Brown – Wave Links Hair Studio 366

Nancy Burris – Jenniffer & Company Hair Salon
164(2)

Olive Benson
131(1), 312(4), 328(1), 329(1), 408(1), 412(1)

Olivia Hughes 314(4), 320(2), 321(3)

Patrick Bradley –
True Perfection Salon, Houston, TX 29(2)

Randee Rick 231

Randy Rick 194, 218(3), 246(1), 257(1)

Renea Smith – Hair Biz, Inc. 408(9), 414(1)

Richard Weintraub –
Yellow Strawberry Global Salon 24(3)

Robert Andrew – The Salon & Spa
103(5), 195(1), 251(3)

Ron Hawkins
Front Cover, 12(1), 18(1), 22(2), 156(1), 160(6),
196(1), 203, 219(2), 221(1), 226, 239(3),
368(1,2)

Salon Visage 212(4)

Sammy Jones 408(11), 414(3)

Sandra Carr – Sheer Professionals Salon 121(3)

Sanita Elliott – Bradcon International,
Norfolk, VA 20(2)

Sharon Thorton – Wilkes /
Dazz Unique Hair Salon 216(4)

Shay – House of Finesse 89(2), 160(1), 227(1)

Shear Pleasure – By Jeffrey Marshall 408(17)

Sheer Professionals Salon
132(1), 163(2), 198(2), 313(7), 323(2)

Sherry Gordon Salon & Spa 409(1)

Shonda Harris – Davis Hair Design 408(3), 412(3)

Shortino's Salon & Spa 23(1,2), 118(3)

Stephan Wake - Focas Salon
16(1), 27(2), 123(3), 223

Sullo Salon & Day Spa 147, 413(3)

Susan Snow 26(3)

Tanya Dickens – Professional Image Salon
165(1), 181(5), 238(6), 409(2)

Tasha Lea – Studio 2000 129(4)

Tawny & Company 22(6), 107(3), 133(3)

Teresa Walker – New Age Hair Salon
313(3), 331(2)

The Brown Aveda Institute 102(6)

The Elite Group Hair Studio/Ft. Lauderdale, FL
28(2), 122(1), 160(4)

The Hairbenders International Design Team
122(2), 147, 195(2), 313(1), 329(2), 408(5)

The Oak Street Hair Group
27(1), 123(1), 205(1), 212(3), 213(5), 227(3)

The Spa at Margo Blue 313(4), 320(1), 321(2)

Tobi Brown – Hair Biz, Inc. 209(2), 214(3), 408(21)

Tobi Brown – Tobi Corp. 230(5), 239(1)

Toni & Guy Advanced Hairdressing Academy
www.Toniguy.com 408(16)

Torie M. Huff – Hair Studio 403 204(2)

Traci Johnson – Total Eclipse Day Spa 217(2)

Ursula Kershaw – Shear Creations by Ursula
89(3), 124(3), 155(4)

Vanis Salon & Day Spa
135(1), 161(1), 216(1), 408(15)

Velma Wooten – By Grace Styling Salon
408(2), 412(2)

Victoria Station Salon 147, 313(2), 327(2)

Vince D'Attilio 161(4), 314(7), 322(2), 323(3)

Wendy Graham – Posses Styling Emporium
314(3), 330(2), 331(3)

Yellow Strawberry Global Salon
119(3), 313(6), 317(2), 408(13)

Zolanda Broom – Images of Hair and Nails
228(1)

"A special thanks to all the professionals who provided their photo images to support the education of future cosmetologists. These images show the rewards of mastering the artistry of hairdesigning."

PHOTOGRAPHY

Artist page(picture number)

Andres Aquino
20(5), 102(1,2,8), 103(1,2,7,8), all background photos on 102 & 103, 208(3), 230(3,4)

Archie Carpenter 89(1), 312(8), 332(1), 333(1)

Brion Price Photography
117, 157, 161(7), 196(2), 230(1), 409(4), 410(3,4), 411(4), 413(2)

Burning House Band 210(1)

Calvin Childs 68(1)

Capitol School of Hairstyling 308

Chip Foust for www.universalsalons.com
22(1,5,8), 29(4), 89(2,3,4), 121(2), 123(2), 124(1,2,3), 125(2,3), 129(3,4), 135(4), 147, 155(4), 159(4), 160(1), 161(2), 165(1) 174, 181(5), 204(2), 207(2,3,4), 209(2), 214(1,3), 216(4), 217(1,2,4), 227(1), 228(1), 230(5), 238(2,4,6), 239(1), 251(2), 313(3), 314(1,3,8), 326(2),327(3), 330(2), 331(2,,3),332(2), 333(3), 338(1), 349(1), 366, 408(2,3,9,12,21), 409(2), 410(1), 411(2), 412(2,3), 413(4), 414(1,4)

Curtis Spratlin
131(1), 312(4), 328(1), 329(1), 408(1), 412(1)

Dexter Cohen20(2)

Don Nyne 160(3)(5), 218(2), 239(2)

Edward Brown 1(3,4),4, 5

Edward Tytel 119(1), 314(2), 316(1), 317(3)

Elite USA Publishing
313(5), 314(6), 324(2), 325(3), 333(2)

Ernest Washington
19(1), 101(2), 102(7), 107(2), 128(1), 133(5), 147

Fromm International
69(2), 135 (6)(9), 147, 164(1), 229(2)

Garland Drake International
371(1), 374, 386, 387, 369(1)

Insights Technical Cutting Guide
Intra-America Beauty Network
www.inspirequarterly.com 1(2), 408(16)

Jack Cutler
22(9), 24(1), 26(3), 135(8), 159(1,2,3), 242(1), 312(1), 314(4), 320(2), 321(3), 324(1), 325(1) 408(8)

Jonathan Martin
8(1), 102(4), 155(2), 314(5)(9), 318(2), 319(3), 328(2), 329(3), 410(2)

Jonathan Roth 251(4)

Marge Nauratil 408(10), 414(2)

Paul Spinak 408(11), 414(3)

Renbow International 78, 79(1)

Robert Sargent
17(1,2), 20(1), 21(2), 23(3), 24(2), 25(1), 28(1,4,5), 29(3), 129(2), 133(1), 151(1,2), 156(2), 181(2,3), 195(3), 217(3), 239(4), 242(2), 400, 408(20)

Ron Rubin 20(4)

Salon Styler.com 82

Scott Bryant 211(2), 251(1)

Sean Sharp 29(2)

The Bell Group,
Albuquerque, NM
116 (gemstones)

Tom Carson
1(1), 7, 16(1), 22(6-7), 23(1-2),24(3-5), 26(1), 27(1-2), 28(2), 29(1), 70(1), 101(1), 102(3,5,6), 103(3-5), 106(1), 107(1,3-5), 113(1,5,11), 118(2-3), 119(2-3), 121(1,3), 122(1-3), 123(1,3), 125(1), 127(1-4), 128(3), 131(2), 132(1), 133(2-3), 135(1-3,5), 147, 154, 155(1), 158, 160(2)(4), 161(1,4), 163(1,2), 164(2,4), 165(3), 181(4), 194, 195(1,2), 198(1,2), 204(1,3), 205(1), 207(5), 208(1), 209(1), 210(2), 211(1)(3), 212, 213(2-5), 214(2), 215(1), 216(1), 223, 227(2-3), 229(1), 251(3), 312(2-3,5,6,9), 313(1,2,4,6-9), 314(7), 317(1,2), 318(1), 319(1,2), 320(1), 321(1,2), 322(2), 323(2,3), 325(2), 326(1), 327(1,2), 329(2), 330(1), 331(1), 408(4-6,13,14-15,17-18), 409(1,3), 412(4), 413(3)

All photographs ©2005 Tom Carson, All Rights Reserved.

William Marvy Company 75(1)

Foreword...

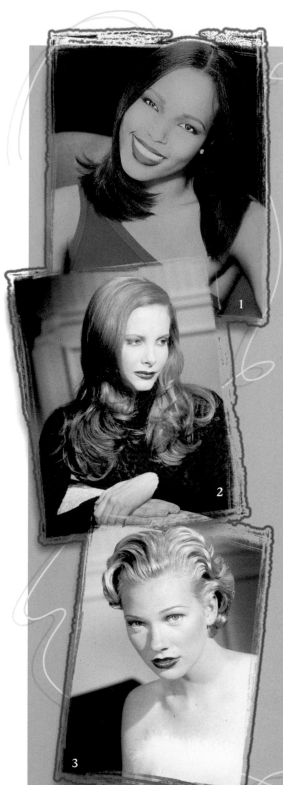

Sir Isaac Newton once said, **"If I have been able to see further, it was only because I stood on the shoulders of giants."** This profound statement represents one of the guiding principles of the Certified Learning in Cosmetology® (CLiC) system. There is much to be learned and discovered by "standing on the shoulders of giants." It is only by studying the discoveries and accomplishments of the leaders who came before us that we can prepare for the future.

The CLiC system provides a broad cosmetology education with a focus on three key areas:
1- A basic cosmetology foundation
2- An introduction to artistic concepts and visual inspiration to nurture creativity
3- Effective interpersonal, sales and retail techniques

Although the cosmetology industry is continually evolving, its basic foundation remains unchanged.
The foundation of cosmetology is an understanding of human biology combined with scientific and mathematic concepts used to create desired results. Building on the basic foundation of cosmetology, artistic concepts and visual inspiration are explored to develop and nurture creativity. Throughout the foundational and artistic learning process, successful interpersonal, sales and retail skills are introduced and practiced. These skills are paramount to the financial success of the professional cosmetologist.

CLiC is a visually exciting and inspirational education system focused on preparing students to be salon-ready upon completion of their studies. Master hairdesigner and international award winner Randy Rick is the creative force behind this revolutionary CLiC system. Always a step ahead, Mr. Rick developed the CLiC system of learning to elevate the artistic and practical skills of today's students. Through the CLiC program, he shares his vast international knowledge and experience with you, the cosmetology professional of the future!

CLiC to a dynamic future in hairdesign!

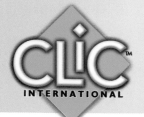

The CLiC Education Team ...

The CLiC Education Team represents more than 100 years of combined cosmetology industry education, experience and wisdom. The team includes international award winners, top educators, stylists, salon and beauty school owners, operations managers and owners/operators of highly successful cosmetology businesses.

Randy Rick
Artist-Teacher-Champion

Having won more than 75 national and international honors and awards, Randy Rick, Vice President of Creative for Empire Beauty Schools, is one of America's most awarded hairdesigners. He is also the former owner of a beauty school, as well as full-service beauty salons and is a graduate of Empire Beauty Schools Teacher's Program.

This background, combined with his artistic genius, makes Mr. Rick uniquely qualified to share his educational vision for the future of the beauty industry. The Certified Learning in Cosmetology system was developed by Mr. Rick in an effort to take standard cosmetology education beyond its current scope providing students at Empire with the best cosmetology education available in the industry. The companion Teacher's Guides were created in conjunction with the Empire Educational Team to help instructors impart the classic principles of the CLiC system.

Starring the CLiC Education Team

Lights! Camera! Action!

"WOW! What a team! You're in great hands with these industry experts. Enjoy your exploration and study of the art of precision hairdesigning."

You are about to begin an exciting journey into the world of cosmetology. The Certified Learning in Cosmetology® (CLiC) system will act as your road map, leading you to reap the rewards of becoming a successful professional cosmetologist.

The CLiC system is designed to enhance fundamental cosmetology education by incorporating artistic inspiration and successful salon service and retail skills. The learning modules cannot possibly cover all vogues, but will always encourage freedom of expression and innovation to adapt to current trends.

This revolutionary system focuses on meeting your educational needs with a solid, competency-based cosmetology curriculum. Each CLiC module is designed to develop manual dexterity, professional perception, tactile sensitivity and the artistic vision used in the field.

The CLiC educational system is presented in individual learning modules, each a complete program. The module system enables you to focus on individual disciplines within the field by offering courses for certified specialization in each field. This ensures the opportunity to learn and develop the skills needed for a rewarding and profitable career in the cosmetology field of your choice.

For additional information, contact:

CLiC INTERNATIONAL®
396 Pottsville/Saint Clair Highway
Pottsville, PA 17901 USA
1.800.207.5400 USA & Canada
001.570.429.4216 International
1.570.429.4252 Fax
info@clicusa.com
www.clicusa.com

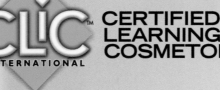

CLiC INTERNATIONAL ™

CERTIFIED LEARNING IN COSMETOLOGY®

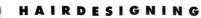

Cast of Characters . . .

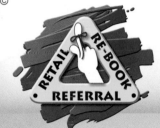

"Hello! My name is CLiCer (pronounced Click-er), and I am your personal tour guide to each of the fields of cosmetology.

In this book, we will be studying hairdesigning. I will lead you and encourage you as we explore the artistic principles, history and techniques of hairdesigning.

Welcome! I'm happy that you will join me for this journey of learning."

Regulatory Alert

Whenever you see the shadow of the **Regulatory Alert** icon, it will remind you and your instructor to check governmental regulations about the subject on the page. The rules and regulations for cosmetology vary according to geographic location. Place a sticker from the back of the book over the shadow if there are governmental regulations that must be followed in your area.

The 3R's

At the conclusion of your services there are three important steps you should consistently follow. **Retail** professional products to your customers for home maintenance. This provides a strong supplement to your income. **Re-book** future appointments to encourage regular visits. Ask for **referrals** to strengthen your customer base. By following the 3R's you will improve your income and profitability as a professional cosmetologist.

CLiCer's Sales Pointers

As you will learn throughout this book, selling and financial skills will be just as important to your success in the salon as your actual hairdesigning knowledge and skills. Whenever you see this icon with CLiCer's hand, pay special attention to the **sales pointers** you are given. Combining sales skills with hairdesigning skills will create a dynamic force for your salon success.

1

The theater is a space shared by performers and audience as living art is created. **Hair fashion is also living art.** In the hands of a skilled stylist, hair becomes a medium of expression — not only of the artistry of the hairstylist, but also, more importantly, of the lifestyle and personality of the client.

The **Hairdesigning Module** will teach you and help you rehearse the skills and techniques of the professional hairstylist. You will become familiar with the tools of the trade, the power and beauty of human biology, and the mathematics that are used to create aesthetically pleasing hairdesigns.

You will master principles of art and design. You will train your mind, your eyes, your hands and your creative intuition to work in harmony.

Through the pages of this book and through your own practice and exploration you will learn how to create hairdesigns that **enhance the appearance and lifestyle of your clients.**

"Learn to see yourself as a performer and an artist. The salon is your theater and hair is your medium."

Table of Contents...

"For information about additional modules, check out the last page of this book."

Table of Contents

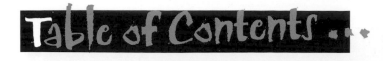

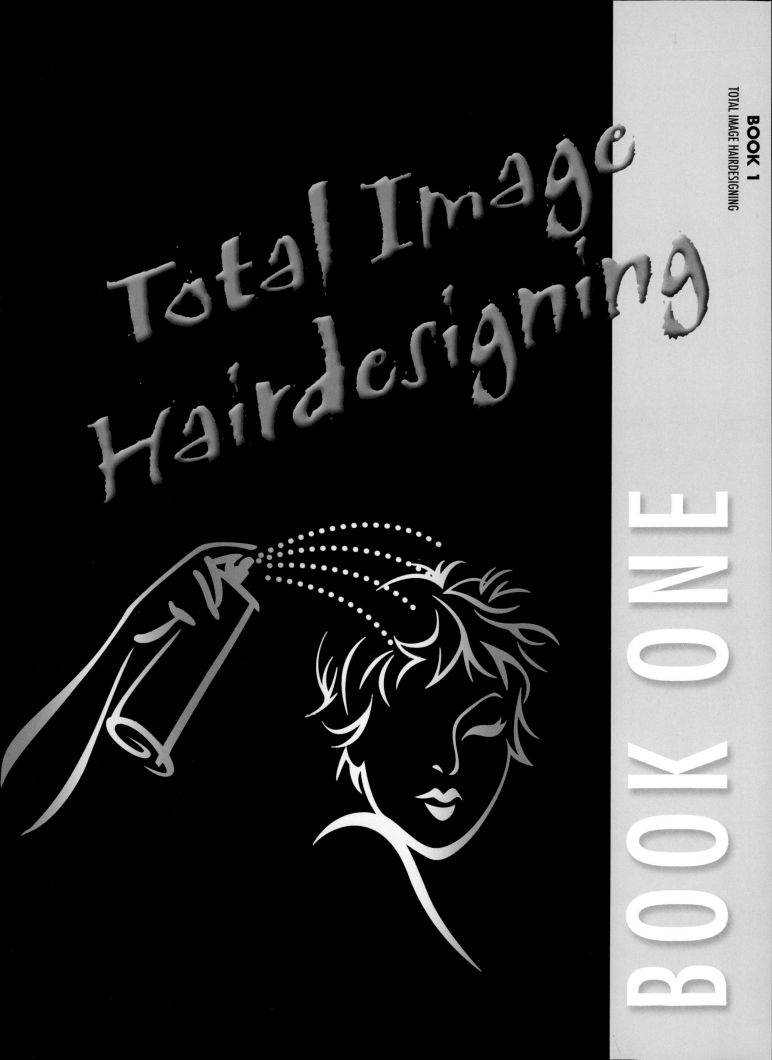

Total Image
Hairdesigning

BOOK ONE

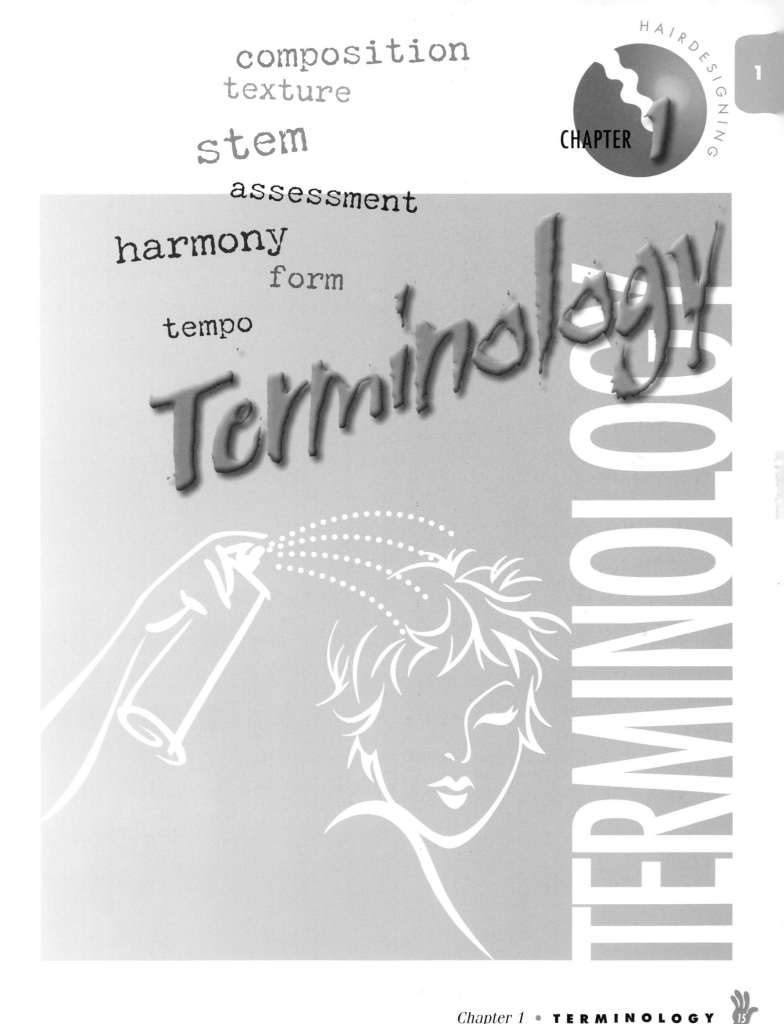

composition

texture

stem

assessment

harmony

form

tempo

Terminology

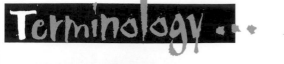
Hairdesigners *are craftspeople who visualize, imagine and construct styles using hair as their medium. They are educators and perpetual students who share knowledge, skills and design interpretations.*

Learning the terminology of hairdesign improves your communication. When using professional vocabulary, clients will value your expertise, and you will gain respect in your industry. As you read this module you will learn how closely related these words are to the world of hairdesigning.

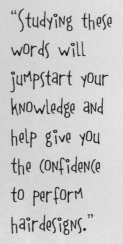

"Studying these words will jumpstart your knowledge and help give you the confidence to perform hairdesigns."

Acceleration

The rate in which line, movement, wave or curl *increases*.

Applications of Hairdesign

The theoretical or practical aspect of design from concept to execution. Elements create the principle idea, which is then implemented to achieve a composition or finished style by arranging individual component parts.

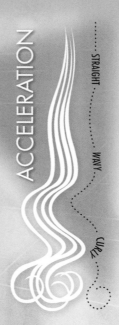

ACCELERATION

STRAIGHT

WAVY

CURLY

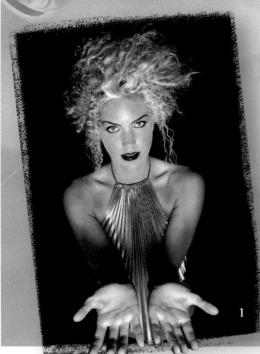

1

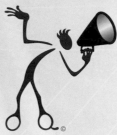

Artistry

Imaginative skill or ability in arrangement or execution.

Assessment

An evaluation in relation to the whole.

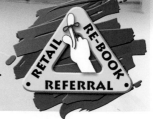

RETAIL · RE-BOOK · REFERRAL

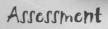

Terminology

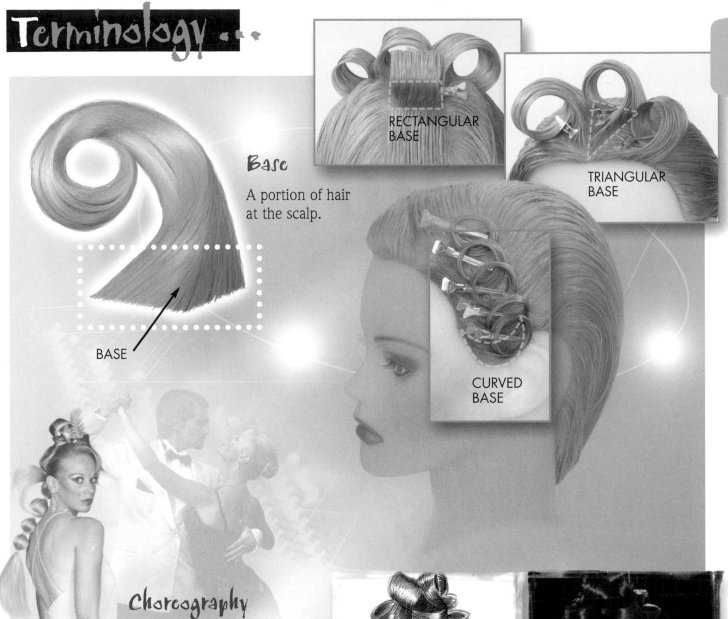

RECTANGULAR BASE

TRIANGULAR BASE

CURVED BASE

Base

A portion of hair at the scalp.

BASE

Choreography

The artistic arrangement of a composition in a hairdesign performance.

1

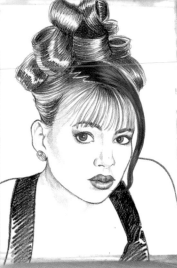

2

Component

One part in the practical application of the whole design.

Composition

The arrangement of components to create a finished hairstyle.

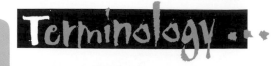
THE INSPIRATION............ ....THE CONCEPT

Concept
1

An idea that combines the theoretical and practical applications of hairdesigning.

Curl

A circle at the ends of the hair.

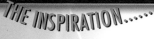

CURL

Cushioning

To compress the hair together with a comb or brush. Also called lacing or interlocking.

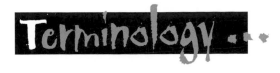

DECELERATION

CURLY · WAVY · STRAIGHT

Deceleration

The rate in which line, movement, wave or curl *decreases*.

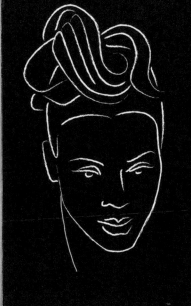

Design Plan

A guide that outlines the elements and components involved in creating the composition of a hairdesign.

1

Detail

The refinement of a hairstyle.

Diameter

The width of an object.

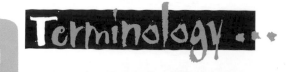

color

line

texture

1

Direction

The path in which the hair flows.

2

Element

An artistic part of a hairdesign. Two or more elements combined create a principle of hairdesign.

4

Emphasize

The act of giving prominence to a component or area of a hairstyle through color, texture or design.

3

Fashion

A style or trend that reflects the time period.

5

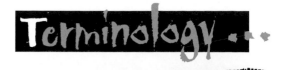

Terminology...

Finishing

The final arrangement of the design.

FOCAL POINT

Focal Point

The main excitement, attraction or action in a hairdesign.

2

Form

The overall outer shape of a hairdesign that makes it identifiable.

Geometric

A measurable figure, line or angle consisting of straight or curved shapes.

Terminology

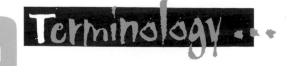

Hairdesign

The artistic
composition
of the hair.

Harmony

The aesthetic placement
of shapes and lines.

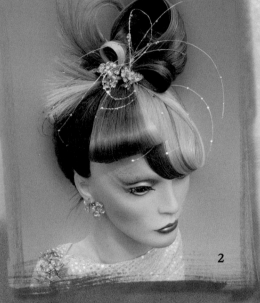

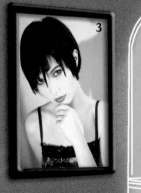

Headshot

A photograph that shows a
hair performer's artistic skill.

Terminology...

Hollow

The concave section of a wave that determines the wave's depth and tempo.

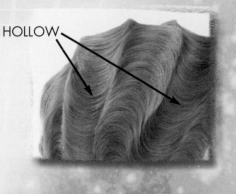

HOLLOW

Illusion

A visual perception causing misinterpretation of an image's actual nature.

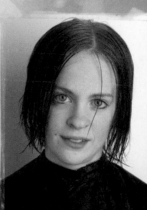

BEFORE 1

AFTER 2

Innovate

To create new and original hairdesigns.

3

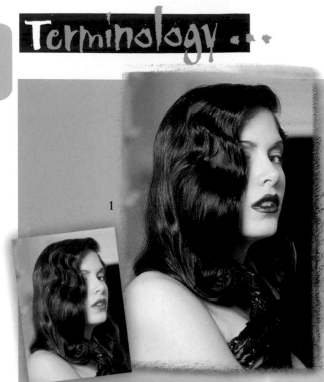

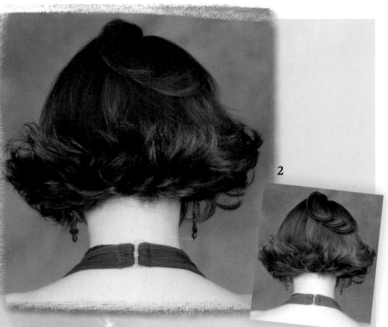

Interruption of Motion

To change direction of a line or movement after it traveled too far in one direction.

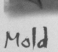

Mold

To draft or sketch a pattern of straight or curved lines into a two-dimensional design. The first step in the chronological order of a design.

Motion

The action of movement, direction or force.

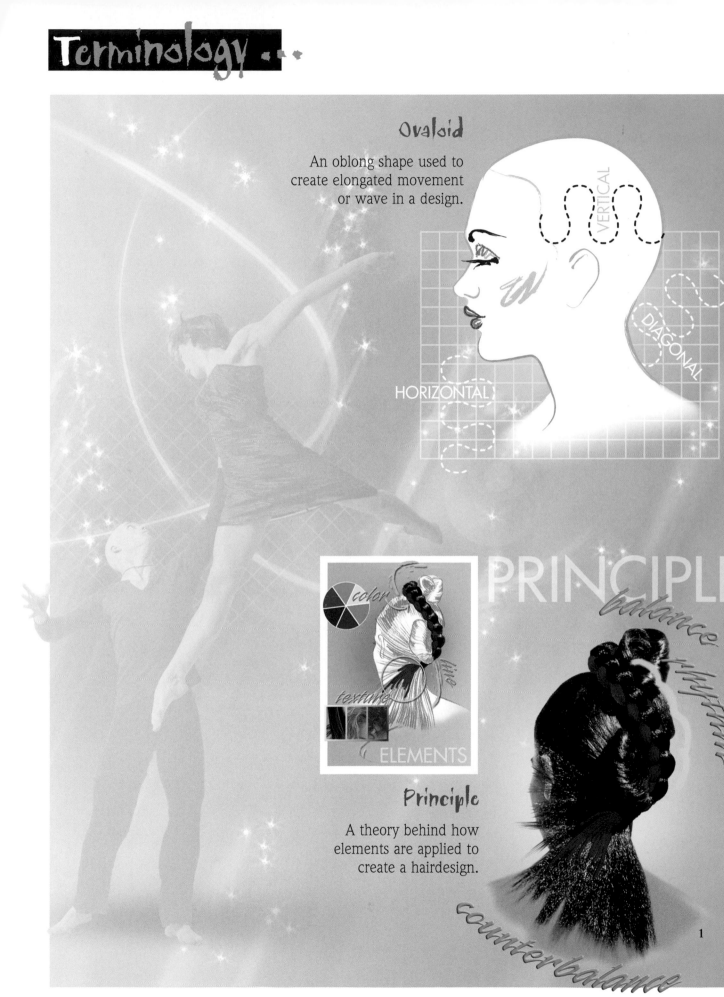

Ovaloid

An oblong shape used to create elongated movement or wave in a design.

VERTICAL

DIAGONAL

HORIZONTAL

color

line

texture

ELEMENTS

PRINCIPLE

balance

rhythm

counterbalance

Principle

A theory behind how elements are applied to create a hairdesign.

1

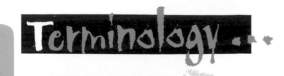

Terminology...

Profile

A view of the head, face or body from the side.

Proportion

To arrange to be harmonious or graceful.

1

2

Repetition

The repeating of elements or components in a hairdesign.

3

Rhythm

A relationship of movement or motion; one part to another that flows.

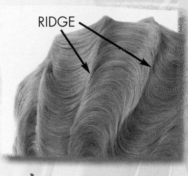

RIDGE

Ridge

The raised section of a wave.

Scaling

The sketching of shapes, sizes and proportions of a design. The second step in the chronological order of a design.

2

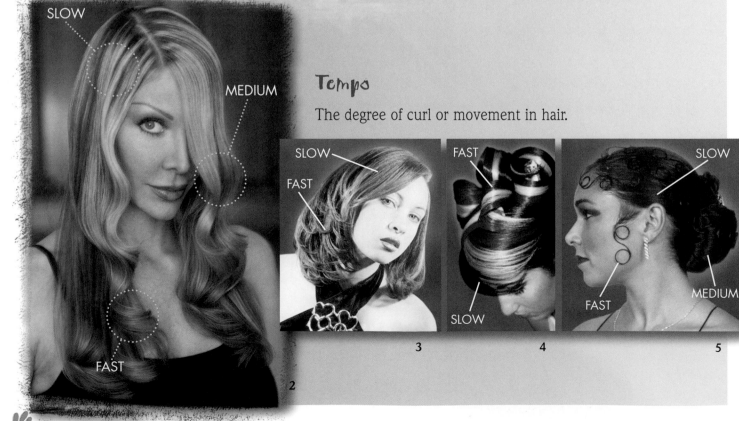

Space

A three-dimensional area in which the hairdesign can move or be formed.

1

STEM

Stem

A section of hair found between the base and the curl. It directs the amount of movement.

SLOW

MEDIUM

FAST

2

Tempo

The degree of curl or movement in hair.

SLOW

FAST

SLOW

3

FAST

SLOW

4

SLOW

FAST

MEDIUM

5

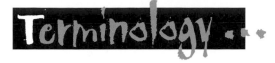

Texture

The visual and tactile quality of hair.

TEXTURE

Vision

An artistic foresight of what will be created.

Wave

A series of curved shapes, consisting of two or more alternating ovaloid shapes. Parts of the wave include the ridge and the hollow.

1

2

3

4

Assessment
Base
Component
Cushioning
Diameter
Direction
Fashion
Finishing
Focal Point
Harmony
Hollow
Innovate
Motion
Ovaloid
Principle
Profile
Proportion
Scaling
Stem
Tempo
Texture

Fill IN THE BLANKS

1. _____ The aesthetic placement of shapes and lines.

2. _____ The visual and tactile quality of hair.

3. _____ To create new and original hairdesigns.

4. _____ The sketching of shapes, sizes and proportions of a design.

5. _____ A section of the hair at the scalp.

6. _____ The width of an object.

7. _____ A style or trend that reflects the time period.

8. _____ A view of the head, face or body from the side.

9. _____ The main excitement, attraction or action in a hairdesign.

10. _____ The final arrangement of the design.

11. _____ The path in which the hair flows.

12. _____ The part of a curl that directs the amount of movement.

13. _____ To arrange to be harmonious or graceful.

14. _____ The degree of curl or movement in hair.

15. _____ An oblong shape used to create elongated movement or wave in a design.

16. _____ One part in the practical application of the whole design.

17. _____ Also called lacing or interlocking.

18. _____ The concave section of a wave that determines the wave's depth and tempo.

19. _____ A theory behind how elements are applied to create a hairdesign.

20. _____ An evaluation in relation to the whole.

STUDENT'S NAME   DATE   GRADE

airformers
brushes
capes
rollers
fasteners
volumizers
irons

Hairdesign Tools

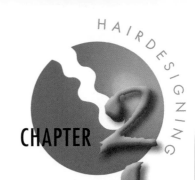

HAIRDESIGN TOOLS

2

Tools are designers' props in the theater of hairdesign. Technological advancements have influenced tools through the years, from cave dwellers' fishbone combs to ionics and ceramics in today's age. This chapter features *some of the tools and equipment* that designers have at their disposal in creating styles.

This chapter includes a brief overview on cleaning and maintenance of tools. To keep tools in good working order, clean and check them frequently according to manufacturer's safety and maintenance instructions. Ask your instructor about your regulatory agency's special requirements.

Tools are an investment in your future. Buy tools from a reputable company that offers **quality**, **service** and **advice** on your purchase. Examine the **warranty** and inquire about additional customer services, like tool repair and replacement.

TOOLS

"Hair fashion evolves with technology. Manufacturers invent new tools or products to creatively challenge and inspire artistic hairdesigns."

Client Protection ...

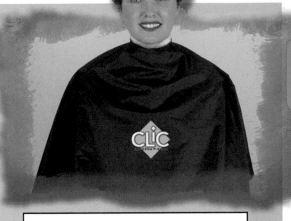

Client Safety *must always come first on a hairdesigner's priority list – even before creating the perfect style. Some equipment may be required by regulatory agencies to protect the client (see Regulatory Alert symbol on this page). Using the supplies listed below shows concern for your client's safety and comfort, helping to ensure client retention.*

Capes are used to shield clients' garments from damage while receiving services. Using a cape or gown to **protect clients' clothing** is called "draping." Capes are available in different materials, lengths, widths and colors, and have a variety of closures including Velcro®, hooks, ties and snaps. Once a cape, smock or towel has come in contact with the client's skin, it must be laundered. Most capes are machine washable, but not all are dryer-safe.

> *It is our responsibility to educate and protect the public; therefore, clients should understand neck strips and towels are used to prevent skin-to-cape contact since capes may be used repeatedly.*

RA

Note: Read the manufacturer's instructions prior to use.

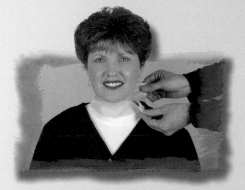

Neck Strips or towels are wrapped around the client's neck to **prevent skin-to-cape contact**. Many regulatory agencies require them to ensure capes do not transmit germs or diseases. Neck strips also help prevent water from running down a client's neck. Neck strips are available in paper or cloth and come in different widths and lengths.

Hairnets are used to **protect roller and design placements** while the client is under the hairdryer. They may also be used to **help hold ear shields and finished styles** in place. Hairnets are available in fine or large weaves.

Ear Shields are used to **protect the client's ears** during the hairdrying process. They are manufactured in paper, plastic and foam.

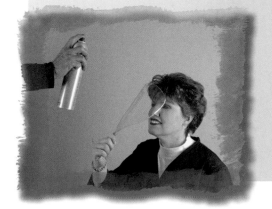

Spray Shields are placed over a client's face at a downward-sloping angle when sprays are being used. They help to **protect the client's skin** from potential allergic reactions, prevent a client's makeup from being disturbed and guard the client from inhaling the excess spray.

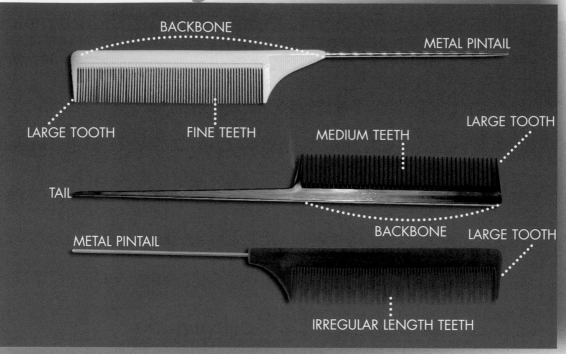

Diagram labels: BACKBONE, METAL PINTAIL, LARGE TOOTH, FINE TEETH, MEDIUM TEETH, LARGE TOOTH, TAIL, BACKBONE, LARGE TOOTH, METAL PINTAIL, IRREGULAR LENGTH TEETH

A Tail Comb, *also called a rattail comb, has several uses:*
- *to distribute, shape and part the hair into sections*
- *to help separate and lift hair when finishing the hairdesign*
- *to weave strands of hair*
- *to control loose ends*

Placement: Professional stylists keep a comb in hand until they are finished using it on a client. When you are not using a comb, place it between your thumb and forefinger, holding it secure with the webbing of your hand.

Teeth: The length and teeth of tail combs vary. Some tail combs have shorter teeth inserted next to longer ones to assist the stylist with cushioning and lacing. Your regulatory agency may prohibit salon use of combs with metal pintails for safety reasons.

Control: Practice holding the comb while manipulating different implements such as rollers, end papers, irons and airformers.

Key Elements:

 Lightweight and durable

 Makes clean, precise partings in a geometric shaping with its tail

Separates and lifts the hair when combing out hairdesigns

Helps control loose ends when setting or curling hair

 Used for cushioning and lacing

RA

Cleaning, disinfection and maintenance of your tools should be performed after every use according to your regulatory authority.

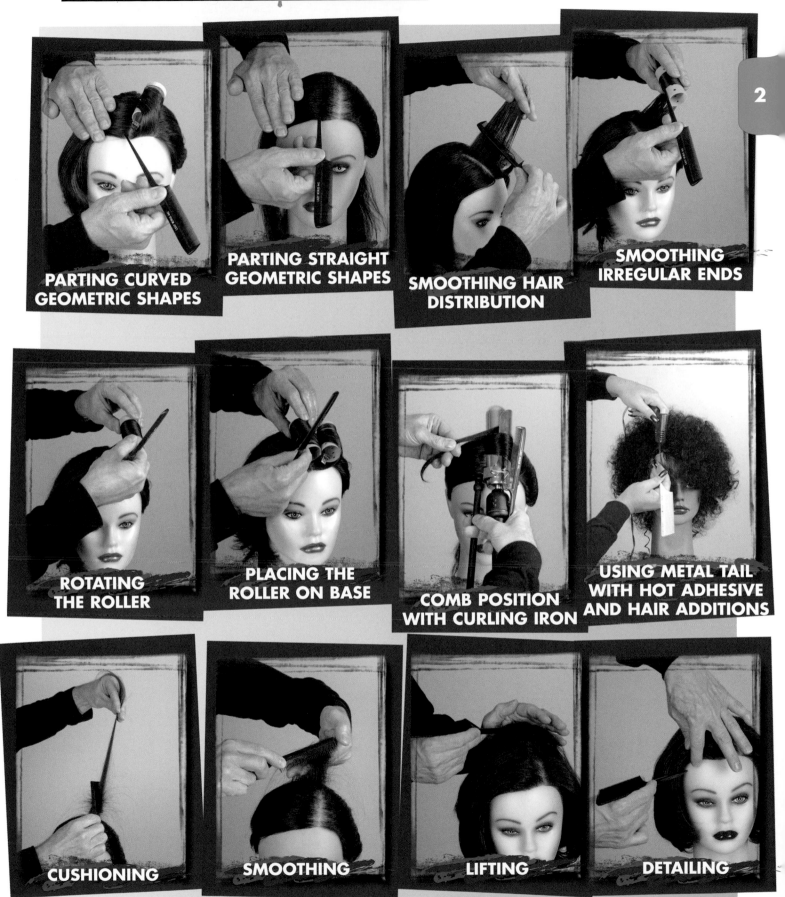

PARTING CURVED GEOMETRIC SHAPES

PARTING STRAIGHT GEOMETRIC SHAPES

SMOOTHING HAIR DISTRIBUTION

SMOOTHING IRREGULAR ENDS

ROTATING THE ROLLER

PLACING THE ROLLER ON BASE

COMB POSITION WITH CURLING IRON

USING METAL TAIL WITH HOT ADHESIVE AND HAIR ADDITIONS

CUSHIONING

SMOOTHING

LIFTING

DETAILING

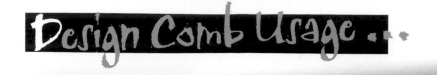

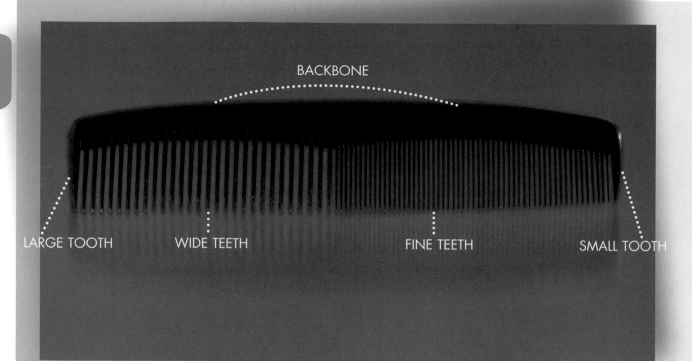

BACKBONE

LARGE TOOTH   WIDE TEETH   FINE TEETH   SMALL TOOTH

The Design Comb *is a large all-purpose comb used to sketch and distribute a two-dimensional design into the hair, as well as comb finished hairdesigns into three-dimensional forms. It is used to create a variety of hairdesigns and is excellent to use for lacing techniques.*

Placement: This comb is held firmly between your fingers and palm.

Teeth: The large teeth are used to sketch and distribute a hairdesign into wet hair. The fine teeth are used to create various types of lacing.

Control: The comb's large size makes it easier to use and manipulate. Practice using the comb to sketch a two-dimensional hairdesign on the clay-covered scalp of a mannequin. Imagine that this comb is your pencil, and use it to draw the design into the clay.

Key Elements:

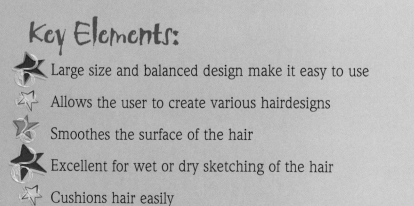

- Large size and balanced design make it easy to use
- Allows the user to create various hairdesigns
- Smoothes the surface of the hair
- Excellent for wet or dry sketching of the hair
- Cushions hair easily

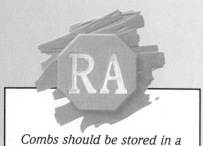

Combs should be stored in a dry sanitizer until needed.

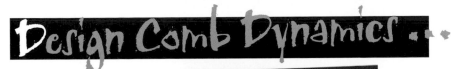

Design Comb Dynamics

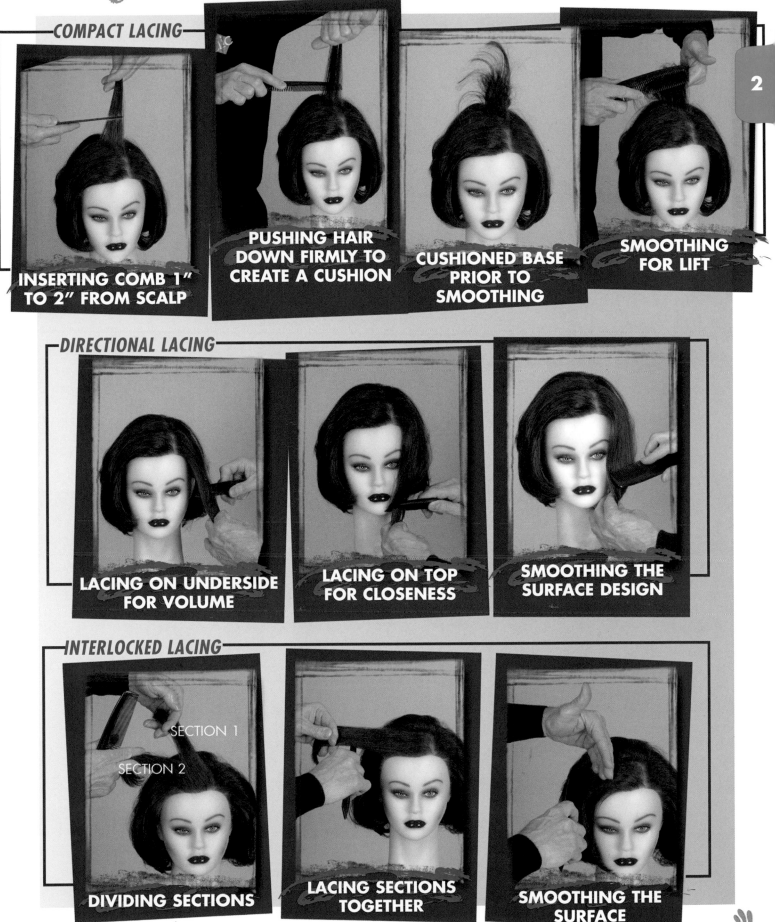

COMPACT LACING

INSERTING COMB 1"
TO 2" FROM SCALP

PUSHING HAIR
DOWN FIRMLY TO
CREATE A CUSHION

CUSHIONED BASE
PRIOR TO
SMOOTHING

SMOOTHING
FOR LIFT

DIRECTIONAL LACING

LACING ON UNDERSIDE
FOR VOLUME

LACING ON TOP
FOR CLOSENESS

SMOOTHING THE
SURFACE DESIGN

INTERLOCKED LACING

SECTION 1

SECTION 2

DIVIDING SECTIONS

LACING SECTIONS
TOGETHER

SMOOTHING THE
SURFACE

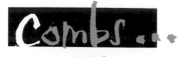

2

Combs *are available in a wide array of colors, materials and styles. Each hairdesigner's choice is dictated by his/her personal sense of function and comfort.*

Coil Combs™ have fine, short teeth that are closely spaced together. This comb creates tightly coiled curl formations when it is inserted into the hair near the scalp area and turned. For best results, use styling gel with this comb.

Cushioning Combs help finish and add dimension and texture to hairdesigns. These combs contain a mixture of longer and shorter teeth to cushion hair as close to the root area as desired. Cushioning combs come in a variety of styles; some have attached lifts.

Pleating Combs made from a variety of materials are primarily used on dry hair. They help create pleats and textures within hairdesigns. Single, double or triple teeth spacing determines how deep the pleats are within the hairdesign.

Finger Wave Combs have wider backbones and wider-spaced teeth than all-purpose combs, making it easier to grip and slide through the hair when creating wave ridges.

Heat-Resistant Combs are designed to resist damage from heat and chemicals. They are made of hard rubber, which is an excellent insulator against heat when used during thermal curling or straightening. Theses combs come in many different styles.

Ruled Combs are versatile tools because they can be used to measure and also create waves, pin curls, shapings and roller sections.

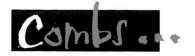

Combs ...

Detangling Combs have wide, rounded teeth to help separate hair before and after shampooing. They cause less snagging while removing tangles from the hair.

Finishing Combs are made from plastic or hard rubber and have teeth of varying lengths and widths. The shorter teeth are used to cushion and smooth hairdesigns. The longer teeth are used to refine the hair's surface when finishing hairdesigns.

Rakes are manufactured of metal or plastic. The long teeth reach to the scalp and lift hair to help comb into a finished hairdesign. Rakes are specially designed for combing curly hair since wide spacing of the teeth allows curls to remain intact while separating them.

Designer Combination Combs have areas with different types of teeth. This practical feature allows a stylist to perform several styling techniques with a single tool.

Cushion Brush Usage...

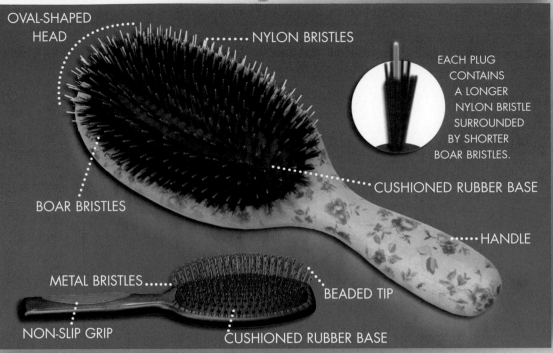

OVAL-SHAPED HEAD

NYLON BRISTLES

EACH PLUG CONTAINS A LONGER NYLON BRISTLE SURROUNDED BY SHORTER BOAR BRISTLES.

CUSHIONED RUBBER BASE

BOAR BRISTLES

HANDLE

METAL BRISTLES

BEADED TIP

NON-SLIP GRIP

CUSHIONED RUBBER BASE

A Cushion Brush has great versatility for use in hairdesigning and is available in many sizes ranging from purse size to professional size. Its bristles can be nylon, boar, metal or any combination. Boar or nylon bristles on cushion brushes relax sets and loosen dirt and debris on hair or scalp before shampooing. Metal bristles on cushion brushes help detangle wet hair after shampooing and eliminate static electricity. This brush type is not recommended for use while airforming.

Placement: To loosen dirt from the scalp prior to shampooing:
- Insert the brush on the scalp at a 45-degree angle.
- Roll the brush onto the scalp (all bristles must come in contact with the head).
- Brush the hair firmly downward from base to ends.

Control:
- Hold the brush firmly in your dominant hand.
- Rotate your wrist slightly as you brush the hair.
- Follow the brush line with your free hand to smooth the hair as you brush.

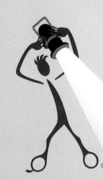

RA

Follow your regulatory agency's cleaning and disinfecting guidelines for each type of tool.

Key Elements:

⭐ Cushion brushes act like shock absorbers. They are gentle on the scalp and hair, helping prevent scalp abrasions and hair breakage

⭐ Boar or nylon bristles are best when used to prepare hair for shampooing

⭐ Use metal bristles to style wigs, extensions, hairpieces and other hair attachments

"Cushion brushes with boar bristles increase the hair's shine."

2

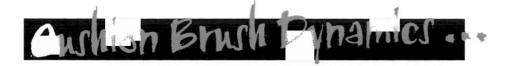

Cushion Brush Dynamics

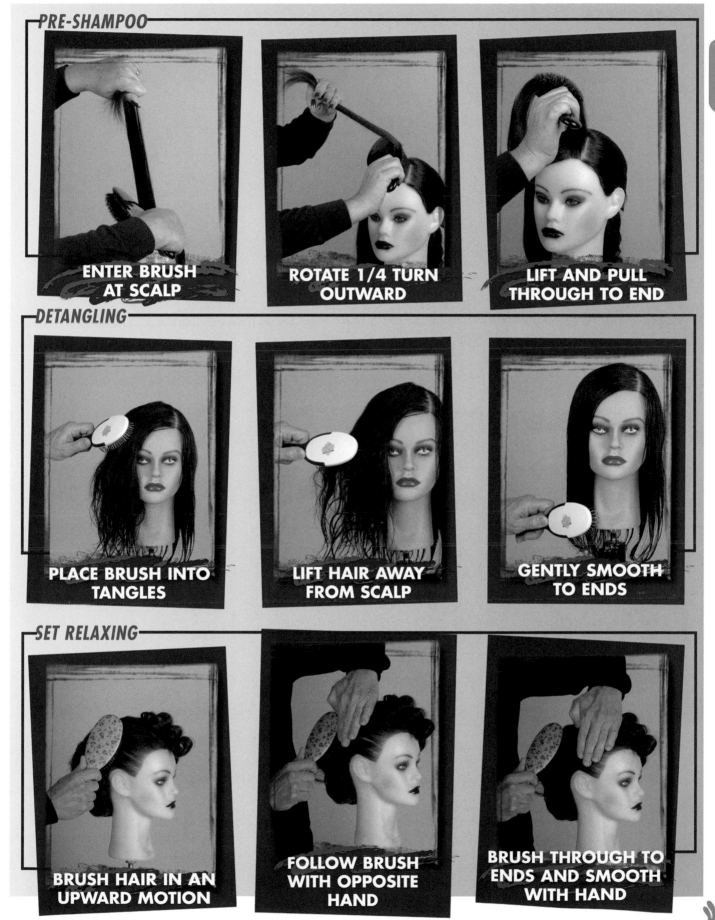

PRE-SHAMPOO

ENTER BRUSH AT SCALP

ROTATE 1/4 TURN OUTWARD

LIFT AND PULL THROUGH TO END

DETANGLING

PLACE BRUSH INTO TANGLES

LIFT HAIR AWAY FROM SCALP

GENTLY SMOOTH TO ENDS

SET RELAXING

BRUSH HAIR IN AN UPWARD MOTION

FOLLOW BRUSH WITH OPPOSITE HAND

BRUSH THROUGH TO ENDS AND SMOOTH WITH HAND

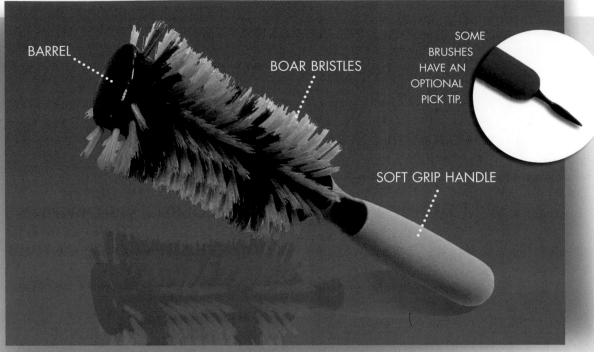

BARREL

BOAR BRISTLES

SOME BRUSHES HAVE AN OPTIONAL PICK TIP.

SOFT GRIP HANDLE

A Natural Boar Bristle Round Brush polishes the hair with each rotation, giving the hair a healthier and shinier look. The bristles are made from boar's hair, which can be light or dark in color. As with all round brushes, boar bristle brushes are available in a variety of diameters.

Placement: The boar bristle brush should be inserted at the base area of the hair to lift and stretch the hair for volume and smoothing **before rotation**. It can also be wrapped around the ends of the hair to form curl patterns like a curling iron.

Control: The boar bristles allow the ends of the hair to wrap firmly around the barrel, offering smoother results and better control. Practice using a round brush to create a variety of volume and indentation base placements.

Key Elements:

⭐ Polishes the hair while adding brilliance to finished hairdesigns

⭐ Natural bristles do not cause split ends or damage the hair

⭐ Smoother results and better hair control

RA

Most boar bristle brushes feature a wooden or cork handle that should not be sanitized by soaking in a cleaning solution. Clean these brushes with soap and water, towel dry and place in a dry sanitizer.

"Be careful not to tangle the hair while rotating the brush close to the scalp."

Round Brush Dynamics

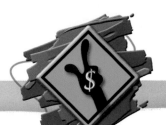

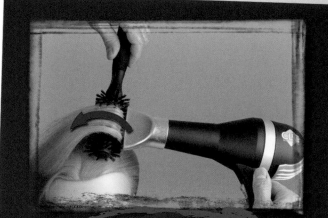

INSERT BRUSH AT BASE AREA. LIFT AND STRETCH HAIR SHAFT FOR VOLUME.

Teach your client how to properly use a round boar bristle brush to achieve smooth, voluminous, shiny hair.

ROTATE BRUSH AT ENDS OF HAIR FOR CONVEX (VOLUME) CURLING. NOTICE CORRECT AIRFORMER PLACEMENT TO THE BRUSH.

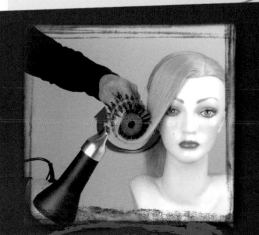

CORRECT POSITIONING OF BRUSH AND AIRFORMER FOR CONCAVE (INDENTATION) CURLING.

"Remember, when the hair turns under, it produces volume. When the ends of the hair turn up, it produces indentation."

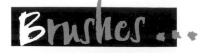

Brushes...

Brushing stimulates blood flow to the scalp, nourishing the hair. Brushes are as varied as the designs they help create. Every hairdesigner will have a personal preference.

Nylon Bristle Brushes are inexpensive brushes for everyday use. They usually have a plastic base and handle. Nylon brushes can be used on the hair before shampooing or after removing rollers from a set. Nylon brushes are easily cleaned by removing loose hair from the brush and soaking in a commercial brush cleaner.

Paddle Brushes can have boar, nylon or a combination of bristles with a base of plastic, wood or cushioned rubber. The paddle brush is used for controlling large amounts of hair. By keeping the cuticle of the hair shaft unruffled, it increases the shine of a finished hairdesign.

Triangle Brushes have nylon, boar or a combination of bristles in a cushioned rubber-backed base. The triangle brush allows the hairdesigner to cushion hair and smooth the finished design. It is good for detailing in tight or difficult areas.

Hot Air Brushes force warmed air through a rounded barrel to create soft curls or waves in slightly damp hair. The hot air brush should not be held in one spot for too long to prevent dehydrating and damaging the hair. Many hot air brushes have soft nylon bristles or stiff nylon pins, are tangle-free and have cool tips. They are available in a variety of diameters and are used for quick, versatile styling. The hot air brush is not to be confused with the brush curling iron, which uses the heat of the barrel to curl dried hair.

"The hot air brush is a popular retail item for busy or traveling clients because of its lightweight design and convenience as a two-in-one styling tool."

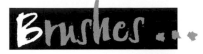

2

Straightening Brushes have two brushes joined together with a spring-loaded handle. These brushes can sometimes be used with chemical straightening agents to relax curl patterns in the hair. Straightening brushes help to relax and smooth the hair when used with an airformer.

Vent Brushes help remove water from hair prior to styling. Its bristles are farther apart with openings in between allowing air circulation to dry hair faster while airforming. They help create direction, movement and lift to the hair. Some vent brushes are double-sided and have shorter bristles on one side to help mold and lift the hair in the scalp area. The larger bristles help smooth and distribute the hair. Vent brushes are usually made of materials that resist heat and chemicals.

Pin Brushes have heat-resistant nylon bristles on a rubber backing which can be removed for cleaning. Pin brushes smooth hair while airforming, reduce friction and eliminate static.

Round Brushes are available in a variety of diameters, materials and colors. Some have a metal barrel, which when used with an airformer mimics the action of a curling iron. The amount of curl is controlled by the size of the brush and how the hair is heated and cooled while it is wrapped around the brush. Some styles feature a retractable pick that aids in sectioning the hair. A round brush is made with nylon, boar and/or ball-tipped bristles. The boar bristle brush is recommended for its quality and the strength and shine it gives hair. The porcupine round bristle brush has longer, nylon bristles that separate and detangle while its boar bristles help direct and smooth hair.

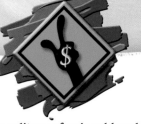

High-quality professional brushes are worth the investment to your clients. They reduce snag and friction while increasing the shine of the hair.

2

Fasteners come in a variety of shapes, sizes and materials. All fasteners hold hair in place whether on a roller, wave ridge or a section on the head.

Bobbie Pins

come in various sizes and match common hair colors in order to make them less noticeable in hairdesigns. They can be used for securing roller placements and for creating and supporting upswept hairdesigns, known in competition as "long hair up." Bobbie pins also secure hairpieces and ornaments in the hair. To obtain the strongest support from bobbie pins, interlock them.

Hairpins

help secure a style by weaving them through and into the hair. They can also be used to help secure bobbie pins by interlocking them with one another. Like bobbie pins, hairpins come in varying colors and sizes to blend in with the hair.

Fantasy Pins

are extra-long, lightweight hairpins that are about twice the size of a standard hairpin. They are typically used in competition work and long hairdesigns.

Single Prong Clips

are preferred for pin curl settings and small area sectioning. They are lightweight and come in short or medium lengths.

Double Prong Clips

may be used in roller and pin curl settings.

Roller Clips

are used in roller placements. They slide inside the roller so the rollers can be set closer together, helping eliminate breaks in the hairdesign.

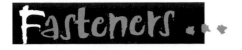

Fasteners...

Sectioning Clips divide large sections of hair, making it easier for the stylist to maintain control. They are manufactured in plastic or metal.

Wave Clips, also called Marcel clips, are usually made of lightweight aluminum. They are used to create strong wave formations by supporting the wave ridge.

Butterfly Clips are often used to secure hot rollers, but they are also ideal for sectioning large amounts of wet or dry hair.

Roller Picks come in two main varieties: plastic-coated steel and nylon. Plastic-coated steel roller picks are stronger and thinner than nylon picks. Roller picks hold rollers in place and lift or separate perm rod bands to prevent creasing the hair.

Hair Tape can be made of paper, nylon or other materials. It is most commonly used on the outer perimeter of the hairline to hold hair in an immovable position.

Hair Forms are artificial materials inserted into hairdesigns to create height or unusual dimensions. Commercial hair forms come in several shapes, sizes and colors. They are normally made of soft net material so the form is pliable and easily pinned. Sometimes referred to as a "rat" or "filler," the hair form is most frequently used in long hairdesigns.

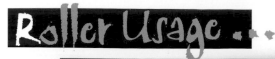
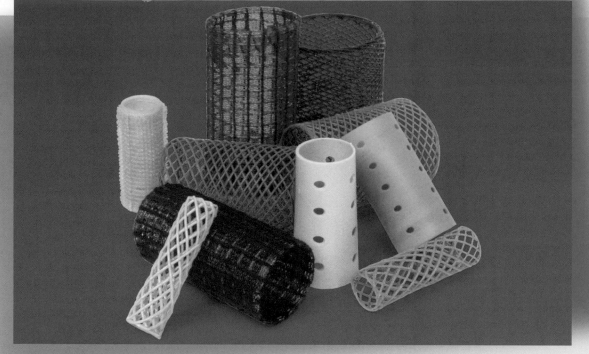

$Rollers$ *play a leading role in creating various hair patterns and textures, from curly to straight.*

Features: Rollers are made of many different materials, ranging from hard plastic to soft Velcro®, and can be secured in the hair with various fasteners.

Placement: Rollers produce a stronger set than styles that are airformed or pin curled. The roller's placement, base control and size all help to decide the degree and amount of curl in a hairdesign. (This is explained in more detail in Chapter 4.)

Key Elements:

 Create different patterns and textures

Can be secured with various fasteners

Available in a variety of diameters, lengths, colors and materials

May be used on wet or dry hair

"Progressive salons today do more soft-setting with airformers and curling irons than hard-setting with wet hair on rollers."

RA

Remove loose hair from the rollers, then clean, disinfect and store according to the guidelines of your regulatory authority.

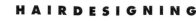

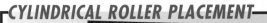

Roller Dynamics...

CYLINDRICAL ROLLER PLACEMENT

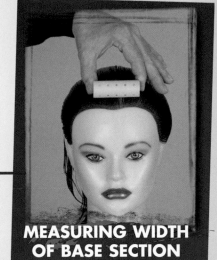

MEASURING WIDTH OF BASE SECTION

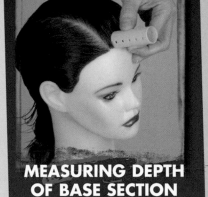

MEASURING DEPTH OF BASE SECTION

FASTENING ROLLER ONTO BASE

CONICAL ROLLER PLACEMENT

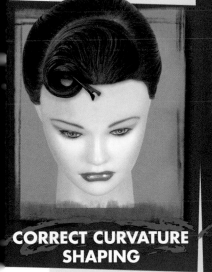

CORRECT CURVATURE SHAPING

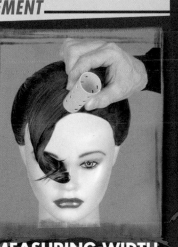

MEASURING WIDTH OF BASE SECTION WITH SMALL END

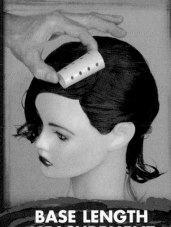

BASE LENGTH MEASUREMENT STARTS WITH SMALL END PLUS LENGTH OF ROLLER

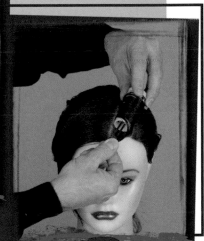

FASTENING ROLLER INSIDE SHAPING

MESH ROLLER PLACEMENT

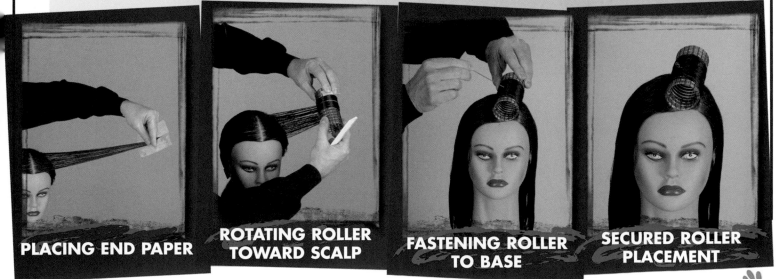

PLACING END PAPER

ROTATING ROLLER TOWARD SCALP

FASTENING ROLLER TO BASE

SECURED ROLLER PLACEMENT

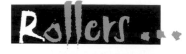

2

Cylindrical Plastic Rollers come in a variety of lengths, diameters and colors and are easy to maintain. They are used to wet set the hair. Because wet hair sticks to the roller easily, cylindrical rollers are also called magnetic rollers. The small holes that run lengthwise on the roller allow for better air ventilation for quicker drying. Cylindrical rollers create straight or curved shapes in hairdesigns.

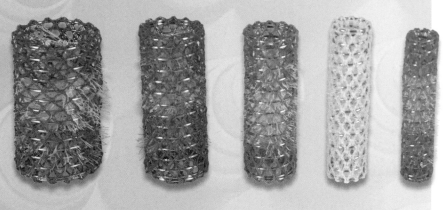

Conical Plastic Rollers are used to create curvature shapes in hairdesigns. They are smaller at one end and fit into triangular-shaped sections better than cylindrical rollers.

Brush Rollers have bristles (which can be made of boar, nylon or plastic) inside flexible outer rollers. Advancements in technology have made these rollers convenient to use in the salon. Always sanitize brush rollers prior to re-using. To clean and sanitize them, remove the brush from inside, clear away loose hair and clean the outer part of the roller before replacing the brush.

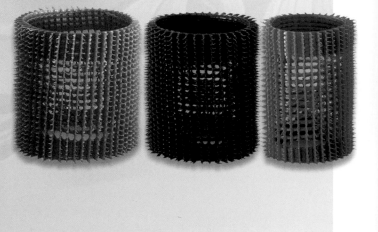

Self-Gripping Rollers are lightweight and color-coded for fast setting. They can be made of Velcro®, ceramic-coated aluminum or other material and are designed to create better airflow to let the hair dry faster. As the name implies, no fastener is required. Self-gripping rollers are used on **dry** or slightly damp hair to create a soft, casual set. Avoid using these rollers on overly wet hair; as the hair shrinks and tightens around the hook and loop surface of the roller while drying, snagging or tangling of the hair during removal may occur.

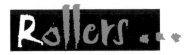
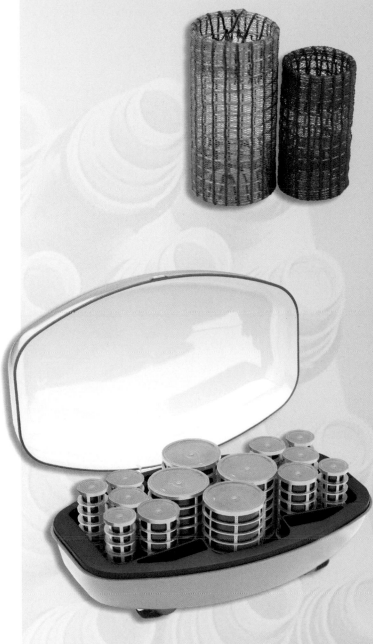

Mesh Rollers are designed for faster drying time when used on wet hair. These rollers require an end paper and a pick to maintain tension. Mesh rollers can be made with plastic- or ceramic-coated metal frames or heat-resistant mesh.

Thermal Rollers can be used on clean, **dry** hair by clients or professionals. They are available in a variety of sizes and diameters to create soft-set hairdesigns. The main types, electric and steam, are quick to use and convenient for travel. They are especially useful when doing fashion photography and runway work.

Electric Rollers are made of hard plastic, have metal inserts and are heated individually on metal spindles. The set of rollers usually comes with metal or plastic fasteners to secure the rollers. Some electric rollers have soft outer coverings of material to help protect the hair and scalp from excessive heat.

Steam Rollers are heated individually on a spindle with steam. Roller sets usually include plastic clamps with the system. Steam rollers and vapor shot irons are **not recommended** for very curly textured hair that has been straightened, since the use of steam on this type of hair may **revert the curl pattern.**

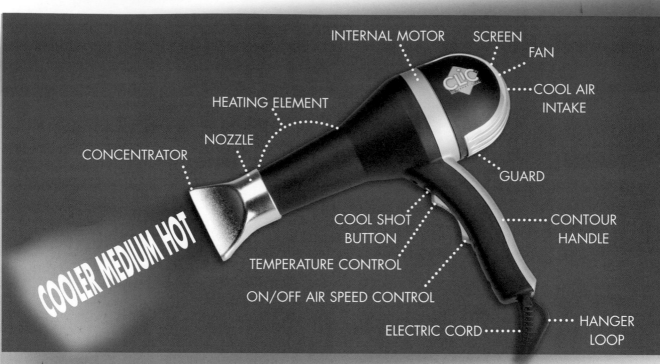

INTERNAL MOTOR   SCREEN
FAN
COOL AIR INTAKE
HEATING ELEMENT
NOZZLE
CONCENTRATOR
GUARD
COOL SHOT BUTTON
CONTOUR HANDLE
TEMPERATURE CONTROL
ON/OFF AIR SPEED CONTROL
ELECTRIC CORD
HANGER LOOP

COOLER MEDIUM HOT

The Airformer dries hair by re-forming hydrogen bonds broken while the hair was being shampooed. Remove most of the moisture in wet hair before beginning the hairdesign, since hydrogen bonds in overly wet hair are too weak to be re-formed. For optimal styling, hair should be evenly damp, about 50 percent dry.

Placement: As the hair dries, controlling the airformer's heat with constant, controlled movement between sections prevents the client's scalp from being burned. Drying in the direction of the hair's cuticle produces smooth, shiny hair. To create curls, direct the heat over and under the brush to reach both the hair's base and ends. Use a rocking motion with alternating heating and cooling to set the curl before removing the brush.

Control: To maintain control of the hair, only airform small sections of the hair at a time. Trying to dry too much hair at once or over-drying will produce inconsistent results and may damage the hair. A concentrator should be kept on the airformer for maximum control and precision. Remember to keep the air intake clear to prevent overheating of the motor.

Note: *For proper body positioning during airformer use, please refer to the airforming design components section of Chapter 4.*

Key Elements:

★ Dries hair quickly by re-forming hydrogen bonds in the hair

☆ Sets the hair when hair is still damp, not dry

☆ Controls and directs air more accurately with a concentrator

★ Relaxing the hair helps curl, and tension on the hair helps straighten

"Remember, the more you close the cuticle, the SHINIER the hair becomes."

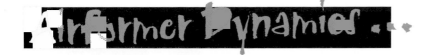

Airformer Dynamics...

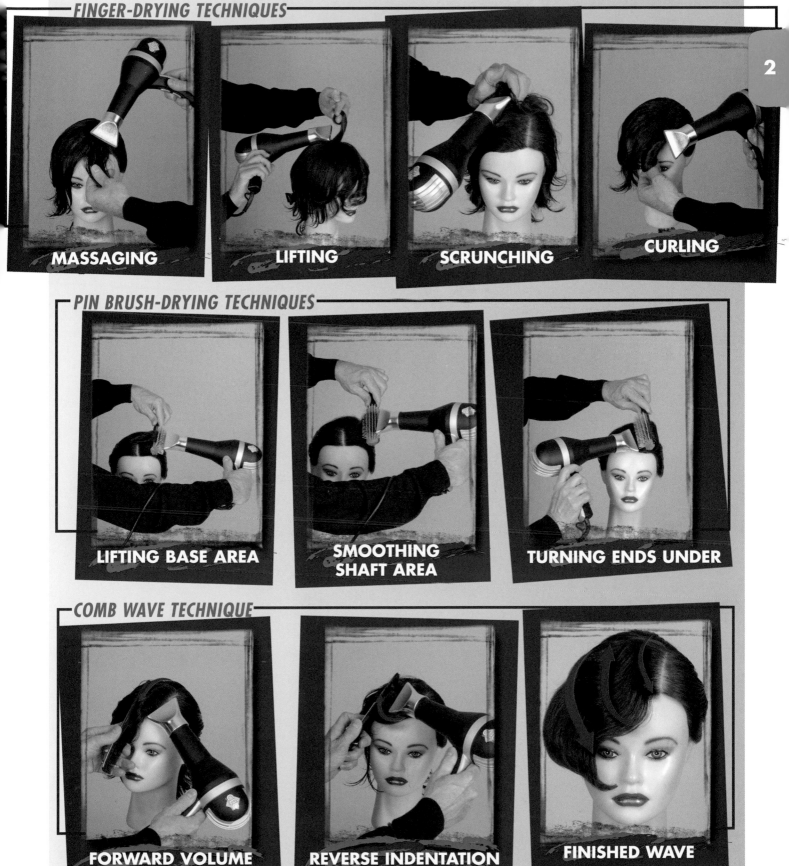

FINGER-DRYING TECHNIQUES

MASSAGING

LIFTING

SCRUNCHING

CURLING

PIN BRUSH-DRYING TECHNIQUES

LIFTING BASE AREA

SMOOTHING SHAFT AREA

TURNING ENDS UNDER

COMB WAVE TECHNIQUE

FORWARD VOLUME C-SHAPING WITH COMB

REVERSE INDENTATION C-SHAPING WITH COMB

FINISHED WAVE

Airformers

Airformers are commonly known as blow dryers outside the world of hairdesign. The airformer creates temporary changes in the shape and texture of wet hair while drying. The varieties of airformers are turbo, conventional and diffuser types.

Turbo Airformers draw air in from the back and propel heated air out the front through a nozzle, with switches to control the heat and airflow. Turbo airformers commonly have a button that produces a cool shot of air for curl setting. Some have an extra long power cord. Advancements in technology have produced turbo airformers with ceramic components for safer, faster drying.

Conventional Airformers draw air into the side and propel heated air out the front nozzle. Some have a swivel power cord and multiple heat settings. Many conventional airformers have a cool shot switch to set curls.

Diffuser Airformers draw air through the back and softly disperse the air flow through the front. They minimize the airflow to retain curls and wave formations within hairdesigns. These airformers have variable speeds and heat controls.

Airformer Accessories

WIDE **MEDIUM** **NARROW**

Concentrators are usually included with the purchase of airformers. A narrower concentrator directs the flow of air with greater heat precision and control.

Bell-shaped Diffusers disperse airflow more softly in multiple directions. They are available with fingers of varying lengths to separate and lift the hair, decrease drying time and maintain more curl in the hair.

Air Bag Diffusers function like bell-shaped diffusers and inflate when in use. They deflate to a compact size for easier travel and storage.

Hair Picks are available with teeth of different lengths and widths. They help smooth, separate and lift the hair while drying. The hair pick is ideal for **curly hair** and creates **smooth styles** by concentrating airflow while combing the hair. This attachment is great to use before a hot iron on the hair.

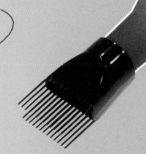

Soft Bonnets attach to airformers to function like traditional hood dryers. They are useful when drying hair set with self-grip or conventional rollers.

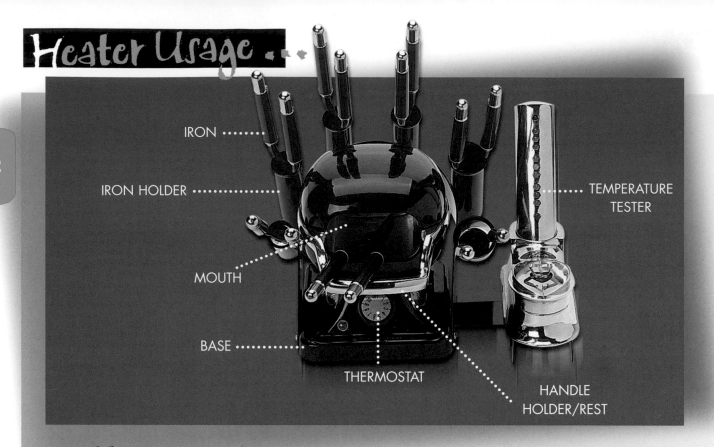

IRON

IRON HOLDER

TEMPERATURE
TESTER

MOUTH

BASE

THERMOSTAT

HANDLE
HOLDER/REST

A Heater is sometimes called a stove. It is used to heat conventional irons and pressing combs. Heaters are available with small or large mouths for heating one or several irons or combs at a time and come with adjustable handle rests. Most heaters have a convenient on/off switch built into the cord.

Features: Accessories for stoves include detachable temperature testers for irons and racks with holders of various shapes and sizes for irons or combs. A thermal carrying case is essential for storing and organizing irons and pressing combs.

Control: No automatic heat regulator exists in a conventional heater. Stoves heat quickly and can reach extremely high temperatures; therefore, testing the temperature of the iron or comb is essential prior to use. Carefully test your instruments using either a commercial heat tester or by manually running the heated comb or iron over a paper neck strip to test for scorching. Commercial heat testers assist stylists in self-regulating temperatures to varying degrees based on the manufacturer's temperature recommendations for each type and texture of hair to be styled.

Key Elements:

⭐ Heats quickly and can reach extremely high temperatures-testing is essential prior to use

⭐ Heats only conventional Marcel irons and pressing combs

⭐ Various attachments and accessories are available

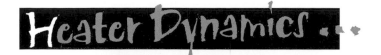

Heater Dynamics

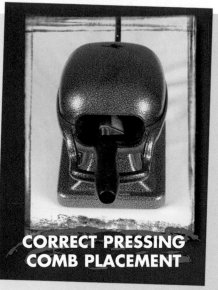

CORRECT PRESSING COMB PLACEMENT

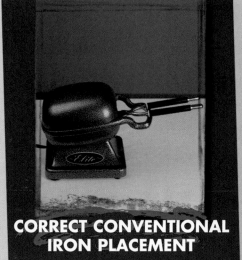

CORRECT CONVENTIONAL IRON PLACEMENT

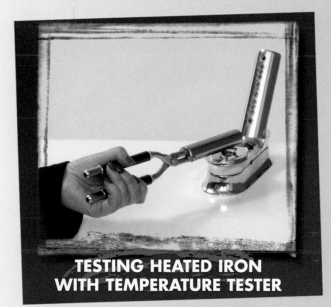

TESTING HEATED IRON WITH TEMPERATURE TESTER

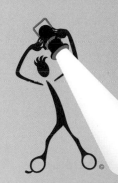

"Exercise caution when using heaters. Never place your hand inside a heater at any time, and always be sure to lift tools by their heat-resistant or wooden handles."

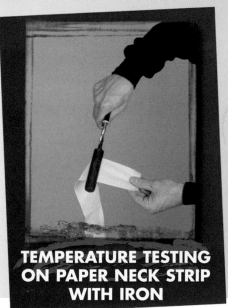

TEMPERATURE TESTING ON PAPER NECK STRIP WITH IRON

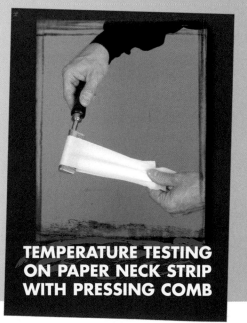

TEMPERATURE TESTING ON PAPER NECK STRIP WITH PRESSING COMB

HANDLE WITH ROTATING SLEEVES

BARREL/ROD

SHAFT

COOL TIP

SHELL/GROOVE

BALANCE POINT

A **Conventional Iron** *is rated in diameter and is available in designs such as beveled, flat, bumper and French.*

Features: Conventional thermal irons can only be heated inside an electric iron heater. Conventional irons should be made from the best quality steel in order to maintain an even temperature. They are available with Marcel-type grips and heat-resistant rotating handles, which should be rotated using only the fingers without any motion from the arm.

Control: The iron's temperature is adjusted by the amount of time the stylist leaves it inside the heater. Adjust heating time for the texture and condition of the client's hair. Less heat is required to thermal style hair that is fine, naturally white, highlighted or colored a lighter shade. An iron should always be tested on a piece of tissue paper or a paper neck strip to verify that it is not too hot for the hair.

Key Elements:

★ Available in various diameters, designs and finishes

★ Temperature **must be controlled by the user**

★ Has rotating heat resistant handles

"To test the temperature of the conventional iron, place the iron against a piece of white paper. If the iron scorches the paper, it is too hot to be used."

Conventional Iron Dynamics ...

CORRECT HAND GRIP – TWO-FINGER PLACEMENT

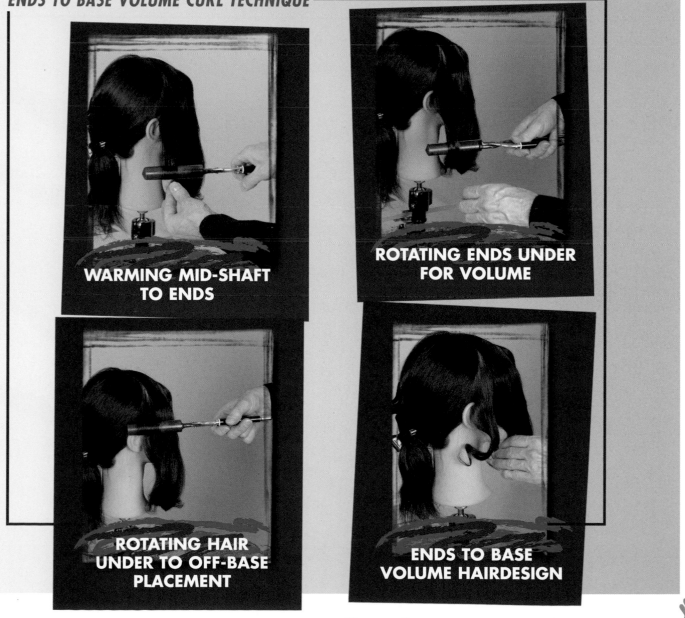

**OPEN IRON—
PALM VIEW**

**CLOSED IRON—
PALM VIEW**

**OPEN IRON—
BACK OF HAND VIEW**

**CLOSED IRON—
BACK OF HAND VIEW**

ENDS TO BASE VOLUME CURL TECHNIQUE

**WARMING MID-SHAFT
TO ENDS**

**ROTATING ENDS UNDER
FOR VOLUME**

**ROTATING HAIR
UNDER TO OFF-BASE
PLACEMENT**

**ENDS TO BASE
VOLUME HAIRDESIGN**

Conventional Marcel Irons *create a variety of hairdesigns based on the style of iron that is used. Some of the different styles are pictured here.*

Flat Irons are available in a variety of widths. The primary function of a flat iron is to straighten curly hair. These irons sometimes have a round back to straighten and bevel the hair in one step for flips or pageboy hairdesigns. These irons can also be pointed to use around the hairline, close to the scalp or to straighten moustaches.

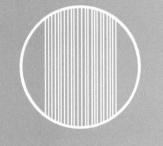

RESULTING HAIR TEXTURE

Waving Irons usually have two or more barrels joined together to form a waver. The diameter and number of the barrels can vary depending on the type of wave formation desired.

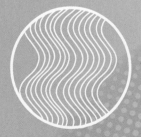

RESULTING HAIR TEXTURE

Conventional Irons ...

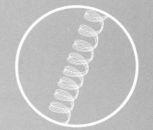

RESULTING HAIR TEXTURE

Conventional Spiral Irons are warmed in heaters and feature a coiled attachment that helps keep spiraled curls evenly spaced on the Marcel-type barrel. Conventional spiral irons have corners or edges that produce crimped or "z"-shaped designs that vary in width and depth. Some feature a shortened shell to hold only the ends of the hair when creating spiral designs.

Curling irons are available in various **diameters**. Diameters can be described using conventional size measurements, letters of the alphabet or coin denominations. Factors influencing decisions when designing with curling irons include the length of the hair, the size of the section, the angle on which the iron is rolled, the diameter of the barrel and the desired style to be achieved.

"Just as a carpenter maintains an assortment of instruments in his tool chest for each type of job, salon designers should have multiple styles of professional irons from which to choose. It is difficult to do all hairstyle variations with only one type of curling iron."

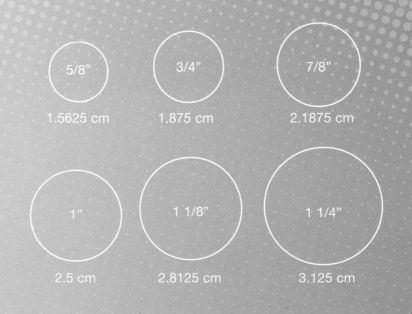

5/8"	3/4"	7/8"
1.5625 cm	1.875 cm	2.1875 cm
1"	1 1/8"	1 1/4"
2.5 cm	2.8125 cm	3.125 cm

2

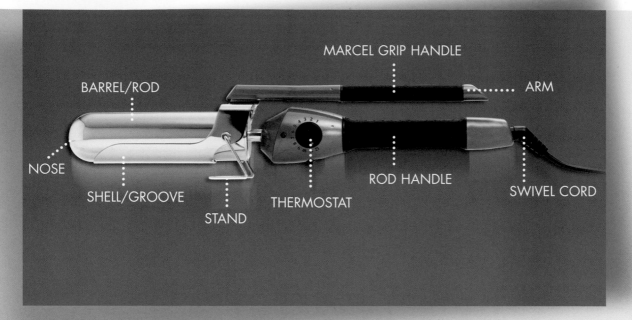

MARCEL GRIP HANDLE

BARREL/ROD

ARM

NOSE

SHELL/GROOVE

STAND

THERMOSTAT

ROD HANDLE

SWIVEL CORD

A Professional Electric Iron *is available in a variety of wattages, some of which may be adjustable. Unlike conventional irons, most professional electric irons have temperature controls.*

Features: The difference between a professional electric iron versus the retail, or "at-home," electric iron lies in the handle and length of the electric cord. Many professional electric irons feature a convenient longer electric cord that does not cross over in front of the client's body. Handles are available in spring tension or Marcel grip (shell/groove).

Control: The Marcel grip handle promotes a more professional image and is preferred by professionals for maintaining better control of the hair. It enables stylists to control the application of heat by transferring the heat evenly from base to ends of the hair.

Key Elements:

★ Available in various diameters, designs and finishes

★ Temporarily curls, waves, straightens and shines hair of any texture

★ Convenient to use

"Never submerge an electric iron into water. Clean the barrel by polishing it with very fine sandpaper or steel wool."

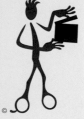

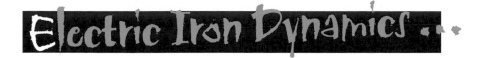

Electric Iron Dynamics...

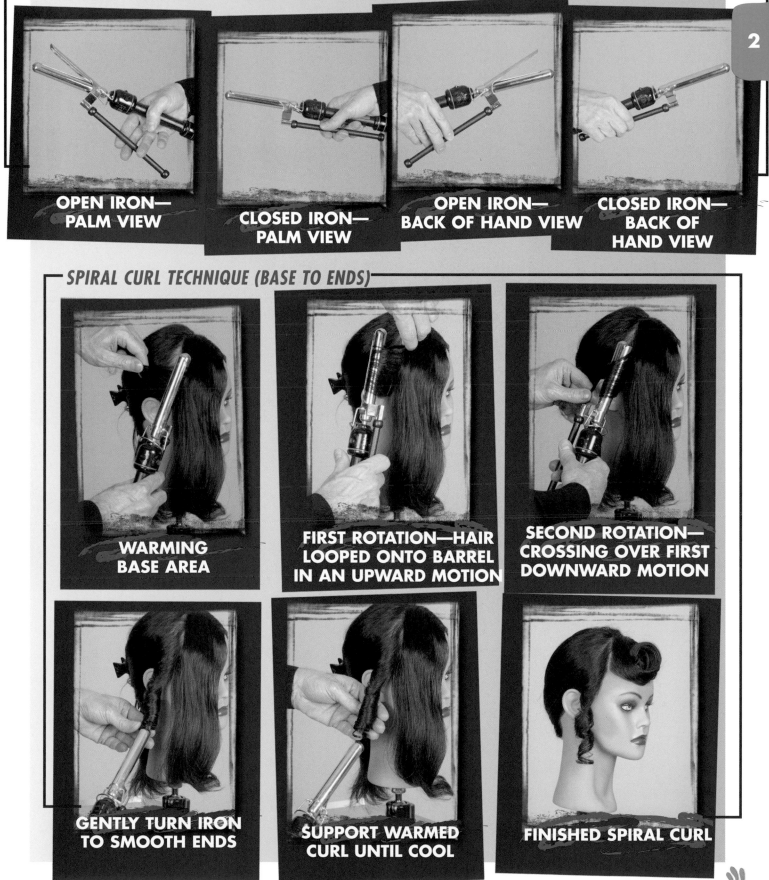

CORRECT HAND GRIP – TWO-FINGER PLACEMENT

OPEN IRON— PALM VIEW

CLOSED IRON— PALM VIEW

OPEN IRON— BACK OF HAND VIEW

CLOSED IRON— BACK OF HAND VIEW

SPIRAL CURL TECHNIQUE (BASE TO ENDS)

WARMING BASE AREA

FIRST ROTATION—HAIR LOOPED ONTO BARREL IN AN UPWARD MOTION

SECOND ROTATION— CROSSING OVER FIRST DOWNWARD MOTION

GENTLY TURN IRON TO SMOOTH ENDS

SUPPORT WARMED CURL UNTIL COOL

FINISHED SPIRAL CURL

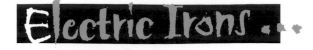

Electric Irons...

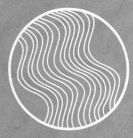

2

Professional Electric Irons *create a variety of hairdesigns based on the style of iron that is used. Some of the different styles are pictured here.*

Flat Irons are available in a variety of widths with either metal or ceramic plates. The primary function of a flat iron is to straighten curly hair. Some flat irons have interchangeable plates that can be used for a variety of effects such as waving, crimping and imprinting.

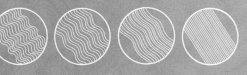

RESULTING HAIR TEXTURES

Waving Irons usually have two or more barrels joined together to form a waver. The diameter and number of the barrels can vary depending on the type of wave formation desired.

RESULTING HAIR TEXTURE

Electric Irons...

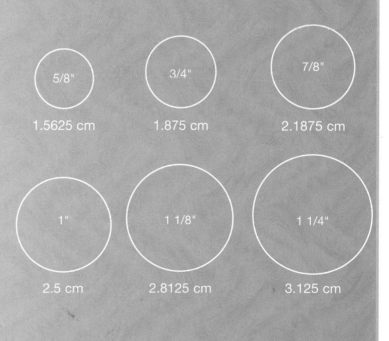

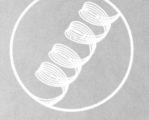

RESULTING HAIR TEXTURE

Spiral Irons that are heated electrically with the use of power cords also feature a specially-designed coil attachment, which helps keep spiraled curls evenly spaced on the barrel. Spiral irons can sometimes have corners or edges that produce crimped or "z"-shaped designs. These angular designs can vary in width and depth. Some electric spiral irons feature a shortened shell to hold only the ends of the hair when creating spiral designs.

Curling irons, whether conventional Marcel-type or electric, are available in various diameters. An example of a typical manufacturer's diameter sizing is listed below. To achieve the style you envision, consider the hair's length, the section size and the angle on which the iron is to be rolled in addition to the diameter of the barrel.

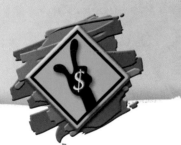

Encourage your clients to invest in a spiral iron, enabling them to more easily duplicate their curly look at home. The barrel's design keeps curls positioned more evenly, resulting in a perfect spiral curl.

5/8"	3/4"	7/8"
1.5625 cm	1.875 cm	2.1875 cm

1"	1 1/8"	1 1/4"
2.5 cm	2.8125 cm	3.125 cm

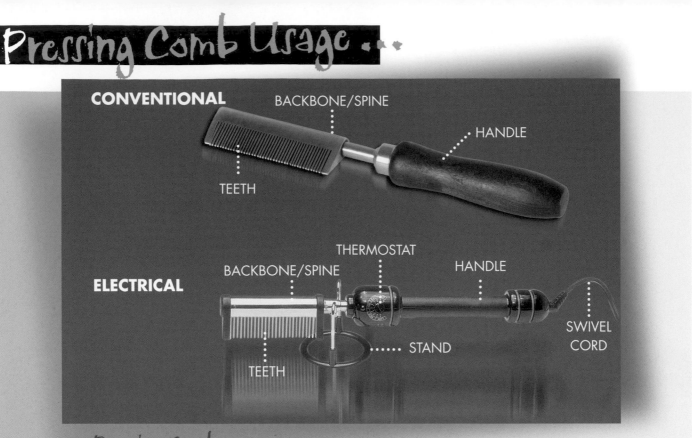

CONVENTIONAL

BACKBONE/SPINE

HANDLE

TEETH

ELECTRICAL

BACKBONE/SPINE

THERMOSTAT

HANDLE

STAND

SWIVEL CORD

TEETH

Pressing Combs are designed to smooth curly hair or create waves of various widths and depths. Pressing the hair is a temporary change that lasts until the next shampoo.

Features: Pressing combs come in various lengths and weights and are manufactured in metals such as copper, brass, steel or a combination of these materials. The teeth can be straight or curved, closely-spaced or far apart. The backbone of the pressing comb may be flat, round, square or curved. Some pressing combs also have short teeth on the backbone to lift the hair close to the scalp, especially around the hairline.

Control: Electric pressing combs are controlled by a thermostat. Some have adjustable temperature controls. More heat is required to straighten coarse hair than fine hair textures. Excessive heat on gray or lightened hair may cause discoloration. **Conventional pressing combs** are heated in a stove and must be heat-tested using a paper neck strip or a commercial temperature tester.

Key Elements:

★ Straightens curly hair or creates waves

★ Different lengths and weights

★ Electric or conventional models

"Any tool heated in a conventional style heater or stove is designed specifically for professional salon use, and should never be given to clients, who have not been trained in proper safety precautions for the use of these tools."

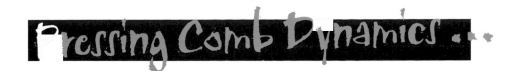

Pressing Comb Dynamics

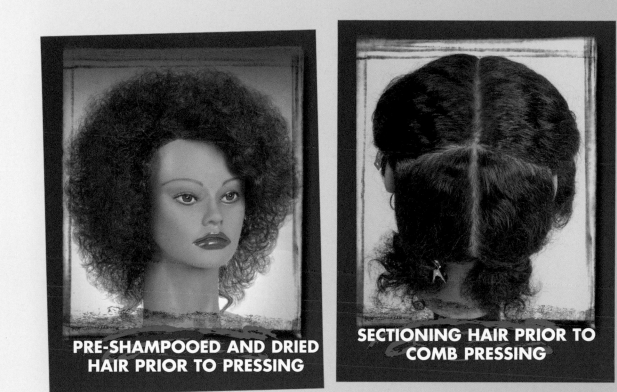

PRE-SHAMPOOED AND DRIED HAIR PRIOR TO PRESSING

SECTIONING HAIR PRIOR TO COMB PRESSING

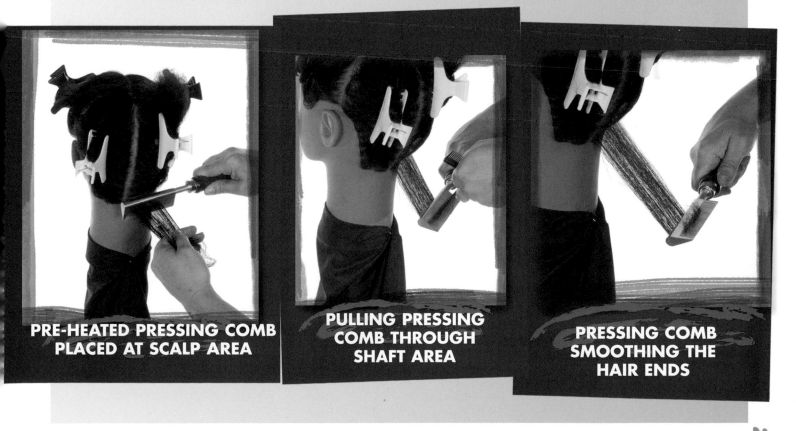

PRE-HEATED PRESSING COMB PLACED AT SCALP AREA

PULLING PRESSING COMB THROUGH SHAFT AREA

PRESSING COMB SMOOTHING THE HAIR ENDS

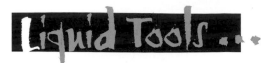

Liquid Tools

Liquid Tools *give stylists the ability to create state-of-the-art hairdesigns by defining the direction of the hair, maintaining a desired form and adding visual texture.*

New products are continually being developed to support the art of hairdesign. While it is impossible to list all liquid tools currently available, the following are most widely used.

Cornrow Creams keep cornrows (also called cane rows) tight, smooth and shiny.

Curl Activators stimulate curl formation and keep the hair from getting frizzy during the drying process. The magnetic elements of these products assist the curl formation by keeping the cuticle uniform while drying.

Curling Waxes help protect the hair shaft during thermal curling. This humidity-resistant wax is applied to the individual sections prior to curl formation. It helps create firm, long-lasting curls.

CURLING WAX

1

Liquid Tools

GLOSSER

"Each hairstyle has a liquid tool specifically designed to help create the right texture."

1

2

PASTE

Fixatives are maximum hold hairsprays generally used to keep finished designs in place. They come in aerosol or pump sprays.

Glossers are used at the end of the design process to help increase shine.

Oil sheens can be used before thermal styling or after the style is finished to help add strength, bounce and shine. They usually contain lanolin, mineral oil, paraffin, or a combination of all three. It is best to use a water-soluble oil sheen that can be removed by shampooing.

Pastes, Clays and Molding Creams make the hair easier to mold, sculpt and shape into a design. These products can be used on either damp or dry hair to create a variety of finishes.

Pomades add shine while protecting the hair and scalp when thermal styling. Most pomade brands are moisture-resistant, helping hold the hair in form.

Pressing Oils are used in thermal styling to help strengthen the hair shaft and prevent scorching. They can be applied to each section of the hair as it is pressed or curled, or massaged into the hair and scalp to maximize protection. Pressing oil is humidity-resistant; this helps the hair remain in its designed shape.

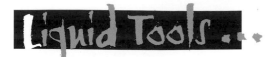

Styling Straighteners are used with the airformer to smooth and straighten hair. Most are humidity-resistant and come in different consistencies such as sprays, mousses and gels.

Thermal Protectants are applied prior to using heat appliances, acting as a thermal barrier to help shield the hair from heat. They are available in spray, liquid and gel forms to add body to the hair.

Working Sprays are light to medium hold hairsprays used throughout the styling process.

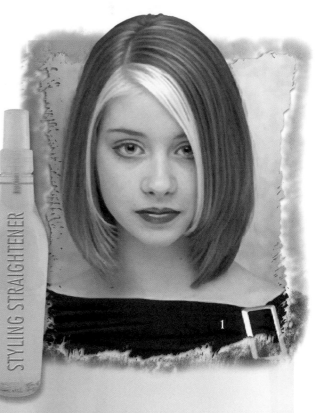

STYLING STRAIGHTENER

1

Wrapping Lotions control wet hair while molding and forming into a hairdesign.

Volumizers create the appearance of increased hair shaft width. Companies sell volumizers as separate products or include them within their styling product formulas.

Your professional recommendation of liquid tools will help clients recreate their hairdesigns at home while increasing your retail sales. Working and finishing hairsprays are the top liquid tools used by hairdesigners and purchased by clients.

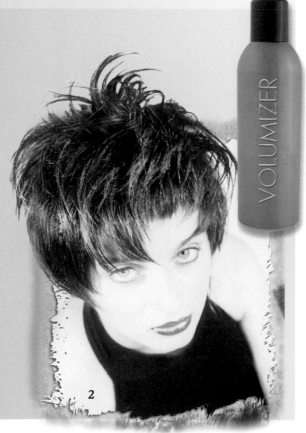

VOLUMIZER

2

Liquid Tools ...

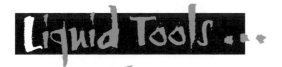

Liquid Tools *are available in varying strengths and control levels. The following guide shows the best use for each type of tool.*

▶ MINIMUM STRENGTH AND CONTROL

Glossers are available in sprays or lotions to create shine, but are not designed for holding control.

Pomades are used for light control and give great thermal protection.

Mousses use a whipped foam consistency to help create volume and definition while allowing some control. Use caution when applying mousse because some brands increase static electricity in hair when airforming.

▶ MEDIUM STRENGTH AND CONTROL

Setting Lotions are used primarily for wet roller setting and airforming.

Glazes may be used on wet or dry hair to hold and shine the hair.

Working Sprays allow stylists to manipulate the hair while finishing the hairdesign.

▶ FIRM STRENGTH AND CONTROL

Cornrow Creams help maintain control of hair while braiding intricate designs.

Gels can be used as a setting or finishing tool to add firm, crisp body to the hair.

Volumizers create firm control while giving the illusion of increased hair mass.

Wrapping Lotions help stylists create firm, smooth styles with strong control.

▶ MAXIMUM STRENGTH AND CONTROL

Fixatives are used for maximum hold and control. They help defy the elements of wind, rain and humidity.

Pastes, Clays and Molding Creams create separations and texture on damp or dry hair.

Styling Straighteners are used with an airformer to help relax curl formations in the hair by helping keep the cuticle flat and closed.

Waxes add shine, accent separations and provide strength and definition to the artistic hairdesign while offering maximum control.

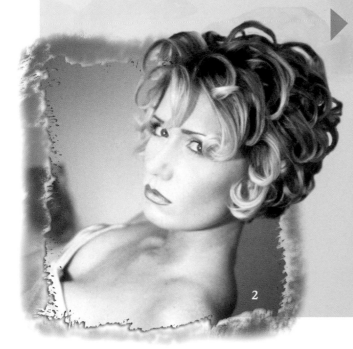

Educational Tools . . .

Mannequins are three-dimensional head forms designers use to reinforce hairdesign principles, develop confidence and perfect their skills before performing them on a client. Even experienced hairdesigners need to learn and practice new techniques throughout their career.

A variety of mannequins help students learn massage, makeup and hairdesigning. Unlike mannequins used for hairdesigning, student competition mannequins have a neck and shoulders. Competing takes practice and discipline but builds experience in learning to recognize and create fine design details.

Mannequin Stands hold a model head form while a stylist practices or demonstrates hairdesigning. Stand designs include the tripod, the tabletop clamp and the adjustable tabletop clamp. Tripod mannequin stands are available with trays and adjustable legs. Clamp versions attach to a table and interchangeable heads control the angle of the mannequin.

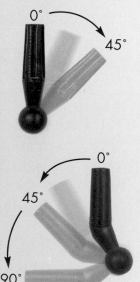

RA

Some regulatory agencies require continuing education for license renewal.

TRIPOD MANNEQUIN STAND

STANDARD TABLETOP CLAMP

ADJUSTABLE TABLETOP CLAMP

INTERCHANGEABLE HEADS

0°
45°

0°
45°
90°

Accessories ...

Professional Quality Traveling Cases are used for travel between hair shows, competitions or client services outside the salon. While in cosmetology school, students purchase cases to hold their tools. Cases are available in various sizes, hard- or soft-sided, with or without wheels.

Pouches are used to store thermal equipment when hot. These thermal-lined pouches organize and protect tools, especially when traveling.

Finger Shields are made of heat-resistant materials and are worn by a stylist to protect the fingers while thermal styling.

Aprons, Lab Coats and Vests are worn by hairdesigners to protect clothing from chemical exposure and create a uniform appearance in the salon or school. They are available in all types of materials, styles, colors and designs.

Sanitation...

Regulatory Agency Law mandates that you maintain safe and sanitary conditions in the salon. It is a salon professional's legal and ethical responsibility to keep all equipment clean and sanitized. Protect your clients and yourself from disease and infection by regularly decontaminating your tools, workspace and hands.

It is important to know which cleaning agents sanitize and disinfect your tools and work area. The following is a brief guide to maintaining a clean workspace.

Sterilizers destroy all living microorganisms on surfaces, harmless or otherwise. This is the strongest and most effective form of sanitation, used in the medical community to sterilize all implements that can penetrate or break the skin. Sterilization is impractical in the salon, since only metal or nonporous tools can be effectively sterilized. Disinfection generally offers the amount of protection against pathogens required in a salon. Always check your regulatory agency requirements.

Disinfectants control or destroy most pathogenic microorganisms on the surface of tools and implements. These strong chemical agents are poisonous and can injure the stylist and the client if they come into contact with hair, skin or nails. The two most common forms of disinfectants are called wet and dry sanitizers. Do not be misled by their names – these cleaners work as disinfectants, **not** sanitizers.

Alcohol and bleach have been replaced with more effective agents, as they may corrode tools or discolor work surfaces. However, bleach remains effective for use in salon laundry. Common forms of disinfectants are quaternary ammonium compounds (quats) and phenols. All containers should be labeled to list the microorganisms for which the product is rated effective. Always add water first and then mix the disinfectant into the water to the appropriate strength required. Most disinfectants work in 10-15 minutes. Prolonged immersion of tools in a solution may damage them. Any item that cannot be disinfected must be discarded.

WET SANITIZERS

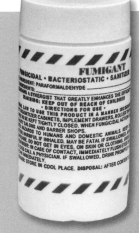

Sanitizers reduce the number of pathogenic microorganisms found on the surface of tools or implements. Common sanitizers are often used to maintain clean work areas and are **not intended to disinfect or sterilize.** Maintain a clean workspace by regularly sanitizing your hands and disinfectings and nonporous surfaces with soaps, detergents or other commercially prepared agents.

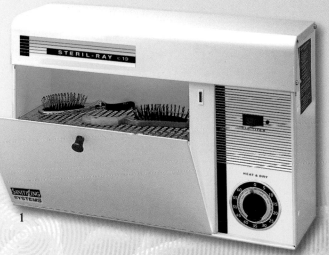

1

DRY SANITIZER

- **Wet sanitizers** are liquid solutions into which tools are submerged for disinfection after their use. Implements must be cleaned before being placed in a wet sanitizer. First, remove hair and use a cleaning solution or soap and water. The solution in wet sanitizers should be changed daily. This category may also include liquid agents which are used to wipe down surfaces and clean tools in the salon.

Implements should not be removed with bare fingers after disinfecting in a wet sanitizer. Instead, use gloves or tongs, and utilize the convenient draining basket inside many wet sanitizers to prevent the skin from contact with disinfectant solutions. Tools that cannot be immersed in a liquid cleaning solution must be wiped down with a disinfectant.

- **Dry sanitizers** are ultraviolet light cabinets where tools such as combs or brushes are placed for sanitizing after being cleaned and disinfected with commercial solutions. Small fumigant tablets placed inside closed storage areas emit a vapor in order to maintain disinfection. However, most are considered harmful and have been banned from salons by regulatory agencies.

Antiseptics, unlike disinfectants, can be **used on the skin** to kill or slow bacterial growth. Antiseptic solutions contain hydrogen peroxide, alcohol, or boric acid in varying strengths but are not effective enough for use on work surfaces or tools.

Personal sanitation is an important part of maintaining a clean work environment. Your hands and clothing must always be kept clean. Sanitize your hands with liquid soap and warm water before and after every client service and after bathroom visits. Waterless hand sanitizers are easy and convenient to use at your personal workstation.

2

Care and Maintenance *of your hairdesigning tools will help ensure they last in accordance with the manufacturer's expected tool life. The type of tool, whether manual or thermal, will determine the proper maintenance procedure to follow to keep tools in good working order. Clean and check your tools frequently, following all safety and maintenance instructions for each type of tool.*

Manual Tools include any non-electric tools such as combs, brushes and rollers. After each use, all manual tools should be cleaned and disinfected according to the requirements established by your regulatory agency.

To clean a manual tool, first remove loose hair and soak the implement in a bucket containing a soap and water solution or professional cleaner. (Be sure to follow all manufacturer's directions when using a professional cleaning agent.) After soaking your tools, rinse them in fresh, clean water, then sanitize and store them.

Some manual tools, such as boar bristle brushes, should not be soaked in cleaning solutions. To avoid swelling and damage to certain types of handles from prolonged immersion in liquid, clean the tool's surface with soap and water, towel dry and disinfect your tools before placing them in a dry sanitizer.

RA

Ask your instructor about additional regulatory requirements or refer to the CLiC Cosmetology module.

Tool Maintenance ...

Thermal Tools should always be unplugged before cleaning. Follow the manufacturer's and your regulatory agency's guidelines on cleaning any heat appliance. Improper care and maintenance will limit the life expectancy of your tools. Below is a brief overview of commonly accepted methods for cleaning most thermal equipment.

Irons and Pressing Combs, whether conventional or electric, can be sanitized by wiping them with a damp cloth containing a soap and water solution. Grease, dirt and chemical buildup on the teeth or barrels of these tools can be removed by adding a small amount of ammonia to the solution for irons, or hot baking soda for pressing combs. Use a light grit sandpaper or very fine steel wool with some mineral oil to remove any remaining carbon or rust.

Airformers require special attention around the air intake area when cleaning; the vent and air filter screen can collect dust and lint quickly. If not removed, debris will block the airflow.

Electric Rollers, Air Brushes and Heaters should be regularly wiped with a damp cloth containing a soapy water solution to keep them in good working order. Be sure that the appliances are unplugged. Always wipe the appliance with a dry cloth after cleaning.

Hood Dryers should be wiped down daily. They have an air filter that requires cleaning regularly. Follow the manufacturer's instructions for proper filter removal and cleaning.

Some important tips to remember for all your electrical equipment:

- Check electrical cords for exposed wires when performing routine maintenance of your equipment.
- Be careful not to overload electrical outlets.
- Never submerge any electrical tools into water or liquid chemicals.

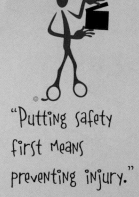

"Putting safety first means preventing injury."

When planning a salon, special attention should be paid to lighting, flooring and climate control. A well-designed salon is a pleasant place to work and a comfortable environment for your clients. Here is an overview of the main areas found in a salon.

The Reception and Retail Area

is where clients form their first impression of the salon, so it is important that this area appears welcoming and friendly. The reception area usually contains a front desk, waiting area, magazine rack, retail shelves and a coat closet. Some reception areas offer refreshments. This is also where appointments are made and financial transactions within the salon occur.

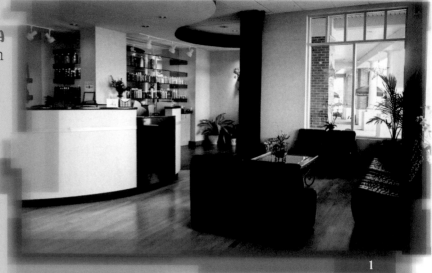

1

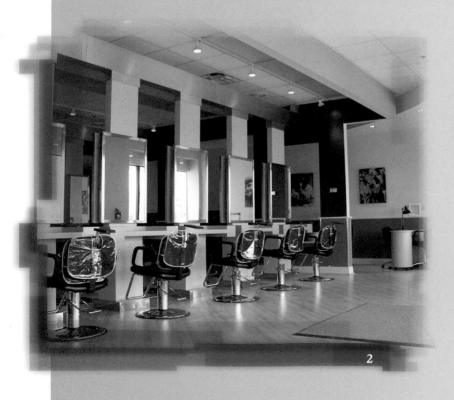

2

The Styling Area

contains workstations. Each station should include a mirror and a styling chair and should allow an efficient amount of working space. Stations need to be kept clean and well-organized. Hydraulic and styling chairs with adjustable height allow hairdesigners to make services more comfortable and convenient for their clients. Roller carts store various types of equipment. Some styling stations have a shampoo bowl attached; others have freestanding shampoo units in a separate area.

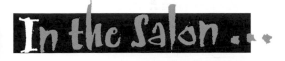
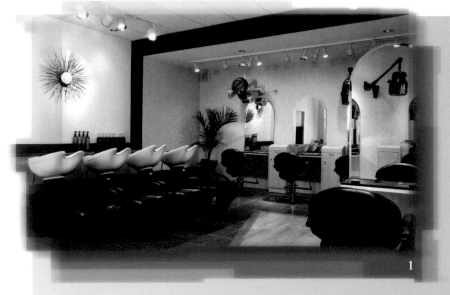

The Shampoo Area

contains sinks and reclining chairs. It should also contain shelves for clean, fresh towels, a covered hamper for dirty linens and a covered trashcan for soiled and used supplies. In certain salon floor plans, the shampoo area is included within the styling area.

The Dryer Area

typically houses a row of conventional hood dryers and may also include manicure tables. Keep this area client-friendly and clean. Current magazines and newspapers should be available for clients to read while under the dryer. Some salons do not have a separate dryer area but include dryers in the styling area.

A **hood dryer**, or air-conditioned dryer, is used to dry the hair and process chemical treatments. Hair is dried by blowing warmed air through the open holes of the dryer's circular, plastic hood. Check the temperature setting while the client is under the hood of a dryer and ensure that he/she is comfortable. Some clients, especially those who have high blood pressure or other physical conditions, may be sensitive to the heat.

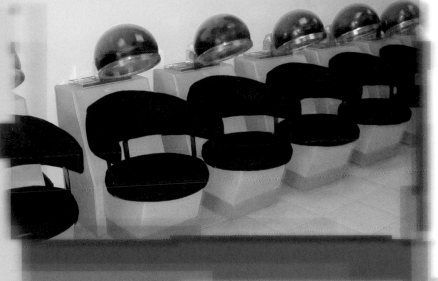

Manicure, Pedicure, Makeup, Massage and Facial Areas

are expected to be included in the layout of a full-service salon. In today's world of one-stop shopping, most clients prefer to have all of their services performed in a single salon. Selling your clients on more than one service can also ensure client retention.

The Dispensary Area

stores supplies used by salon staff members. This room or area should have a sink for staff members to wash their hands between client services. The staff's personal items may also be stored in this area.

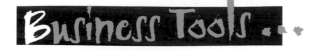

2

The Salon Appointment Book is a fundamental time management tool used to track several stylists' schedules at once. Be aware of other staff members' timing when sharing a client for multiple services. Symbols easily identify multi-serviced clients at a glance. Different colors or icons can be used to **record each service** next to the client's name; i.e., red for a chemical service and blue for haircuts. Use colored pencils instead of markers so changes can be made if necessary. Allow extra time for consultation when booking a new client.

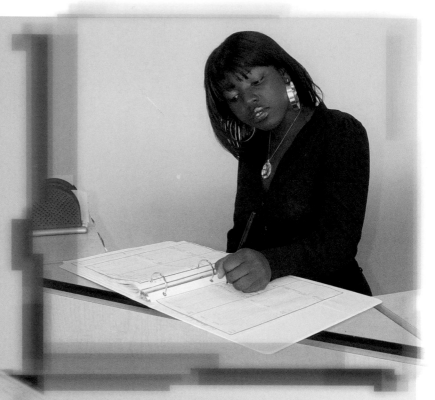

Client Profile Cards are questionnaires clients complete during their first visit to the salon. Useful information requested includes:
- client's name
- home and e-mail addresses
- home and work phone numbers
- how the client learned of the salon
- client's interest in various services the salon offers

This tool helps define the client's wants and needs. Helping clients complete the card in a private area of the salon provides the perfect opportunity to ask about health issues, medications and anything else that might affect cosmetology services. Clients can be sensitive about revealing personal information, so be careful to **protect client confidentiality**. Computer software programs designed for the salon industry will help protect and organize this important information gained during a client consultation. Thorough, accurate record keeping avoids mistakes and builds good client relationships.

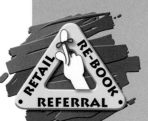

Use profile data to:
- thank clients for their referrals
- send appointment reminders
- offer a discount on a future visit

"Personal information is contained on these cards, so the utmost care should be taken to protect client confidentiality."

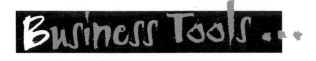

Business Tools ...

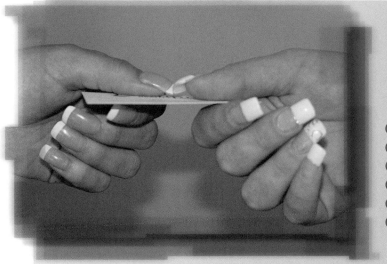

2

Appointment and Business Cards

play a crucial part in marketing your services to clientele. Appointment cards serve as friendly and convenient **reminders** of your client's next hair appointment and include:

- the salon name
- phone number
- e-mail and standard mail addresses
- hours of operation
- hairdesigner's name
- space for the date and time of the client's next appointment

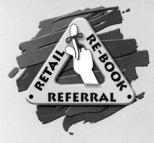

For the most professional appearance, have a printer typeset your name on both appointment and business cards. If your salon does not offer individual cards for each stylist, customize salon cards by clearly printing or stamping your name and hours on the back. Hairdesigners should always carry an ample supply of business cards. Everyone you meet is a potential client or business contact.

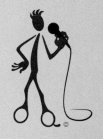

"Make your business card trendy and eye-catching. Your card creates a lasting impression on potential clients, so make it a good one!"

Gift Certificates and Cards

are effective tools for promoting additional salon services. They can also be used to thank a client for a referral or remember a special event in a client's life. Certificates and cards **attract new clients** during the holidays. For instance, a "Two for One" haircut special is a creative way to bring couples into your salon around St. Valentine's Day.

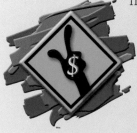

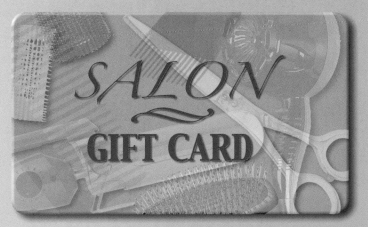

SALON GIFT CARD

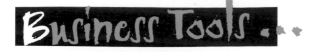

Salon Imaging Systems are computer software programs originally created for cosmetic surgeons to help clients visualize the expected results and later adapted for use in salons. Imaging systems use a client's digital photograph to preview different hair colors, hair lengths, hairdesigns and makeup applications. Hairdesigners use this tool to consult with the client to create and apply the desired look. Some programs make changes appear three-dimensional so a client can see how a style will appear from various angles.

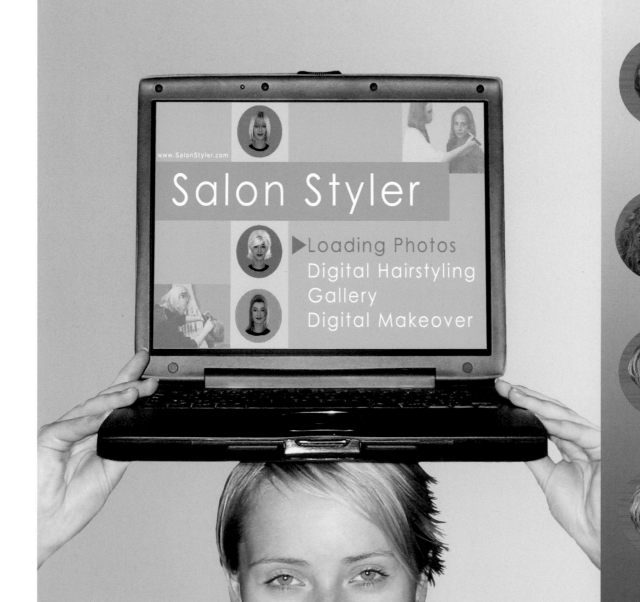

www.SalonStyler.com

Salon Styler

▶Loading Photos
Digital Hairstyling
Gallery
Digital Makeover

Now that you have learned about the tools and equipment used in hairdesigning, here are some exciting Web sites you can visit to learn more about the world of cosmetology. To learn more about us and other cosmetology groups and associations, visit CLiC International: www.clicusa.com.

Industry Associations & Organizations:

American Association of Cosmetology Schools (AACS)
www.beautyschools.org

American Beauty Association (ABA)
www.abbies.org

Behind the Chair
www.behindthechair.com

CLiC INTERNATIONAL
www.clicusa.com

Cosmetic, Toiletry, and Fragrance Association (CFTA)
www.ctfa.org

Cosmetology Advancement Foundation (CAF)
www.cosmetology.org

Cosmetology Educators of America (CEA)
www.beautyeducators.org

Cosmoprof International
www.cosmoprof.com

The Day Spa Association (DSA)
www.dayspaassociation.com

The Professional and Beauty Association (PBA)
www.probeauty.org

The International SalonSpa Bussiness Network (ISBN)
www.salonspanetwork.org

Locks of Love
www.locksoflove.org

Look Good Feel Better
www.lookgoodfeelbetter.org

National Accrediting Commission of Cosmetology Arts & Sciences (NACCAS)
www.naccas.org

National Cosmetology Association (NCA)
www.salonprofessionals.org

Organisation Mondiale de la Coiffure (OMC)
www.omchairworld.com

The Salon Association (TSA)
www.probeauty.org

The Spa Association (SPAA)
www.thespaassociation.com

Beauty Shows:

Americas Beauty Show (ABS)(Chicago Midwest Beauty Show)
www.americasbeautyshow.com

International Beauty Show (IBS), New York
www.ibsnewyork.com

Premiere Beauty Show
www.premiereshows.com

Industry Magazines:

American Salon
www.americansalonmag.com

Modern Salon
www.modernsalon.com

Salon Today
www.salontoday.com

European Web Sites:

Beauty Jobs Online
www.beautyjobsonline.com

Comité International Desthétique et de Cosmétologie (CIDESCO)
www.cidesco.com

Dermascope
www.dermascope.com

Esthétique Spa International
www.spa-show.com

International Esthetic, Cosmetic and Spa Conference
www.magda.com

Professional Beauty
www.professionalbeauty.co.uk

Spa and Resort Expo and Conference
www.spaandresortexpo.com

2

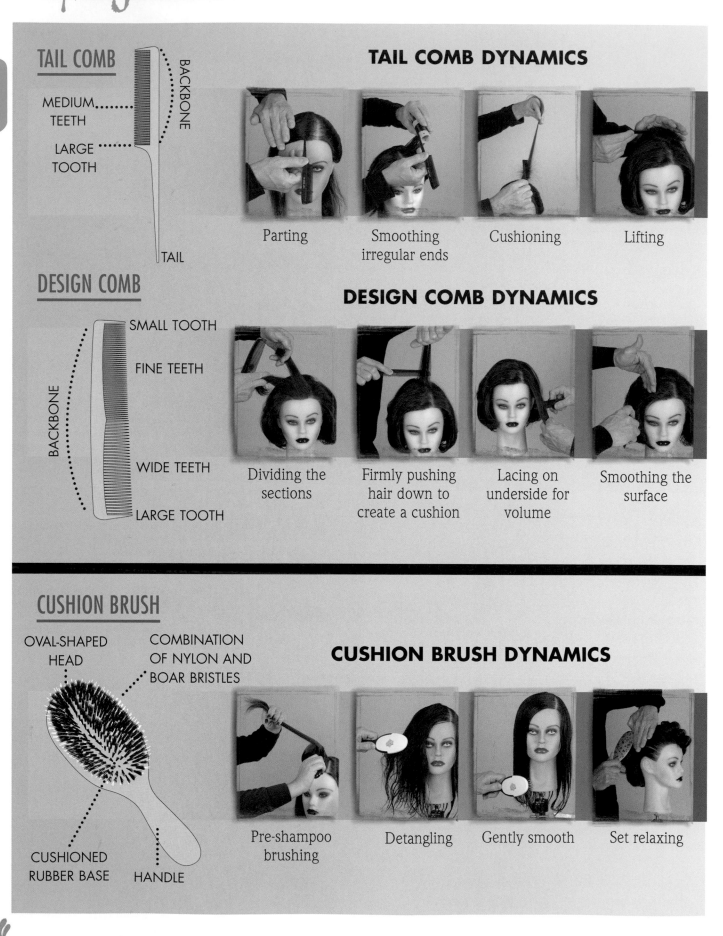

TAIL COMB

BACKBONE
MEDIUM TEETH
LARGE TOOTH
TAIL

TAIL COMB DYNAMICS

Parting

Smoothing irregular ends

Cushioning

Lifting

DESIGN COMB

SMALL TOOTH
FINE TEETH
BACKBONE
WIDE TEETH
LARGE TOOTH

DESIGN COMB DYNAMICS

Dividing the sections

Firmly pushing hair down to create a cushion

Lacing on underside for volume

Smoothing the surface

CUSHION BRUSH

OVAL-SHAPED HEAD
COMBINATION OF NYLON AND BOAR BRISTLES
CUSHIONED RUBBER BASE
HANDLE

CUSHION BRUSH DYNAMICS

Pre-shampoo brushing

Detangling

Gently smooth

Set relaxing

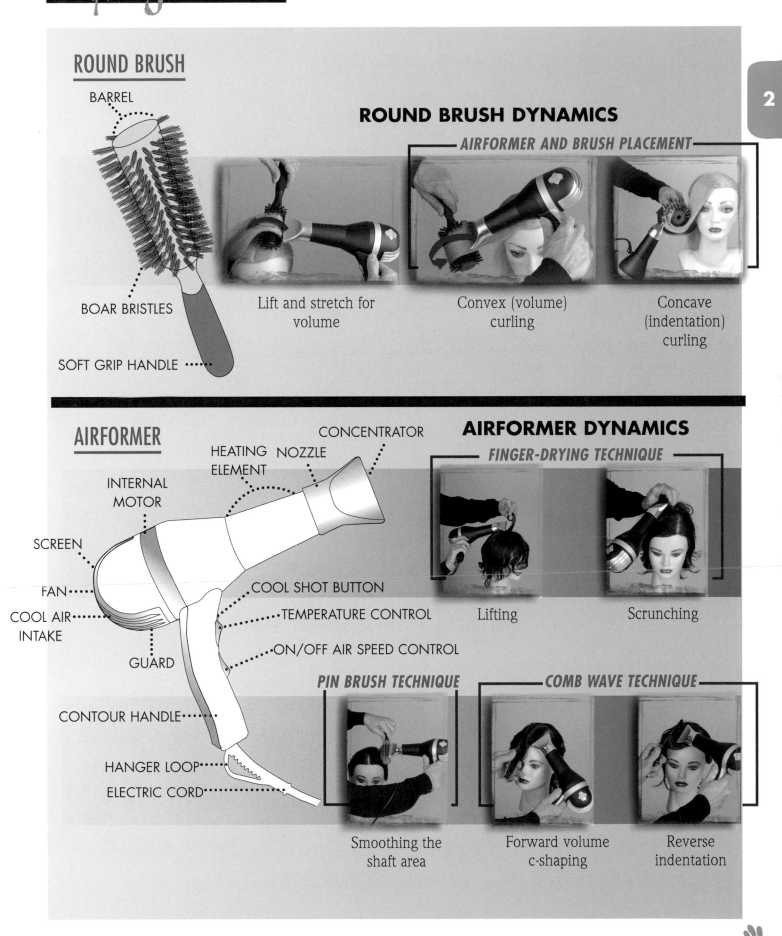

ROUND BRUSH

- BARREL
- BOAR BRISTLES
- SOFT GRIP HANDLE

ROUND BRUSH DYNAMICS

AIRFORMER AND BRUSH PLACEMENT

Lift and stretch for volume

Convex (volume) curling

Concave (indentation) curling

AIRFORMER

- CONCENTRATOR
- HEATING ELEMENT
- NOZZLE
- INTERNAL MOTOR
- SCREEN
- FAN
- COOL AIR INTAKE
- COOL SHOT BUTTON
- TEMPERATURE CONTROL
- ON/OFF AIR SPEED CONTROL
- GUARD
- CONTOUR HANDLE
- HANGER LOOP
- ELECTRIC CORD

AIRFORMER DYNAMICS

FINGER-DRYING TECHNIQUE

Lifting

Scrunching

PIN BRUSH TECHNIQUE

Smoothing the shaft area

COMB WAVE TECHNIQUE

Forward volume c-shaping

Reverse indentation

2

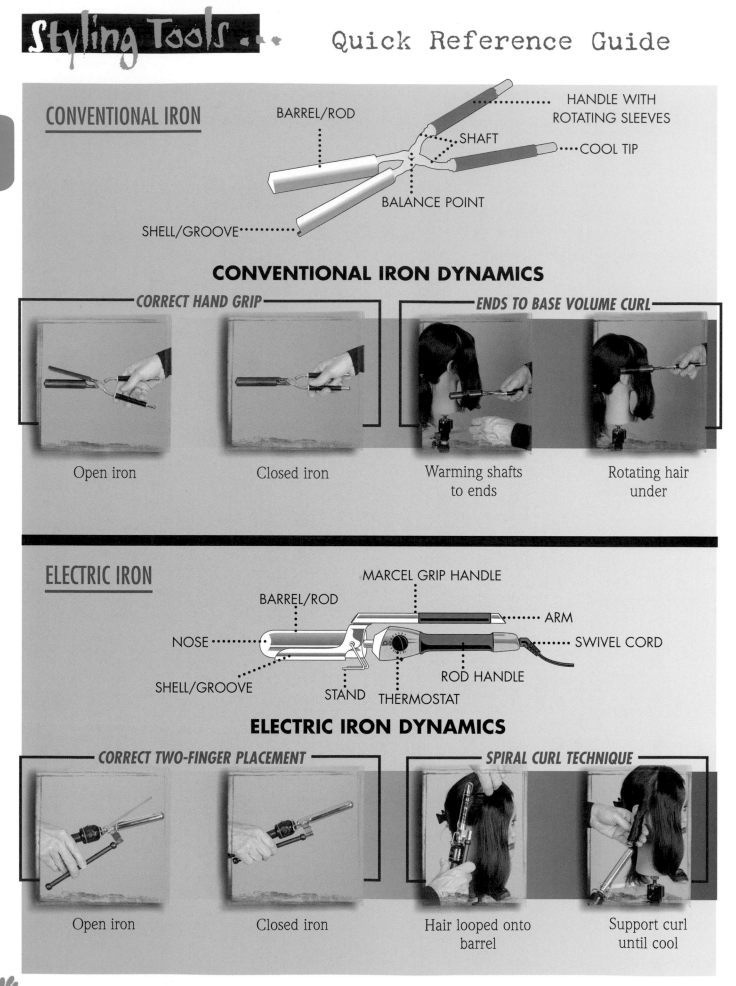

CONVENTIONAL IRON

BARREL/ROD

HANDLE WITH
ROTATING SLEEVES

SHAFT

COOL TIP

BALANCE POINT

SHELL/GROOVE

CONVENTIONAL IRON DYNAMICS

CORRECT HAND GRIP

ENDS TO BASE VOLUME CURL

Open iron

Closed iron

Warming shafts
to ends

Rotating hair
under

ELECTRIC IRON

MARCEL GRIP HANDLE

BARREL/ROD

ARM

NOSE

SWIVEL CORD

SHELL/GROOVE

ROD HANDLE

STAND

THERMOSTAT

ELECTRIC IRON DYNAMICS

CORRECT TWO-FINGER PLACEMENT

SPIRAL CURL TECHNIQUE

Open iron

Closed iron

Hair looped onto
barrel

Support curl
until cool

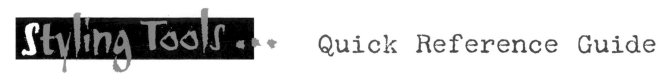

2

CONVENTIONAL PRESSING COMB

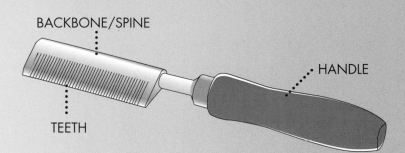

BACKBONE/SPINE

HANDLE

TEETH

PRESSING COMB DYNAMICS

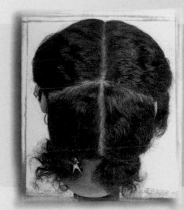

Sectioning

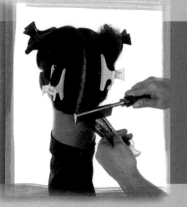

Placing preheated
comb at hair in
scalp area

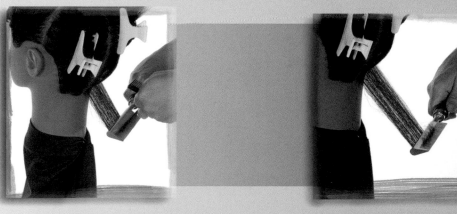

Pulling through
shaft

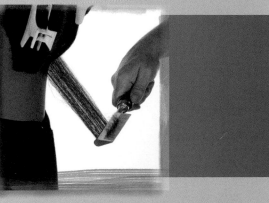

Smoothing hair
ends

FILL-IN-THE-BLANKS

Antiseptics
Butterfly
Client Profile
Concentrators
Cornrow
Cushion
Disinfectants
Fixatives
Hair Form
Heater
Imaging
Maintenance
Marcel
Neck Strips
Paddle
Pressing
Single Prong
Steel Wool
Tail
Waving Iron

1. _____ combs make clean, precise partings in a geometric shaping.

2. _____ are used between the cape and a client's skin.

3. _____ cards are confidential records of services performed on clients.

4. _____ combs are used to straighten hair.

5. Prolong the life of hairdesign tools with routine _____.

6. _____ systems show clients a preview of how a finished hairdesign will look on them.

7. _____ handle grips are preferred by professional hairdesigners.

8. _____ brushes are used for controlling large amounts of hair.

9. _____ are hairsprays used to hold completed hairdesigns.

10. _____ clips are often used to hold electric rollers in place.

11. _____ control the growth of pathogenic microorganisms on the surface of tools.

12. To create height or unusual hairdesign dimensions, insert a _____.

13. A stove used to warm irons and pressing combs is also called a _____.

14. _____ are used on skin to kill bacteria.

15. _____ brushes are used to relax sets or prior to shampooing.

16. _____ add more heat precision and control to the airformer.

17. _____ creams help maintain control of hair while braiding intricate designs.

18. A multi-barreled tool used to create movement is a _____.

19. _____ clips are used to secure pin curl placements.

20. Irons should be cleaned with fine _____.

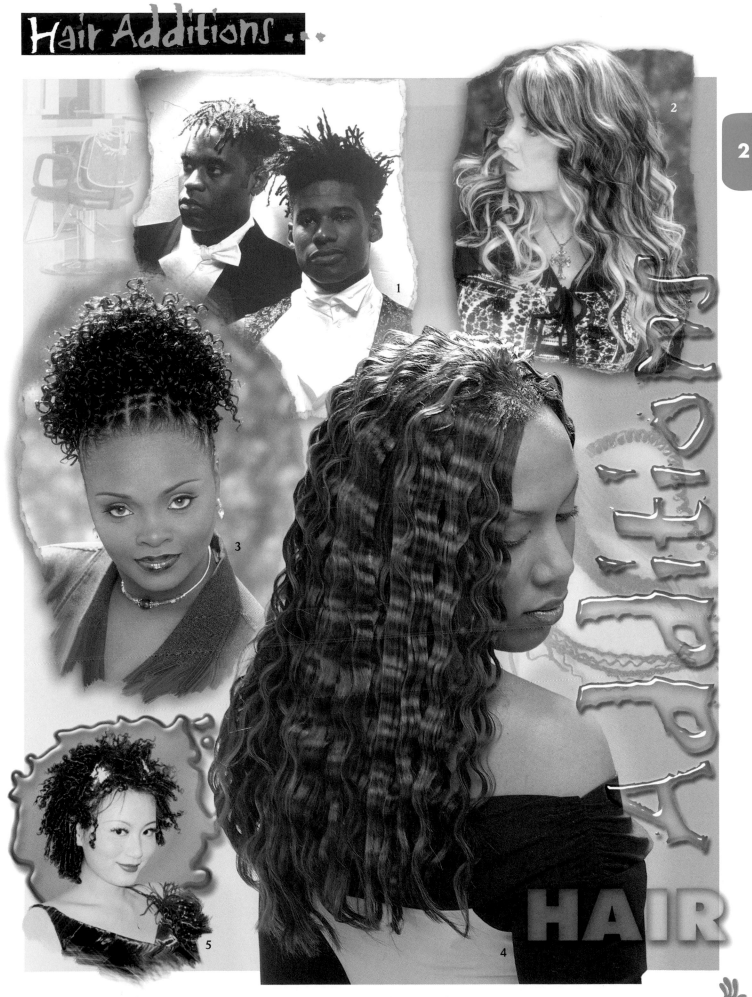

Hair Additions *services are used to increase volume, add length and create a variety of special effects. For clients who wish to instantly modify their look, hair extensions are considered fashion accessories, providing color and texture to accompany any fashion personality. Wigs and hairpieces help clients who may have experienced hair loss or simply desire a dramatic new look. The techniques for the art of hair additions selection, application, maintenance, and removal are found in Chapter 9.*

Many tools used in hair extensions, cranial prostheses (wigs) and hair replacement have been created exclusively to assist in the attachment process. A pattern called a **template** is used as a guide to form a custom made wig or hairpiece. Here is a brief overview of tools used either to make templates or to assist in the application of hair additions services.

▶ MEASUREMENT AND TEMPLATE-MAKING TOOLS

A Tape Measure calculates the circumference of a client's head, the hair's length and the size of thinning areas on the scalp.

A Standard Marker or Grease Pencil aids in measuring and marking areas on a template.

Wig Blocks are head forms used to support wigs and hairpieces for styling, sizing and storage. They are made from wood, plastic foam or a cloth-covered filler. Special hairless massage mannequins may also be used when designing hairpieces or wigs to ensure proper placement of the style's focal point in relation to the features on a face.

Hair Additions...

▶ **EXTENSIONS**

Extensions are available in varying lengths, colors and textures ranging from straight hair to dreadlocks. Extensions can be purchased pre-bonded or individually. (When hair is not bonded by any material, it is held together by elastic bands.) Commercially prepared hair can be clipped-in, bonded with adhesive or sewn together along a seam into wefts. The best cap wigs are hand-tied to closely mimic actual human hair growth patterns. A "capless" wig is formed by sewing wefts into a circular pattern in an open, breathable framework.

Some manufacturers mix an assortment of hair and fiber types in their final products which will affect the way hairdesigners work with them. Before purchasing, verify whether the material to be used is 100 percent human, animal, synthetic or a blend of hair and/or synthetic fiber.

Synthetic Hair is offered in various colors, lengths and textures. Because synthetic fiber is made of man-made modacrylic material, it retains its shape after shampooing, requires minimal care and is less costly than human hair. Synthetics come with pre-determined color, texture and style to match the client's hair and cannot be chemically altered to any great degree. Heat styling appliances may damage the fiber. Since liquid tools containing alcohol or certain oils alter the appearance and texture of synthetic fibers, they require special cleansers and styling agents.

Natural Human Hair is more durable than synthetics and is available in a variety of colors, lengths and textures. It is cut, cleaned and sanitized prior to use. The chemicals used during the manufacturer's cleaning and sanitizing process can damage the cuticle, alter the natural color and affect the overall condition of the hair. Many commercial strands have been re-colored to the desired shade. Because of these factors, always shampoo natural human hair products to test for colorfastness and apply a conditioning agent prior to use to keep naturally harvested human hair soft and pliable.

Animal Hair goes through a cleaning and sanitizing process similar to that used on human hair, and is usually used for hair additions only when blended with other hair or synthetic fibers. This hair is widely available from the yak, horse, camel, sheep, boar, goat, or rabbit (angora), but the natural white color of yak hair is widely preferred as a base for hair additions in fantasy colors.

Yarns can be manufactured from cottons, nylons, polyesters or any combination of these. This fiber is used to create braids, dreadlocks, and other integrated hairpieces.

APPLICATION TOOLS

A **Tail Comb** helps divide and section hair for hair extension placements. The tail can be used for holding sections of hair in place prior to applying a hair addition.

Sectioning Clips are used to separate hair for the application of extensions.

A **Wire or Pin Brush** has flexible teeth to easily brush over and through hair additions to help eliminate static electricity, smooth the hair and remove tangles without damage.

A **Razor, Scissors and Thinning Scissors** help cut and blend hair additions into the natural hair. A razor is often used to create softer edges. Thinning scissors may be used on hair additions to eliminate bulk in the design.

Bonding Agents are used to attach hair additions to the existing hair, a mesh cap or other bases. Bonding agents, also called adhesives, glue or fusions, are available in stick, liquid, gel or spray form. Solid adhesive sticks are warmed with a heated applicator gun prior to their application or removal. Some manufacturers suggest the use of needle nose pliers to crack or loosen an adhesive seal during hair additions removal. Use only the alcohol or oil based **solvent recommended** by the bonding agent's manufacturer to prevent adverse chemical reactions and damage to the hair or scalp.

Double-Sided Tape made especially made for hair additions is another method of attachment. Practice is required in the proper application of double-sided tape in strips to cover the entire base surface. Failure to do this will limit the amount of adhesion for maximum durability. After application, the tape must not be exposed to water until the agent has cured.

Thread can be manufactured in cotton, nylon or a combination of the two. Match the thread color to the client's hair and/or the color of the hair additions. Commercial thread cutters are used to keep thread from fraying and weakening the integrity of the extension.

Hair Additions ...

A Curved Needle is used to sew hair extensions to existing hair or other materials such as nets or weave caps. The needle should be curved to protect the client from harm during its use in the application of hair extensions.

Weave or Mesh Caps are used to create the bases of attachments. They are usually made from nylon, cotton, polyester or a blend of these materials. A good weave cap should be breathable and inexpensive.

Hairnets in fine or wide mesh may be substituted for weave or mesh caps for "integration," which utilizes some of the client's hair without completely covering it.

The Weaving Pole Machine is comprised of any number of spindle poles to hold thread and natural hair or synthetic fiber while making wefts or tracking (a process of creating a base to which hair is attached). A weaving pole machine is usually placed in an elevated position beside a client. Machine-made wigs are generally less expensive than those that are hand-tied.

A Braid Sealer is a commercial product designed to cut, shape and fuse the end of a synthetic fiber plait below the elastic band and prevent loose or frayed ends. Some braid sealers may contain adhesive, heat, or a combination of both and are also used to join the client's existing hair to extensions.

The Latch Hook has a bent end used to catch and loop extensions or wefts through the base of a client's hair that has been braided into cornrows.

FILL–IN–THE–BLANKS

Adhesive Sticks
Applicator Gun
Bonding Agents
Braid Sealer
Conditioner
Curved Needle
Double-Sided
Grease Pencil
Hairnets
Human Hair
Latch Hook
Pin Brushes
Prosthesis
Solvents
Tape Measure
Template
Weaving Pole
Wefts
Wig Block
Yak

1. _____ are adhesives used to attach a hair addition to existing hair or a mesh cap.

2. To avoid injuring clients while sewing additions to existing hair, use a _____.

3. _____ are used to loosen adhesives and remove hair additions.

4. _____ are hair or fibers sewn together along a seam.

5. Maintain the shape of hairpieces by storing them on a _____.

6. Calculate the circumference of the head with a _____.

7. A machine used to hold hair or fiber for creating wefts is a _____.

8. A guide used to form a custom wig or hairpiece is a _____.

9. _____ is a type of animal hair commonly used in additions.

10. To fuse plaited additions with natural hair, use a _____.

11. A tool with a bent end used to attach additions to cornrows is a _____.

12. To preheat a bonding agent and secure hair additions, use an _____.

13. _____ made of mesh help integrate natural hair with additions.

14. _____ should be tested for colorfastness prior to use.

15. To keep naturally harvested hair soft and pliable, use _____.

16. _____ tape is applied in strips when attaching hairpieces.

17. _____ are used with a heating gun for the attaching process.

18. _____ have flexible teeth to remove tangles without damage.

19. Another term for a wig is a cranial _____.

20. Mark areas on a template using a _____.

STUDENT'S NAME   DATE   GRADE

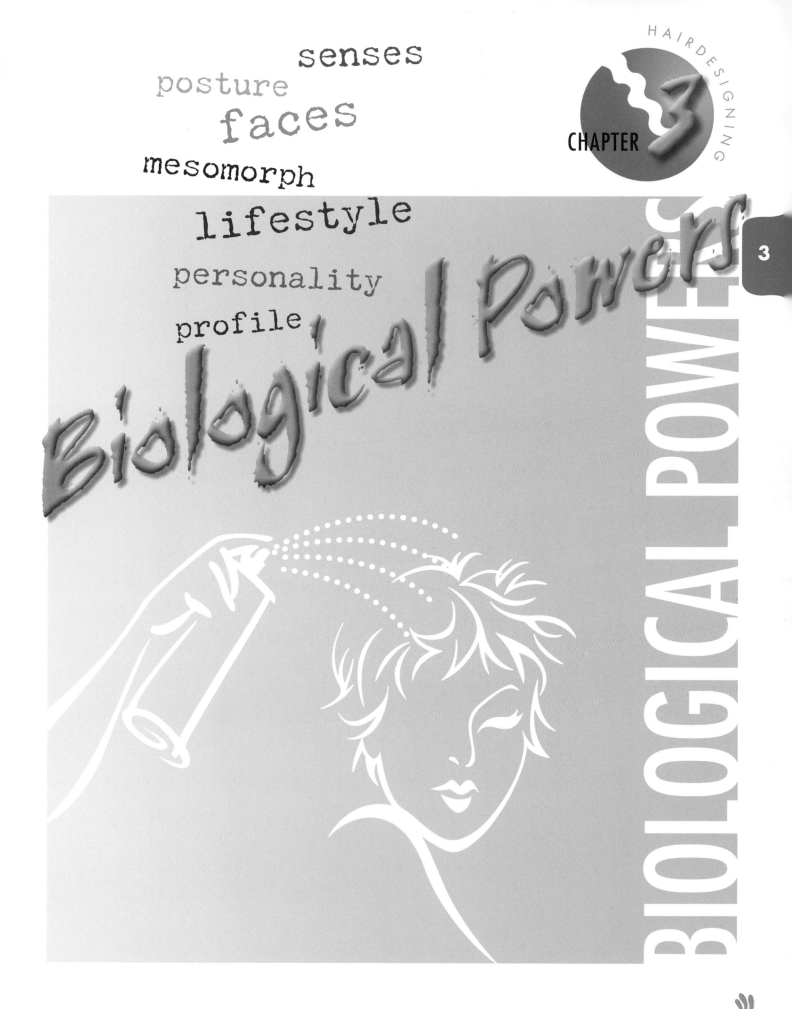

senses

posture

faces

mesomorph

lifestyle

personality

profile

Biological Powers

BIOLOGICAL POWERS

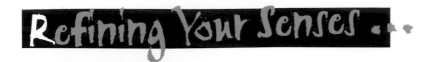

Refining Your Senses

By expanding your knowledge of hairdesign, the ability to use your inborn talent and skill grows. The first step toward becoming a more knowledgeable and artistic hairdesigner is to heighten your senses.

As you step into the theater of hairdesign, challenge yourself to **see**, **listen**, and **feel** more intensely.

"Many people LOOK, but do not see...
LISTEN, but do not hear...
and TOUCH but do not feel!"

▶ EXERCISE

Look at the picture to the left, and list everything you see. When you finish the Hairdesigning module, return to this page and make another list of everything you see. Compare lists to observe how much you have learned. Keep practicing!

NOW

LATER

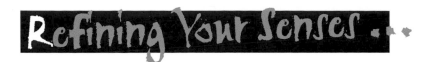

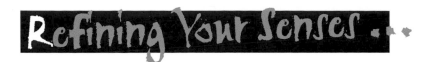

► **EXERCISE**

Look at the picture to the right, and list everything you see. When you finish the Hairdesigning module, return to this page and make another list of everything you see. Compare lists to observe how much you have learned. Keep practicing!

NOW

_____

_____

_____

_____

_____

_____

_____

_____

LATER

_____

_____

_____

_____

_____

_____

_____

_____

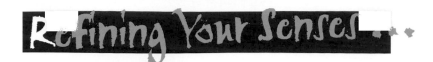

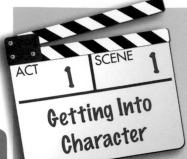

ACT **1** SCENE **1**

Getting Into Character

3

Hairdesigners *use four of the five senses (sight, hearing, touch, and smell) to assess clients and create artistic expressions. From the moment the client arrives, the **senses** are employed, reading the client in anticipation of creating a unique, complementary hairdesign that will add to the client's total image. Honing the **use** of these senses brings a greater level of expertise in the art of hairdesigning.*

Sight: The sense of sight allows you to analyze your client from head to toe. Examining **colors** and **textures** of the hair and the client's overall appearance is just the beginning. The professional stylist needs to go deeper to mentally visualize the **form, direction,** and **balance** the hairdesign will take, the effects of a design on the **facial shape,** and the finished design's impact on the **client's lifestyle.**

Hearing: The things your client **says,** along with what you **see,** will affect your hairdesign. **Listen** attentively for your client's **needs** and **desires,** making adjustments according to the design plan.

Touch: As your hands touch your client's hair, scalp, and face, you learn about the hair as well as the client's underlying bone structure. You also learn about your client's **comfort levels.** Pay attention to how the client reacts as you perform services. A **gentle touch** is required on **sensitive** individuals.

Smell: **Memories** associated with smell are the **strongest** and most **enduring**. Create an atmosphere that is positive for your client, and you will see the rewards in both financial and personal ways.

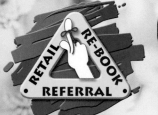

RETAIL · RE-BOOK · REFERRAL

Refining Your Senses...

Look at the big picture when planning a hairdesign for a client. Start with an assessment, which is an evaluation in relation to the whole. Examine your client from head to toe, and listen attentively to his/her wants and needs. This chapter covers the *biological areas* hairdesigners use to assess their clients.

The **Biological Areas of Client Assessment** include:

- Lifestyle
- Fashion Personality
- Body Proportions
- Body Type
- Posture
- Face Shape
- Facial Features
- Head Shape
- Hair Structure
- Hair Texture
- Hair Growth Patterns
- Individual Considerations

Professional stylists need to examine each of the biological areas and consider how they will influence the hairdesign plan. Rely on your senses to determine each area during a client assessment. See the Success Dynamics module for more consultation dialogue.

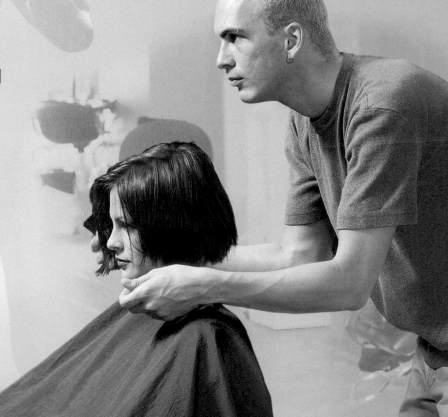

Michelangelo saw his statue of David in the block of marble. Stroke after stroke he removed what stood in the way of revealing his masterpiece. Your masterpiece is waiting. Use your inborn sensory ability to create hair artistry.

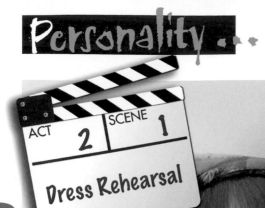

ACT 2 SCENE 1

Dress Rehearsal

3

aah!

Use your senses to assess the client's lifestyle and personality.

An actor shows the audience a character's lifestyle and personality through costume, makeup, body language and facial expressions. The audience focuses on the actor's face, watching for cues on mood, thoughts or feelings. The actor's success is measured by the audience's approval and applause.

hmmm...

oooooh!

A hairdesigner shows his/her artistic skill through a hairdesign that reflects the client's lifestyle and personality. The audience for your artistic work includes the people your client interacts with in his/her life. Your success is measured by the client's repeat business and recommendations to his/her friends and family.

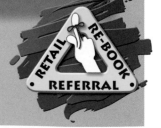

RETAIL · RE-BOOK REFERRAL

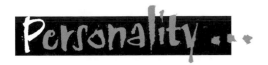

Personality ...

Active

Is your client extroverted, outgoing, and active?

Does your client appear to be **extroverted** or **reserved?** Do mannerisms tell you anything? What is the client wearing? Is **appearance** of vital importance to his/her professional success? Is flexibility of style important? What do you **see?**

As you question your client about lifestyle, likes and dislikes, needs and desires, do the answers you **hear** agree with what you **see**, or do they differ? Are you **listening?**

When you first **touch** your client, are you getting any indication that you are too rough? What is the **texture** of the client's hair? Has the client had recent chemical processes performed? **Feel** the information.

Outgoing

1

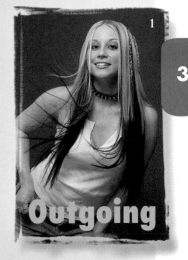

Reserved

"As you develop skill at using your senses, your hairdesigns will become as unique as the client."

Dramatic

2

Casual

Active

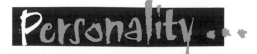

Personality...

A client's fashion personality sets the stage for creating a hairdesign that coordinates well with the **total look**. Understanding the latest trends in fashion will help your hairdesigns become more artistic. Four basic fashion descriptions identify each personality style for men and women.

The **Sporty** woman tends to wear unstructured or softly tailored clothing. Fresh, friendly, and often athletic, she prefers hairstyles that are uncomplicated or wash-and-go.

The **Classic** woman leans toward clean, simple lines and finely tailored elegant or sophististicated clothing. Sleek, well-groomed hairstyles are favored by this elegant and refined fashion personality.

1

3

4

2

SPORTY   CLASSIC

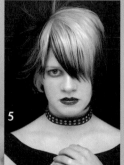

5

6

DRAMATIC

The **Dramatic** woman likes high fashion clothing, form-fitting suits, and other severely tailored ensembles. Like the Classic, the Dramatic fashion personality wants a hairdesign that is sleek and well-groomed but has angularity or asymmetry.

ROMANTIC

The **Romantic** woman is the quintessential ideal of femininity. She loves delicate details and soft, flowing fabrics. Hairdesigns that include graceful curls or soft, curvy layers are her dominant choice.

7

8

Some individuals have more than one fashion personality. These people enjoy change and adapt to the occasion or their mood of the day.

3

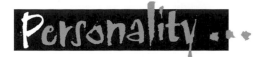

Personality ...

The **Sporty** man prefers straighter cut suits and unstructured jackets. Sportswear made with textural fabrics suits him. The best hairdesigns for this fashion personality are free-formed and easy to maintain.

SPORTY

2

3

The **Classic** man prefers simple, dignified suits, wears khakis and polo-style shirts for casual wear, and avoids extremes in color, cut, and style. He likes conservative hairdesigns that have clean lines.

1

4

CLASSIC

ROMANTIC

5

6

DRAMATIC

The **Dramatic** man typically wears clothing well, preferring European or designer clothing and the latest sportswear. An angular, trendy hairdesign would suit him.

7

The **Romantic** man is sometimes a flamboyant dresser. He prefers European cut suits with relaxed fit pants, enjoys fine fabrics and designer sportswear. Hairdesigns with soft lines fit his personality best.

8

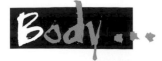

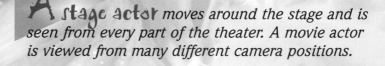

ACT **3** SCENE **1**

Casting

A *stage actor moves around the stage and is seen from every part of the theater. A movie actor is viewed from many different camera positions.*

Your client will be moving before his/her own audience and will be observed from all angles. When creating a design, keep in mind the entire **body proportion**, not just what can be seen above the waist in the salon mirror. Your client's hairdesign should look great from all angles.

Proportion means that every part fits with the whole. Every arrangement must look harmonious or graceful, complimenting your client's individual traits. The hairdesign should appear neither **too large** nor **too small** in comparison to the biological proportions of the body.

1

2

3

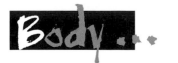

Body...

Body Proportion *has been carefully studied and detailed in its properties by art historians, who consider the human body to be the highest form of art.*

Leonardo da Vinci created an artistic composition called *The Vitruvian Man*, named after the Roman architect Marcus Vitruvius (ve-trü-vE-es), who translated the human body's measurements into a method used for creating symmetry in art and architectural design. The drawing became commonly known as the *Canon of Proportions*, and is symbolic of the human body's artistic balance and proportion. In our industry, it is recognized as an essential influence in hairdesign.

Leonardo da Vinci

"Just as a performer reads a script, checks out the stage and prepares for the performance, you must learn how to read your client, take note of their body type and size and prepare to perform with hair as your artistic medium and nature as your stage."

Leonardo da Vinci's Vitruvian Man

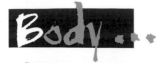

Body...

In art design, *the biological proportions of the body are measured using the length and width of the head. Your role as a professional hairdesigner is to determine the most flattering style for your client's overall features. Through practice you will develop your intuition for evaluating and balancing proportions to more closely resemble an artist's ideal.*

The ideal body proportions:

- An **adult's height** is equivalent to 7 or 8 head-lengths.

- The maximum **shoulder breadth** is approximately 2 head-lengths.

- **Torso length** is equivalent to the height of 2 heads.

- The **waist** should equal twice the size of the neck.

- In the human body the **central point** is naturally the navel.

- **Leg length** (hip to toes) is slightly more than half of the body.

- The span from **elbow to wrist** is equal to the size of the foot.

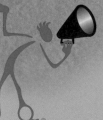

"For a truly personalized approach to hairdesign, add elements complementary to your client's occupation or fashion personality to complete his/her signature style."

1

Use these approximations to assess your client's body proportions in your mind. A person will rarely fit these proportions perfectly. For example, sizes will vary among males and females.

Noticing if your client has smaller or larger body areas (for instance, shorter legs or wider shoulders) than the ideal measurements is the first step in determining what hairdesigns will be most appropriate for the shape of his/her body.

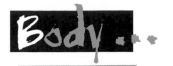

Body...

A child's body proportions *are quite different from those of an adult.*

In comparison to his/her limbs, the torso and head are larger on a child. A typical child's head is rounder and larger in proportion to his/her body than an adult's. A child's facial features appear condensed. The eyebrows rest midway between the chin and crown, the chin and nose are not very prominent, while the eyeballs are almost adult in size.

As a child matures, the body and facial proportions begin to adjust. The facial features move up and the jaw expands as the teeth develop. A child's eyes have moved midway up the face by early adolescence.

Parents often do not consider body proportions when selecting hairstyles for their children. Professional hairdesigners should recommend hairstyles that are appropriate for children as their bodies grow and mature.

► EXERCISE

Practice making hairdesign recommendations to parents of the children pictured on this page. Take turns playing the parts of hairdesigner and parent.

Good proportion
of hair to face

1

2

Tap into a lucrative retail market by recommending hair care and styling products made especially for children or adolescents.

Hair too short for
large head

3

Too much hair
for a small body

4

Too much hair
for face

5

Body...

People are all different

shapes and sizes. In the 1940s, American psychologist William H. Sheldon created Soma Body Types to generally classify physical body proportions (soma is the Greek word for body). A person may possess the characteristics of all three types, but will be predominantly one type.

As you greet a client, briefly assess his or her body from both the front and side. Viewing the body in its entirety will help the hairdesigner create a hairstyle that fits the total picture.

All people will fit into one of the three major body types: the **endomorph**, the **ectomorph** and the **mesomorph**.

"A person cannot change his or her genetic predisposition toward a certain body type, but body condition can change through diet, exercise and physical activity."

▶ Mesomorph (athletic and muscular)

The mesomorph (me-ze-morf) has a **naturally athletic build**. As long as the mesomorph is active, he/she usually has few weight problems. The mesomorph's **shoulders are wider than his/her hips.**

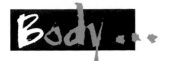

▶ Endomorph (generously rounded or stout and stocky)

The endomorph (en-de-morf) has a **rounded body with short limbs**. Many endomorphs have small hands and feet. This body type is prone to weight problems. The **hips are wider than the shoulders**.

▶ Ectomorph (thin and lean)

The ectomorph (ek-te-morf) has **long, narrow bones and a straight, narrow frame**. This body type has no muscular bulk; instead, the muscles are long and thin. Ectomorphs usually have a low body fat ratio and are sometimes underweight. Notice the ectomorph's **hips and shoulders are equal in width**.

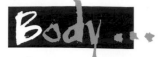

Body...

*Your clients' biological proportions are an essential part of their **total image**. Consider the individual's height, weight and body shape. Accent or counterbalance these important factors as described here to provide a well-proportioned, harmonious end result. Strive to achieve the illusion of a more perfect body proportion by combining clothing and hair fashions that camouflage feature flaws and bring balance to your client's shape.*

Mesomorph

Emphasize this client's muscular physique by creating softer hairstyles. Since this type has a broad upper body and narrow hips, never choose blouses with boat necks or busy patterns that are meant to be tucked. Add volume to the lower half of the body to counterbalance the top by using clothing with heavier or patterned fabric that flares from the waist and hip area.

Endomorph

Balance the endomorph's rounder body image with a fuller or more angular hairdesign, taking care to allow enough length in the style's design to bring the body and head into proportion. Select angular or unbroken vertical lines in clothing with monochromatic (one-color) themes, dropped waistlines, and looser fit.

Ectomorph

Length and volume of the hairdesign should be proportionate to the height of this Soma type. Choose closer styles for a smaller lean frame, or soften a long angular body with fullness or curl. Avoid vertical patterns and solid colors which elongate the body and accentuate lean lines. Consider waist-length jackets that add bulk and define the midsection.

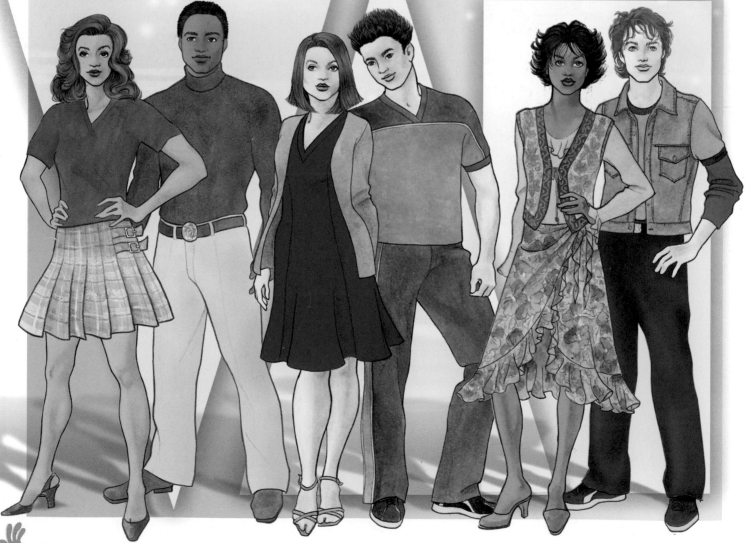

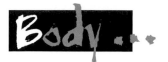

Body...

Once you have determined your client's body type, *consider how the client's biological body structure will affect the hairdesign.*

A long and voluminous hairdesign on a short woman will overpower her body size. On a tall woman, a short, cropped hairdesign will make her head look out of proportion with the rest of her body.

▶ EXERCISE

Identify out of proportion hairdesigns for the body shapes below. Suggest corrections for each out of balance condition.

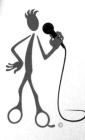

"A well-balanced hairdesign is in proportion to the face and body."

For more information about proportion, see Chapters 4 and 5, the Mathematics and Science of Hairdesigning.

1

2

3

4

5

6

7

8

9

10

11

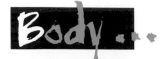

POSTURE

Good posture keeps the bones aligned and allows the muscles, joints and ligaments to function properly no matter what activity is being performed. As with body shape, a client's posture influences the hairdesign plan. By understanding a client's stature, stylists can create hairdesigns that flatter.

During the initial assessment of your client, **examine** his/her body from the **profile** view to look for figure flaws. Consider the upper and lower body proportions and how they relate to one another. Check the position of the client's **head in relationship to his/her shoulders**, then examine the client's **spinal curves**. A forward angle or tilt of the head, sloping shoulders or tilted hips could indicate postural defects. Record any concerns on the client's profile card.

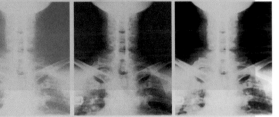

Postural Problems

Scoliosis is an unnatural **side-to-side curvature** of the spine. Indicators of scoliosis are uneven shoulder positions or leg length differences.

Clients with scoliosis should be cautioned against having asymmetrical hairdesigns which accentuate the unevenness of their frames. Recommend soft, flowing curls or waves to flatter the client's body shape.

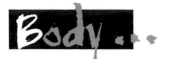

Flat back syndrome is the **absence of normal spinal curves**. This may be seen in clients who have degenerative arthritis or have had corrective surgery for scoliosis. It causes the body to stoop forward, and in extreme cases, makes standing difficult.

Try hairdesigns with curls and waves to soften the body's angular features.

Lordosis, or **swayback**, is an exaggerated **inward curvature of the lower back**. The appearance of a protruding stomach and buttocks are common indicators.

Hairdesigns that flow in straight, vertical movements will counterbalance the vertical curves in the client's body shape.

Kyphosis, or **roundback**, is an exaggerated outward curvature of the upper back, which causes the shoulders to stoop forward.

Sweep hair back in the direction of the occipital bone to counterbalance forward movement of the shoulders and outward curvatures of the upper back.

A **dowager's hump,** associated with osteoporosis, is caused by degeneration of the upper spine. Its symptoms look similar to kyphosis, with a forward positioning of the head and **stooped shoulders**.

Angular hairdesigns that have height in the crown will help counterbalance the rounded spine. If a client has medium to long length hair, use the hair to fill in the visual gap between the neck and shoulders.

Face

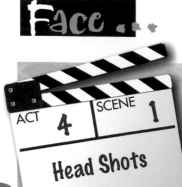

ACT **4** SCENE **1**

Head Shots

3

⫸ Identifying Facial Shapes

Now that we have considered the body, we can focus on the face. The position and prominence of facial bones determines facial shape. Knowing your client's facial shape is crucial in recognizing how to balance the hairdesign.

Square

Rectangle (oblong)

Round (circle)

Diamond

Triangle (pear)

Inverted Triangle (heart)

Oval

To determine facial shape, draw the hair away from the face and neck, allowing full view from hairline to chin and from ear to ear. Mentally trace the perimeter of the face. Is it wide or long? Where is the widest area? Which facial feature is the most appealing, and which is the least? Let this general impression guide you as you visualize the seven face shapes.

"Trace the outline of your face onto a mirror. What face shape do you have?"

THE FACETS OF BEAUTY

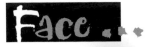

3

Artistic performers and magicians create illusions — hairdesigners do too. Working their magic on clients, they create the illusion of a more proportioned face.

The **Oval** face shape has an ideally balanced vertical and horizontal proportion for hairdesigning. It tapers in a gentle slope from the widest portion, the forehead, to the narrowest portion, the chin.

Although cultural differences bring their own definition of what is beautiful, stylists strive to create the illusion of an oval face on all other face shapes with hairdesigning. Undesirable features may be made less noticeable, while enhancing desired attributes.

"When you use the art of hairdesign to change the features on a client's face, you are practicing the magical art of illusion."

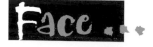

3

"There is beauty in everything; not everyone can see it." *Confucius*

The **Round (Circle)** face is almost as wide as it is long. It typically features a wider middle zone, shorter chin and rounded hairline. Balance the round face with angular hairdesigns.

The **Square** face shape is equal in width and length. The outer lines are straight vertically and horizontally. Add excitement in a hairstyle to draw the eye away from the strong jawline and frame the forehead line to soften it.

The **Rectangle (oblong)** face shape is longer than it is wide. A person with this face shape often has prominent cheekbones, a long, angular chin and a high forehead. Add curvature to the design and shorten the face using a fringe in the forehead or chin area.

ROUND

1

SQUARE

2

RECTANGLE
(Oblong)

3

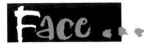

INVERTED TRIANGLE
(Heart)

The **Inverted Triangle (heart)** is widest at the forehead and narrowest at the chin. Balance with fullness around the jawline and soft waves at the forehead.

The **Diamond** shape has a narrow forehead and jaw. The face is angular and typically has prominent cheeks. Divert attention from angular features with a style that skims the cheekbones or adds fullness above or below the cheeks to counterbalance.

The **Triangle (pear)** face shape features a narrow forehead and wide chin. Add softness in the hairstyle around the jawline or fullness above the eyes.

"Look and see: Studying face shapes is an art. Without mastering the dynamics of this art, you may place the incorrect hairdesign on your client."

1

DIAMOND

2

3

TRIANGLE (Pear)

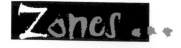

Zones

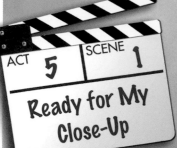
3

Zone 1

Zone 2

Zone 3

Facial Features

Once you have determined your client's face shape, focus on the facial features. The features of the three facial zones help define how the hair will be designed.

You can use the hairdesign to disguise less attractive facial features, emphasize others, or focus on the entire face. Plan the total effect and decide which will have center stage—the hair or the face?

▶ EXERCISE

To help plan the most attractive hairdesign, the stylist mentally divides the face into **three zones**.

- The **first zone** is between the hairline and eyebrow line.
- The **second zone** is between the eyebrow line and the tip of the nose.
- The **third zone** is between tip of the nose and the chin line.

With a ruled comb, measure the three zones for length and width individually and then combined.

"The best hairdesign emphasizes a person's great facial features while altering or concealing the appearance of weaker ones."

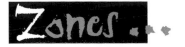
"The wisest mind has something yet to learn."

George Santayana, Spanish-American philosopher and poet
(1863-1952)

Zone 1

The Forehead *varies in length and width from person to person. Consider this zone when determining whether a fringe should be added to the hairdesign.*

Styling suggestions

for emphasizing or concealing the forehead:

- **Narrow forehead** – Style the hair away from the outer edge to add width.

- **Wide forehead** – Help minimize with a soft fringe on the outer corners.

- **Short forehead** – A slightly off-center part creates the illusion of length.

- **Long forehead** – Add an elongated fringe.

- **Wrinkles or scars** – Minimize with a soft fringe.

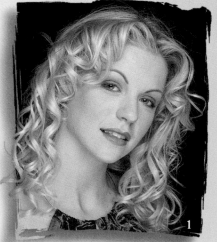

Wide forehead – soft corner fringe
1

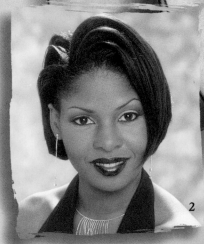

Short forehead –
off-center part creates length
2

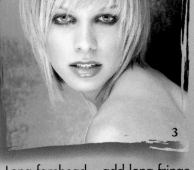

Long forehead – add long fringe
with minimal volume
3

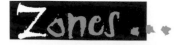
Zones

"The face is the mirror of the mind, and eyes without speaking confess the secrets of the heart."

Saint Jerome, biblical translator and monastic leader
(374 AD-419 AD)

Zone 2

The Eyes are the most expressive facial feature and often the focal point of the overall design. Sometimes the client may need a hairdesign to correct close- or wide-set eyes. The effect of age around the eyes may also be diminished with a well-designed style.

Styling suggestions

for emphasizing or concealing the eyes:

○ **Wide-set eyes –** Add a partially lifted fringe area to make the eyes appear closer together.

○ **Close-set eyes –** Add width in the temple area to make eyes appear farther apart.

○ **Droopy eyes –** Minimize by creating volume and lift in the frontal design area.

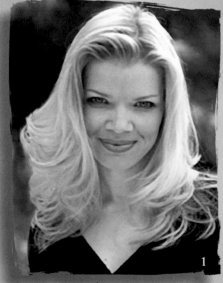

Wide-set eyes –
add partially lifted fringe

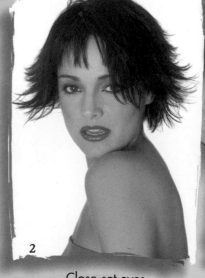

Close-set eyes –
add width in temple area

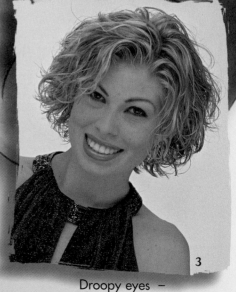

Droopy eyes –
use lift in the hairdesign

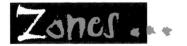

"Reason is sight. Instinct is touch. Intuition is smell."

Mason Cooley, American aphorist (1927-)

The Nose is often the most prominent facial feature because of its size and location at the center of the face. The nose's shape can either strongly influence or be influenced by the hairdesign.

Styling suggestions
for emphasizing or concealing the nose:

- **Large nose** – Minimize by keeping volume in the forehead and crown areas and adding softness in the frontal area.

- **Small nose** – Draw attention away from the nose by sweeping the hair off the face.

- **Flat nose** – Keep hair close on the sides or extending outward from the face.

- **Long nose** – Minimize with a softly layered style.

- **Crooked nose** – Select a hairdesign that flows asymmetrically across the face.

Small nose –
sweep hair off face

The Ears' size and position will influence your client's hairdesign options. Small ears can be exposed in shorter cuts and larger or protruding ears are usually covered either partially or completely. Be aware of eyeglasses and high- or low-set placement of ears within Zone 2 when deciding whether or not to reveal the entire ear.

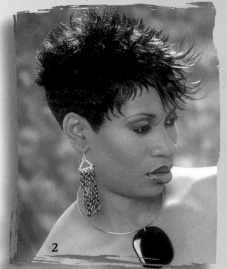

Flat nose –
style sides close or away from face

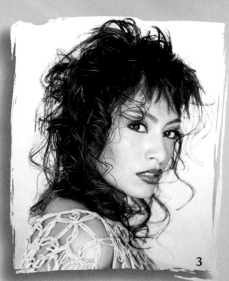

Long nose –
soft layers

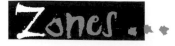

"If one's mouth always wears a smile, one will always feel young."

Chinese proverb

Zone 3 The Mouth, Chin and Jaw

Zone 3 is perhaps the most important area to consider in the design of a complimentary hairstyle.

The **mouth** is often a good feature to emphasize. Its size, shape and balance should all be taken into account when planning the hairdesign. The **chin** is only the frontal portion of the jaw. Look at it from front and side views to see its shape and size. The **jaw's** shape should influence the length, width and angularity of a style.

Styling suggestions

for emphasizing or concealing the chin:

- **Large chin** – Add length and volume in the nape area or fullness falling above or below the chin line.

- **Small chin** – Raise the hair in the crown area for softness and depth perception.

Styling suggestions for emphasizing or concealing the jaw:

- **Square jaw** – Design the hair with curved elements to frame the face and soften the appearance of an angular line.

- **Round jaw** – Use asymmetrical or angular lines.

- **Long jaw** – Add fullness below the jawline to minimize the jaw's length.

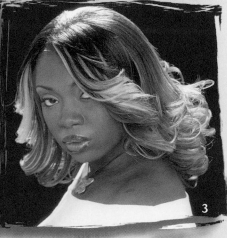

Small chin – add height in crown to counterbalance

Square jaw – frame face with curves to soften angles

Round jaw – use asymmetry or angles for contrast

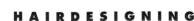

3

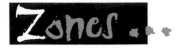

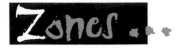

"Order is the shape upon which beauty depends."

Pearl Buck, Nobel Prize-winning novelist (1892-1973)

Gateway to the Body

The Neck and Shoulders *are also considered in planning hairdesigns to help stylists properly proportion the style to the body beyond the three facial zones.*

Styling suggestions
for emphasizing or de-emphasizing the neck and shoulders:

- **Long, thin neck –**
  Requires length and fullness on a horizontal plane.

- **Short, wide neck –**
  Add strong diagonal lines to the hairdesign.

- **Rounded shoulders –**
  Minimize by adding length or fullness at the back of the head.

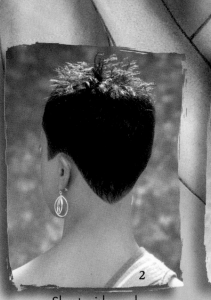

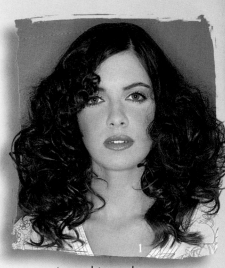

Long thin neck –
add length and horizontal fullness

Short wide neck –
use strong diagonal lines

Rounded shoulders –
add length or fullness in back

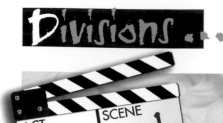

3

The Cranial Divisions

Just as every person's face has a different shape, the skull can have different shapes too. Hairdesigns should create the illusion of an evenly shaped head. The Cranial Divisions help hairdesigners to quickly spot the shape of a client's skull. All three divisions can be viewed by examining the profile (side view) of a person's head. Every angle, including the client's profile view, is important in planning a balanced hairdesign.

1   **2**   **3**

1   **The Facial Division** includes the frontal outline of the head from the tip of the nose to the outer corner of the eye. The ideal outline of the facial division is the straight profile. It has an approximately 10-degree, outward-sloping angle from hairline to nose and an angle of the same degree moving inward from nose to chin.

10°

2   **The Parietal Division** is defined by the outer corner of the eye to the back of the ear. This area may vary from person to person depending on the position of the ears in relation to the eyes. Ideally, the upper tip of the ear should align with the corner of the eye, and the lower tip of the ear should align with the lip line (the middle of the lips).

10°

3   **The Occipital Division** includes the area from the back of the ear to the occipital bone (the back of the skull). Like the parietal division, the size and shape of the occipital bone varies from person to person. The ideal bone shape is evenly rounded from the top of the skull to the neck.

Straight Profile

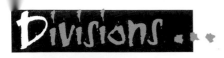

Divisions...

Styling suggestions for counterbalancing profiles in the facial division:

Concave Profile – A concave profile has a protruding chin and forehead, which gives the impression of a receding nose. Counterbalance these prominent features by adding soft, upward movement at the nape and moving hair gently away from the forehead and chin area.

Concave profile

Corrective style for concave profile
1

Convex Profile – A convex profile is typified by a receding chin and high hairline, which makes the nose area protrude. To minimize this rounded profile, style the hair with fullness moving toward the forehead and jawline, adding volume if necessary to counterbalance a flatter crown area. A male client can mask a recessed chin line by growing a full beard.

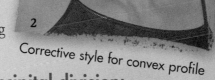

Corrective style for convex profile
2

Convex profile

Styling suggestions for the occipital division:

Flat occipital bone – Add volume in the occipital division.

Prominent occipital bone – Add volume in the crown area or below the occipital bone to soften the appearance of a pointed head.

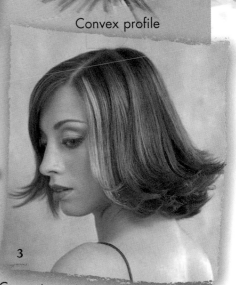

Corrective style for prominent occipital bone – add volume in nape area
3

▶ EXERCISE

Examine the profiles of two classmates or friends. Identify the three cranial divisions. Then compare how the shapes of each head are different, and how you would style the hair to balance their features.

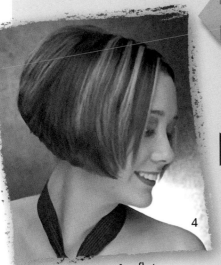

Corrective style for flat occipital bone – add volume in crown or back of head
4

Divisions

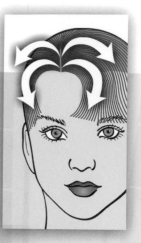

Parts *divide the head and are used as elements within a hairdesign.*

A natural part is a visible line on the scalp with the growth patterns of the hair naturally falling on either side of the line.

Making parts for the hairdesign

To design a part for the finished hairdesign, the hairstylist needs to consider the facial shape and areas that require rebalancing. The eye follows the focal point created by a part line, so if the natural part does not flatter the client's facial features, a part with better placement can be chosen and manually inserted into the hairdesign.

The natural growth patterns that form parts in the hair can be difficult to design around if they are very pronounced.

▶ EXERCISE

To find a natural part, smooth the hair away from the face and gently push the hair forward with the palm of your hand. The hair will divide and fall into a natural part line. Be aware that clients can have more than one natural part line. Select the part line which is complimentary to the client's face shape.

Choosing placement of a part

Side parts are used to balance face shapes or make the hair flow to one side or the other. A side part may be used to develop height in a hairdesign in order to elongate the face.

Center parts create the illusion of length on round and square faces. The eye is naturally drawn up and down the center parting which helps to minimize width. Since a center part accentuates nose length or width, avoid using center parts on a client with a prominent nose.

Off-center parts combined with a soft fringe around the hairline draw the eye toward a strong design element, such as color or textural changes.

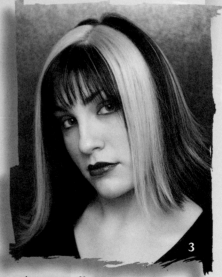

1

To create a side part, insert the comb above the pupil of either eye, and draw the comb straight back.

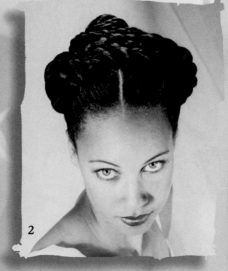

2

When creating a center part, insert the comb at the hairline in line with the nose.

3

Place an off-center part either with natural separations in the fringe area or deliberately to attract attention to a specific hairdesign area.

3

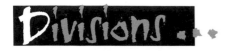

Diagonal parts are used with prominent facial features or to counterbalance angular diamond, triangle and inverted triangle face shapes.

Zigzag parts create drama and interest; the more changes in direction of the diagonal parting, the smaller the zigzag pattern.

Radial parts in hairdesigns attract attention by emphasizing the shape of the client's head.

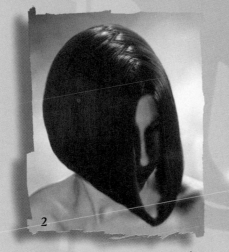

1

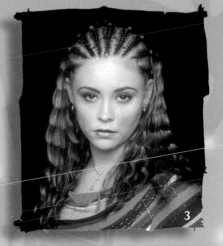

3

For a diagonal part, insert the comb at the front hairline above the pupil of either eye and draw the comb back diagonally across the head.

To create a zigzag part, insert the comb at the front hairline and draw the comb on a diagonal line in one direction and then the other.

Begin a radial part from a predetermined axis point and radiate in an outward direction while following the curvature of the head.

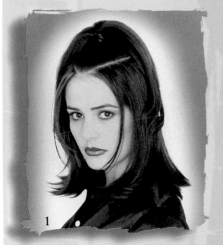

Curved parts are used to round an angular or square face shape. This type of part in the horizontal plane will also minimize a high forehead or receding hairline.

Parts in the frontal area of the head create fringes. A triangle is the classic parting used for angular schoolgirl style fringes.

4

"Because a part divides the head form, stylists need to check for ratio and place parts to balance the finished hairdesign."

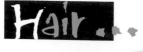

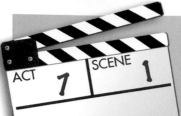

Leading Role

3

After assessing your client's personality, body and face, direct your focus to the hair. The biological qualities of the hair include its structure and texture.

CUTICLE
MEDULLA
MELANIN
(PIGMENT)

CORTEX

HAIR SHAFT

Structure

The chemical elements in hair are **carbon, oxygen, hydrogen, sulfur** and **nitrogen**, which combine to form the protein **keratin**. The portion above the surface of the scalp is called the **hair shaft**, which is composed of three parts. The **cuticle** is the outer, protective layer, responsible for sheen and porosity. The **cortex** is the middle layer, providing elasticity, the pigment melanin, and 90 percent of the hair's total bulk. The **medulla** is the innermost layer and is not present in all hair textures.

The head's skin, called the **scalp**, can be quite sensitive to temperature variations and chemicals in hair care products. The portion of the hair below the scalp is called the **hair root**. The three structures of the hair root are the papilla, bulb and follicle. The **papilla** receives the blood supply and stimulates hair growth. The **bulb** is the hollow covering of the papilla. The **follicle** is the cavity that contains the hair root.

The follicle's angle determines the natural flow of the hair. Hair flowing in the same direction is called a hair stream. A **whorl** is a circular pattern of follicles found at the crown or along the hairline. A person may have more than one whorl in his/her hair pattern.

ROOT

FOLLICLE
BULB
PAPILLA

"The technical name for the study of hair—its diseases and care—is TRICHOLOGY."

RA

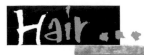

Curly Hair takes the form of a narrow oval.

Follicle Shape

The follicle's shape may determine the hair's **tempo**, which is its degree of curl or movement. Hair assumes the curve, shape and size of the follicle as it grows out. A **flat-shaped** (narrow oval) follicle produces **curly** hair. An **oval-shaped** follicle produces **wavy** hair and a **round-shaped** follicle produces **straight** hair. An individual can have all three shapes of follicles, but one shape is usually dominant.

The degree of natural wave pattern in the hair may be independent of the hair texture. However, extremely curly or coiled hair is often fragile and usually fine in texture.

Coarse texture is more commonly resistant and found in hair that is straight.

Straight Hair takes the form of a circle.

Follicle Shape

Wavy Hair takes the form of a large oval.

Follicle Shape

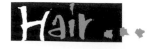

Hair...

The hair's biological tempo, *whether curly, straight or somewhere in between, provides the degree of natural curl or movement.*

Straight hair has a slow, or **decelerated** tempo, whereas curly hair has a fast or **accelerated** tempo. The tempo is accelerated as the rate of curl increases down the length of the hair shaft. The tempo decelerates as the rate of curl decreases down the length of the hair shaft. A **moderate** tempo produces a consistent wave pattern between the two extremes.

Texture *is the visual and tactile quality of the hair (how it looks and feels). The hair's biological or natural texture is determined by its tempo and concentration.*

Here are various hair tempo examples.

Textures of any diameter (fine, medium or coarse) can be used in hairdesign to balance face shapes, features and head forms. **Curly** (accelerated) tempo textures help to offset angular lines of **rectangular** or **square** shapes and features by drawing the eyes away from the face. **Straight**, smooth (decelerated) tempo textures add angular lines to **round** shapes and features while drawing attention toward the face.

Develop a design plan with the texture of the client's hair in mind. Respect the biology of the hair's structure and use it to your advantage. While some styles will work with any texture of hair, successful hairdesigners capitalize on fine hair's ability to create soft wisps or fringe, or utilize the natural bulk of coarse hair for styles that require volume.

Hair that is rough, curly or layered reflects less light than smooth, straight hair which reflects light like a mirror. Altering the natural texture of the client's hair to suit a specific style is covered in Chapter 4.

Combinations of various textures will **create interest.** Too many textures within a hairdesign can **overwhelm** it. The best designs generally use only two or three texture combinations and/or changes in tempo.

1

2

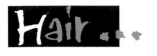

Hair ...

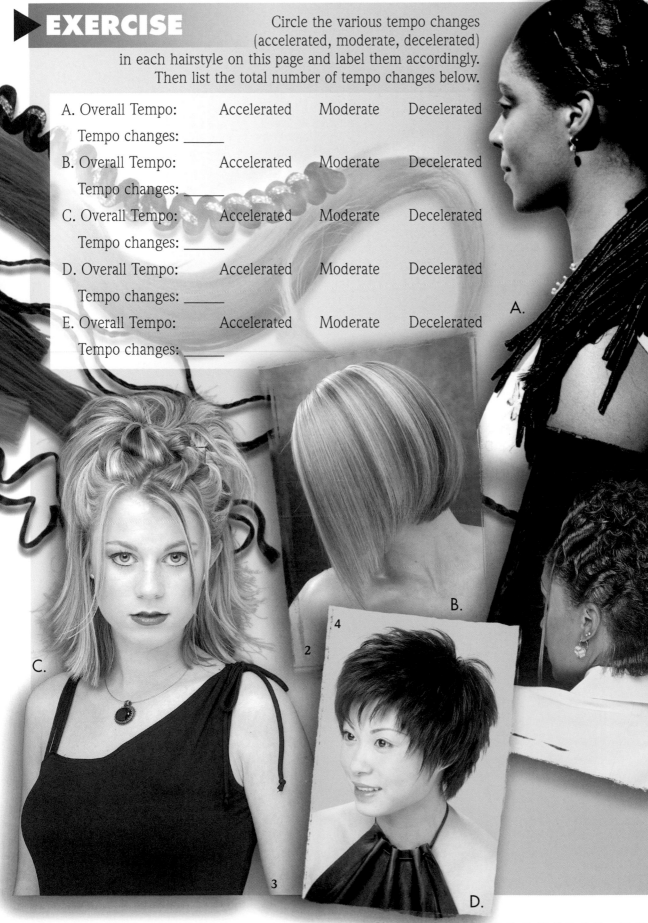

► **EXERCISE**   Circle the various tempo changes (accelerated, moderate, decelerated) in each hairstyle on this page and label them accordingly. Then list the total number of tempo changes below.

A. Overall Tempo: Accelerated   Moderate   Decelerated

Tempo changes: _____

B. Overall Tempo: Accelerated   Moderate   Decelerated

Tempo changes: _____

C. Overall Tempo: Accelerated   Moderate   Decelerated

Tempo changes: _____

D. Overall Tempo: Accelerated   Moderate   Decelerated

Tempo changes: _____

E. Overall Tempo: Accelerated   Moderate   Decelerated

Tempo changes: _____

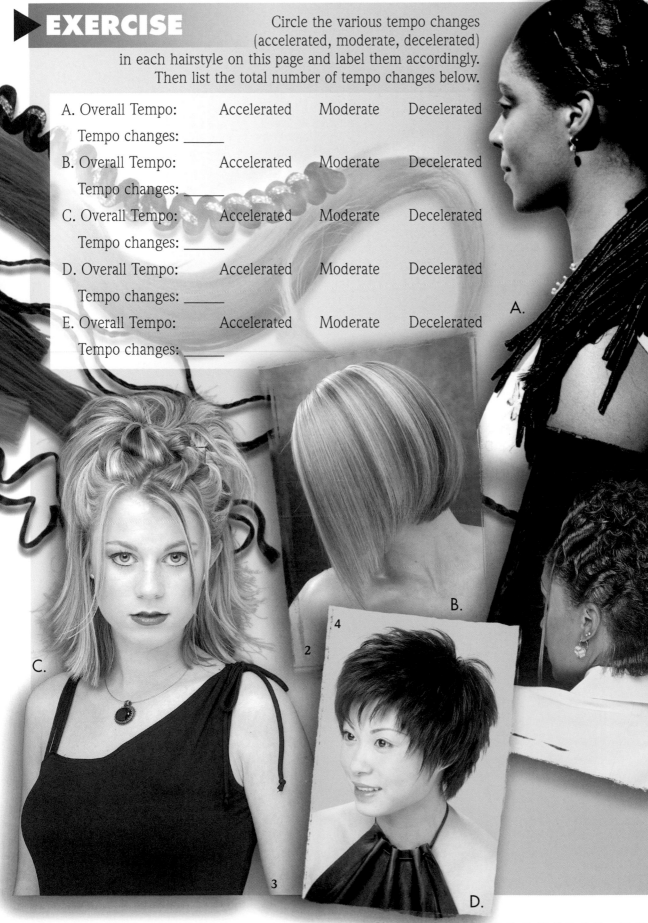

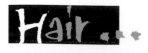

The Concentration *or overall thickness of the hair is determined by density, diameter and distribution.*

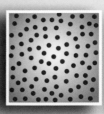
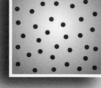
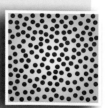
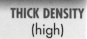

THIN DENSITY
(low)

MEDIUM DENSITY
(average)

THICK DENSITY
(high)

Density is the amount of follicles and hair per square inch (2.5 cm). Density tends to vary in relationship to natural hair color. The average number of hair follicles on a scalp is 100,000. Natural blondes have a **thick** (high) hair density with an average of 140,000 follicles on their scalp. People with naturally black hair have a **medium** (average) density, or about 110,000 follicles. Natural redheads tend to have a **thin** (low) density, since they have only 90,000 hair follicles.

Diameter of the hair shaft refers to the degree of thickness present within a single hair strand. All hair types and textures can be **fine, medium** or **coarse** in diameter. Coarse hair has a large diameter and is therefore thick. Medium hair is considered the average diameter/thickness. Fine hair has a small diameter and is therefore thin. The structure of fine-textured hair can at times lack the medulla. Coarse hair tends to have a thicker and larger amount of cuticle in comparison to hair of fine or medium diameter.

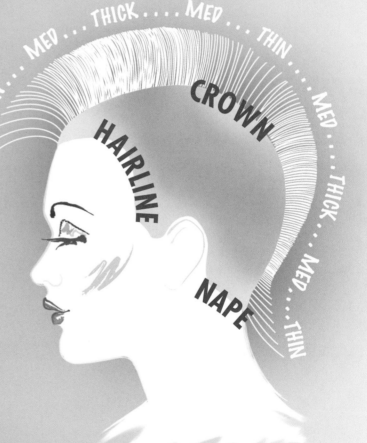

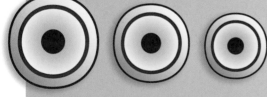

COARSE   MEDIUM   FINE

Distribution is the variance in density around the head. An even density of the hair in all areas of the scalp represents a **balanced** distribution. An **unbalanced** hair distribution means that some areas of the scalp have a thicker or thinner density. The thinnest regions for hair distribution are usually the hairline, crown and nape areas, but can vary for each person.

Concentration is usually dictated by genetics and the natural hair color, but there are **exceptions**. For example, although redheads as a whole generally have a thinner hair density, some cultures with red hair have a very thick concentration of hair on the head. The same can be said for blondes or brunettes of different nationalities or ethnicities.

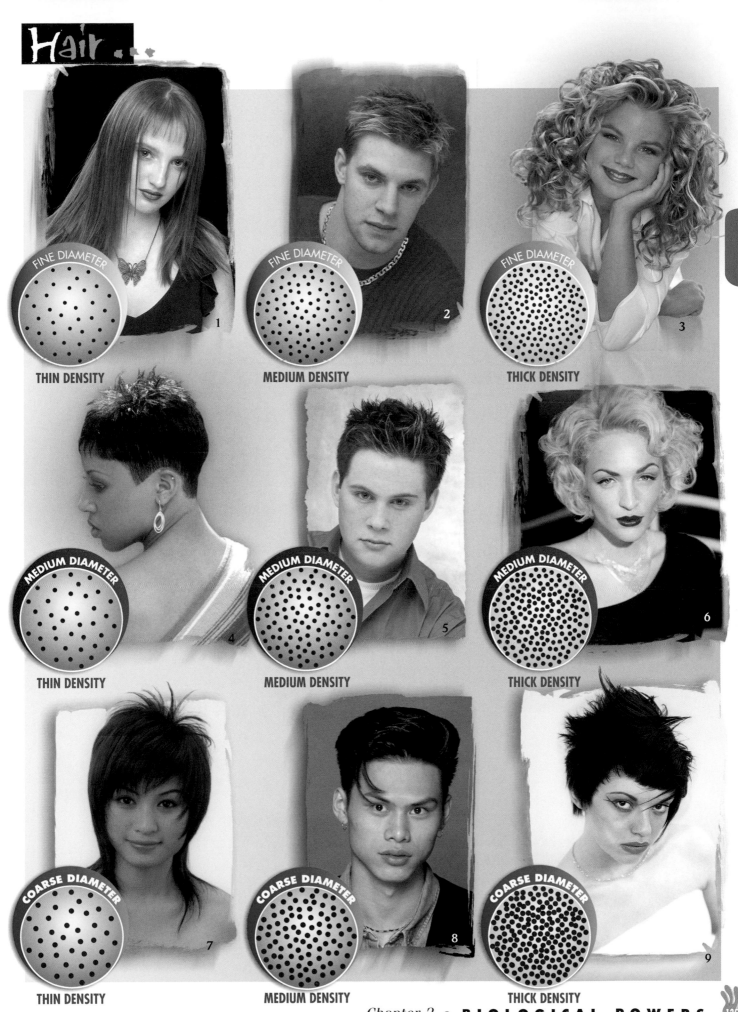

Hair...

FINE DIAMETER
1
THIN DENSITY

FINE DIAMETER
2
MEDIUM DENSITY

FINE DIAMETER
3
THICK DENSITY

MEDIUM DIAMETER
4
THIN DENSITY

MEDIUM DIAMETER
5
MEDIUM DENSITY

MEDIUM DIAMETER
6
THICK DENSITY

COARSE DIAMETER
7
THIN DENSITY

COARSE DIAMETER
8
MEDIUM DENSITY

COARSE DIAMETER
9
THICK DENSITY

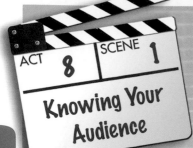

ACT 8 SCENE 1

Knowing Your Audience

3

Accommodating All Clients

Each of your clients will have different needs. Ask how you can assist them. Clients with special needs will generally tell you what is required. The following will help to ensure that you are prepared to accommodate the needs of all your clientele.

Clients with Allergies

To prevent any potential allergic reactions to chemicals or products, ask your clients if they have any allergies before beginning a service. Allergies cause the immune system to **overreact** to a normally harmless substance.

Hypersensitivity to chemicals affects two out of ten people, causing mild to severe reactions during or after treatment. Mild symptoms include localized reactions such as rashes, itchy, watering eyes and slight congestion. Moderate reactions travel throughout the body such as nausea, dizziness and weakness. Severe reactions include difficulty breathing or unconsciousness. Even though clients **may not be aware** of any allergies, pay attention to your clients' comfort and **watch for symptoms**, especially during chemical treatments.

Visually- or Hearing-Impaired Clients

Visually-impaired clients may have difficulty seeing into a regular mirror. Invest in a magnifying mirror to help them see the finished hairdesign. For a client without vision, offer to read the salon's services list or have one printed in Braille.

To ensure that you **communicate** and **understand** the needs of a hearing-impaired client, keep a notepad and a pen at the workstation. Clients with hearing aids may want hairstyles covering their ears. Keep in mind when shampooing or styling that most auditory appliances are moisture-sensitive.

Clients in Wheelchairs

When working with a client in a wheelchair, sit at eye level during your consultation. Remove the shampoo or styling chair and back the client's wheelchair into its place to **service your client in his/her chair.** Protect the client's clothing with **extra draping** if necessary. You may need to be seated, particularly when working in the nape area of the client's hair. Remember to develop a hairdesign suited to your client's ability to maintain the style at home.

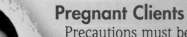

Pregnant Clients

Precautions must be taken in the salon to support the needs of an expectant client. She may be very temperature sensitive or need assistance moving into and out of the chair.

A pregnant client should also be educated on what changes her hair is going through. She produces about 25 percent more **estrogen** than normal, which causes the hair to rest and prevents normal shedding (about 35-40 strands per day). When the mother delivers her baby, the estrogen level drops off almost immediately. This **sudden change** causes all of the hair that has waited to shed to fall out and is known as **postpartum alopecia.**

The effect of shedding is delayed sometimes in a nursing mother, as her estrogen level remains higher than normal. Some mothers are unaware of this natural occurrence and think they may be losing their hair. Help them feel prepared by giving them hair care tips and information about post-natal hair loss. Create a hairdesign to camouflage thinner areas and reduce the weight pulling down on the hair by adding layers or shortening the hair's length. New mothers often switch to a low-maintenance hairdesign.

Clients Managing Hair Loss

Hair loss can be a natural or imposed occurrence for many people at different stages in life. By age 35, some degree of hair loss is apparent in 40 percent of the population. Medical conditions or prescriptions, pregnancy, genetic predisposition, and improper nutrition can all cause some degree of hair loss. A client with male pattern baldness, characterized by a horseshoe shaped recession from hairline to crown, may groom his beard more closely to maintain proportion.

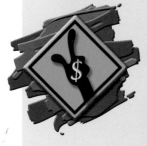

Medications can cause thinning or a complete loss of hair. An inadequate diet can cause hair loss and affect the tone of the hair (loss of pliability and shine). Vegetarians and **dieters** can be prone to hair loss. You cannot diagnose or treat any medical problems, but you can offer support and **recommend** appropriate products.

Cancer patients undergoing **chemotherapy or radiation** may experience hair loss. This treatment attacks fast-growing cells in the body (about 90 percent of all scalp hair cells), which can cause hair to fall out. Help your client maintain a **positive self-image** during this process by recommending a hairpiece, wig or shorter hairstyle that emphasizes his/her favorite feature. See Chapter 9.

Eyeglasses add a whole new dimension to hairdesign. Styles change, but one rule remains: glasses should complement a person's features and not be used as a stand-alone statement.

A balance must be found when styling hair for a client wearing glasses. Eyeglasses influence hairstyle decisions rather than the hairdesign dictating the choice of eyeglasses. Consider shape, size and color of the eyeglass frames **in addition to** the length of the client's middle facial zone, high or low placement of the ears and width of the face and nose.

Average facial width proportion is determined by visualizing five eyes across the head. Ideally, the width of the frames from one end piece to the other should equal the width of the head. The client's eye should be in the center of the frame from top to bottom and the frame should follow the brow line.

Round frames will draw too much attention to the roundness of the face.

Angular style for rounded features.

Square face types should choose frames with minimal width and rounder edges to offset an angular jawline.

Square frames echo the square face instead of helping to soften it.

If your client is fortunate enough to have an oval face, she/he can wear almost any style of frames.

Tall, square frames over-emphasize the long lines of a rectangular shaped face.

Rounded style for angular features.

Individual Considerations ...

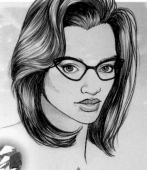

To best flatter your client's features, a tactful discussion is helpful in suggesting hairstyle and accessory tips they may not have considered. It is important to recognize general **eyeglass proportion** rules and how they relate to hairstyling for your client.

Cats' eye frames that flare upward are not flattering to an inverted triangle shaped face.

Inverted triangle/heart face shapes need rounded frames that angle outward for balance.

De-emphasize width across cheekbones with smaller frames and rounded edges for a diamond shaped face.

- Rounded facial features are offset by angular style eyeglass frames.

- Glasses with opposing contrast in shape from the face give a sense of balance to the face. Long, angular faces can be softened by a pair of oval or round glasses.

- Glasses should not overpower or be too small for the face.

- Frame colors should match or be a shade darker or lighter than skin tone.

- Consider the client's eyeglasses in relation to his/her fashion personality when designing a hairstyle.

A diamond shaped face does not need the width of the cheekbones to be emphasized with a wide frame.

Aviator style frames call attention to the bottom heaviness of the triangle/pear shaped face.

Eyeglass styles that are wider than long with decorative edges on the top frame will flatter a triangle or pear shaped face.

"Strive to strike a balance for the client between face, eyeglass frame and hairstyle."

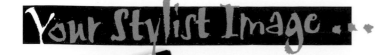

Your Stylist Image...

3

"Creating good habits now will help prevent bodily injuries later."

A Stylist's Posture

Hairdesigners communicate to their clients through body language. Using correct body posture communicates confidence to clients, but most importantly, it helps prevent long-term back, neck or shoulder injuries.

A **good working posture** means placing your **weight evenly on both feet** and aligning your **head directly over your shoulders**, with your **shoulders directly over your hips** and your **hips directly over your knees and feet.**

Salon furnishings are manufactured to allow you to adjust and move your clients without having to stoop or lean while you work. Get in the habit of using correct posture in your regular work activities.

▶ EXERCISE

Standing for long periods of time can become tiresome for the body. You will feel a lot fresher if you take some time between clients to stretch, restore and revitalize.

B-R-E-A-T-H-E

Taking the time to breathe voluntarily rather than involuntarily is crucial for reducing tension.

- Sit comfortably, preferably away from others. Block out outside noises.

- Relax your entire body. Focus only on your breath, and work toward breathing through your nose. Make each inhale and exhale long, deliberate and deep.

- Do this for five minutes a day and feel the benefits. This is powerful!

Head and Neck Rolls

Try this exercise as a quick, easy tension reducer.

- Stand still and erect or sit comfortably with feet on the floor and your back straight.

- Inhale, and then as you exhale, gently drop your chin toward your chest.

- Inhale and slowly roll your left ear toward your shoulder, dropping the opposite shoulder toward the floor to maintain alignment. Hold the pose, and exhale as your neck releases.

- Breathe fully and gently as you drop your chin back down to your chest and repeat the stretch on the right side to loosen these muscles.

3

Shoulder Shrugs

This relaxing stretch helps improve flexibility in the upper back, shoulders and arms while relieving tension in the neck and shoulders.

- Stand still and erect.
- Start moving your shoulders from back to front, making small circles in a fluid motion. Repeat ten times.
- Reverse the circular motion of your shoulders, rotating from front to back for ten repetitions.
- Modify this stretch by lifting the arms until they are fully extended to the sides and rolling back to front and front to back. Make increasingly larger arm circles.

Side Stretch

This stretch strengthens the arms, waist, and upper body, and helps align the spine.

- Stand straight with feet about hip-width apart, and extend the crown of your head up toward the ceiling.
- Keep your feet stationary, and inhale as you raise your arms overhead, palms together. Exhale, relaxing your shoulders.
- Keep shoulders relaxed and inhale. As you exhale, bend from the waist to the left. Hold for a few breaths, inhaling and exhaling easily.
- Return to center on an inhale. Exhale as you bend to the right. Breathe gently as you briefly hold the pose on this side.
- Return once again to center on an inhale, exhaling as you drop your arms gently down to rest at your sides.
- Repeat at least twice; you will notice a deeper stretch the second time around.

"your arms will 'tell' your brain which way they need to move in order to give them a good stretch!"

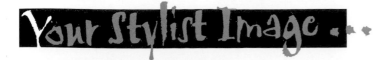

Your Stylist Image ...

Hair Performers

The salon is your stage and the clients are your audience. Your appearance and actions reflect on the professional workmanship you perform.

You present yourself as a beauty professional to the general public. Clients want to know you care about your appearance and what you do. They see your image as a direct application of your skill in hairdesign and cosmetology.

Conveying the right image to clients includes proper care and maintenance of your hands, hair, skin and clothing. View yourself in a full-length mirror and ask: Is this how I want to be perceived? Do I present the right image? Am I a good representative of the beauty industry? Like your skills, your image and hairstyle should be continually updated and refined.

▶ EXERCISE

Check your image: Rate yourself on a scale of 1-10 (10 being the best) of these important professional image criteria. Your answers will indicate areas for improvement.

_____ My hair and clothes are in proportion to my body type.

_____ My hairstyle is well-kept and reflective of current fashion trends.

_____ My clothes represent my fashion personality.

_____ My wardrobe is stylish and properly maintained.

_____ My hands are clean and neatly manicured.

_____ My hair, body and breath are free of offensive odors.

_____ I smile and greet people warmly, speak clearly and maintain eye contact.

_____ I treat others in a mannerly fashion, with dignity and respect.

_____ I do not smoke or have food in the styling area.

_____ I base my clients' designs on their needs, not mine.

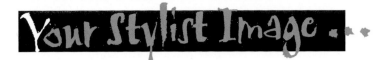
Your Stylist Image...

EXERCISE Personality Quiz

As a professional hairdesigner, you interact with different people every day. Like you, each of your clients and coworkers have their own personality. Identifying your personality style will give you cues on how to strengthen weaker personality traits and communicate better with others. Answer the five questions below to find your personality type.

1. I get annoyed waiting for my client's hair to dry.　　A. Untrue　　B. Somewhat True　　C. Very True
2. I interrupt people in the middle of their conversation.　　A. Untrue　　B. Somewhat True　　C. Very True
3. I get upset waiting for my next client to arrive.　　A. Untrue　　B. Somewhat True　　C. Very True
4. My coworkers tell me I talk too quickly.　　A. Untrue　　B. Somewhat True　　C. Very True
5. I enjoy competition.　　A. Untrue　　B. Somewhat True　　C. Very True

Now score your test. Give yourself one point for all of the times you answered "A," two points for all of the times you answered "B," and three points for all the times you answered "C." Add the total points and compare your results with the guide below.

Scores of:　　**5 - 7**　　Type B personality
　　　　　　　　8 - 10　　Combination of both personality types
　　　　　　　　11 or more　　Type A personality

TYPE A
If you have a Type A personality, reinforce positive traits like your abilities to **work well under pressure** and **show ambition**. Try to think of ways to balance weaker traits by being more patient or listening more attentively.

COMBINATION
If you have a combination of the personality types, focus on your positive qualities like your **well-balanced attitude** and **flexibility**. Practice strengthening weaker traits by working cooperatively or improving timeliness.

TYPE B
If you have the traits of a Type B personality, focus on strong characteristics like your **cooperativeness** and **calm demeanor**. Address weaker traits by being more proactive or decisive.

"Please visit our Success Dynamics Module for more information on developing your people skills."

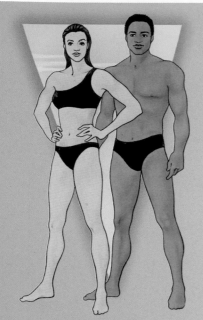
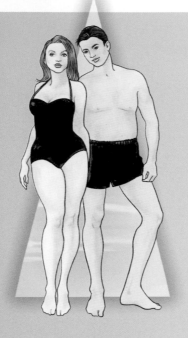
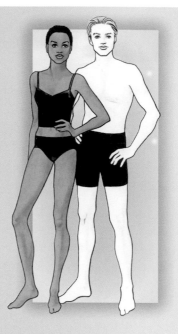

MESOMORPH
Athletic build with wide shoulders and narrow hips.

ENDOMORPH
Rounded body with short limbs and wide hips.

ECTOMORPH
Long, straight frame with hips and shoulders equal.

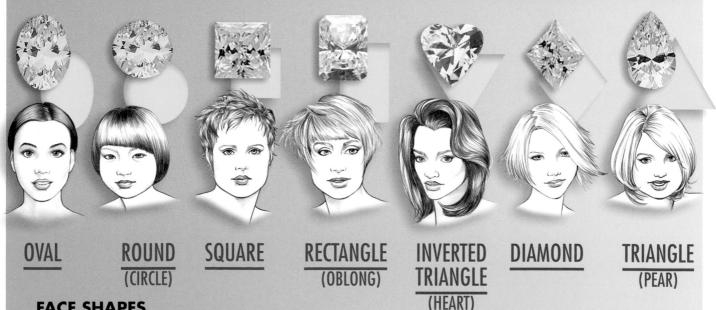

| OVAL | ROUND (CIRCLE) | SQUARE | RECTANGLE (OBLONG) | INVERTED TRIANGLE (HEART) | DIAMOND | TRIANGLE (PEAR) |

FACE SHAPES
There are seven basic facial shapes.

- **Oval** – Balanced horizontally and vertically; forehead slightly wider than chin.
- **Round** – Wide with a curved jaw and hairline; circle perimeter shape
- **Square** – Equal in width and length; angular.
- **Rectangle** – Longer than it is wide; oblong.
- **Inverted Triangle** – Wide forehead and narrow chin; heart-shaped.
- **Diamond** – Narrow forehead and jaw; prominent cheekbones.
- **Triangle** – Narrow forehead and wide chin; pear-shaped.

3

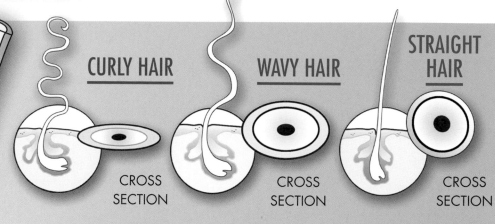

CUTICLE

MEDULLA

CORTEX

HAIR SHAFT

ROOT

FOLLICLE

BULB

PAPILLA

CURLY HAIR

CROSS SECTION

WAVY HAIR

CROSS SECTION

STRAIGHT HAIR

CROSS SECTION

3

HAIR SHAFT

Located above the surface of the scalp; composed of three layers: the **cuticle** (the outer, protective layer; determines sheen and porosity), the **cortex** (middle layer; gives hair elasticity and contains the pigment melanin), and the **medulla** (innermost layer).

HAIR ROOT

Located below the scalp; composed of three parts. The **follicle** is the cavity containing the root. The **papilla** receives the blood and stimulates hair growth. The **bulb** is the hollow covering of the papilla.

FOLLICLE

The hair follicle's shape determines its **tempo** (degree of curl or movement). **Texture** is the visual and tactile quality of the hair (how it looks and feels).

DENSITY

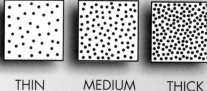

THIN (LOW) MEDIUM (AVERAGE) THICK (HIGH)

DIAMETER

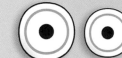

COARSE   MEDIUM   FINE

DISTRIBUTION

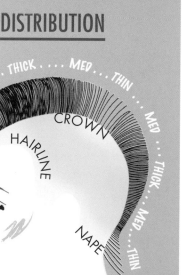

THIN ... MED ... THICK ... MED ... THIN

CROWN

HAIRLINE

MED ... THICK ... MED ... THIN

NAPE

CONCENTRATION

Density is the amount of follicles and hair per square inch.

Diameter is the thickness or thinness of a single hair strand.

Distribution is the variation in density around the head.

3

FACIAL ZONES

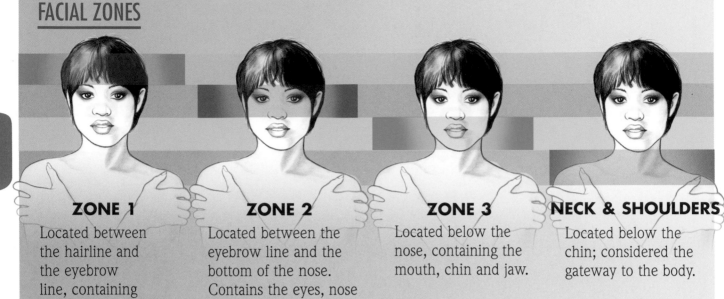

ZONE 1
Located between the hairline and the eyebrow line, containing the forehead.

ZONE 2
Located between the eyebrow line and the bottom of the nose. Contains the eyes, nose and ears.

ZONE 3
Located below the nose, containing the mouth, chin and jaw.

NECK & SHOULDERS
Located below the chin; considered the gateway to the body.

CRANIAL DIVISIONS

FACIAL DIVISION
Includes the frontal outline of the head from the tip of the nose to the outer corner of the eye. Ideal outline is the straight profile, a 10-degree angle sloping outward from hairline to nose and inward from nose to chin.

PARIETAL DIVISION
Defined by the outer corner of the eye to the back of the ear. Ideally, the ear should align between the middle of the lip and the corner of the eye.

OCCIPITAL DIVISION
Includes the area from the back of the ear to the occipital bone. The ideal head shape is evenly rounded from the top of the skull to the neck.

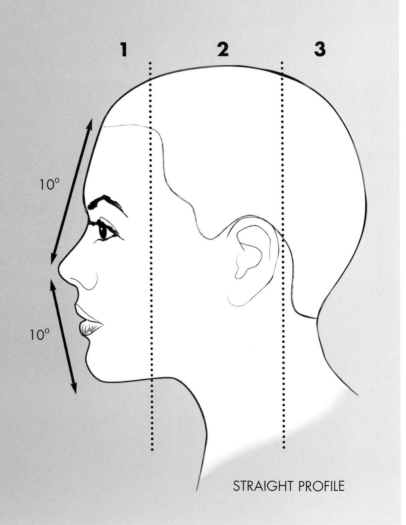

STRAIGHT PROFILE

Hair Tempo ... Quick Reference Guide

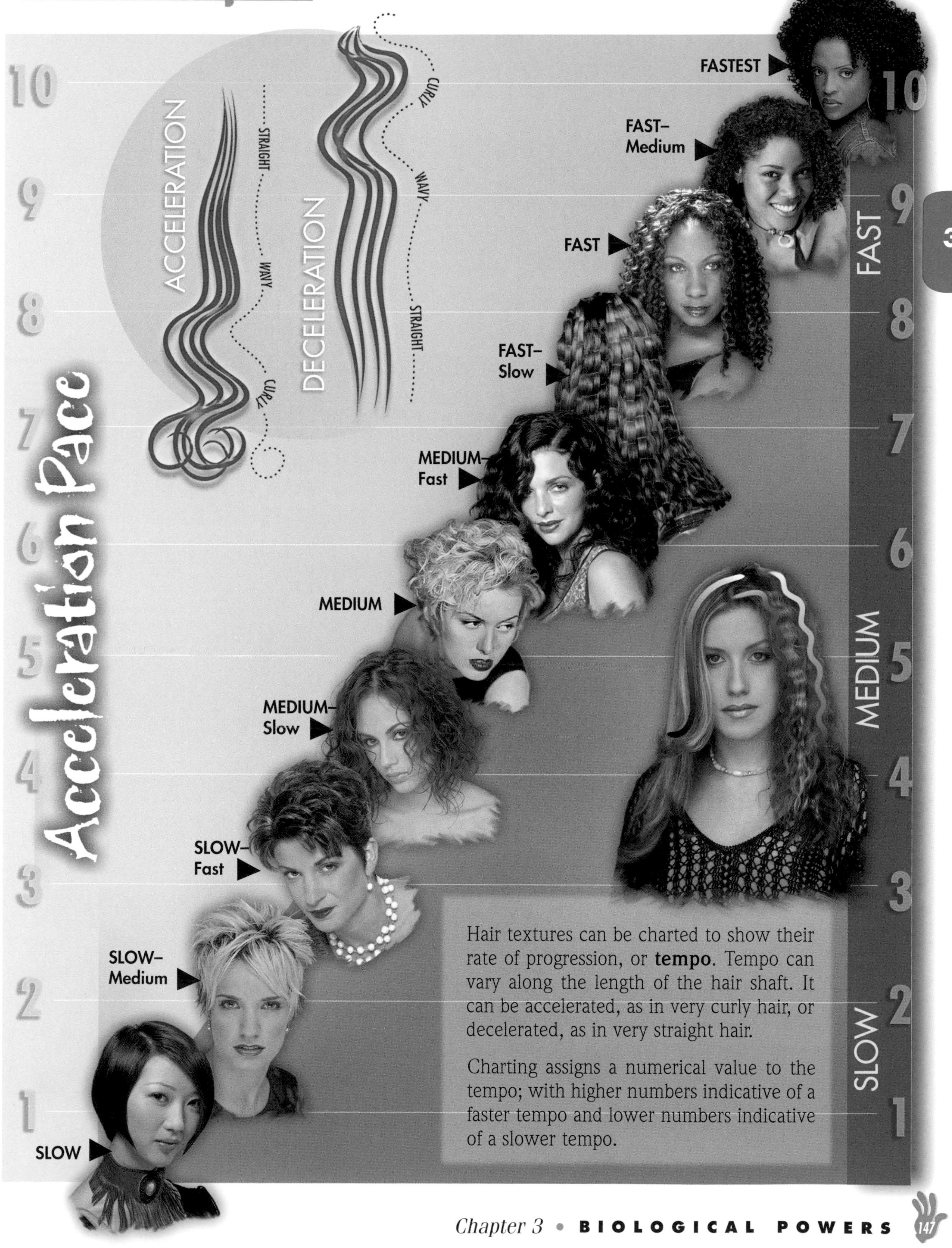

Acceleration Pace

10

9

8

7

6

5

4

3

2

1

ACCELERATION

DECELERATION

STRAIGHT

WAVY

WAVY

CURLY

CURLY

WAVY

STRAIGHT

FASTEST ▶

FAST– Medium ▶

FAST ▶

FAST– Slow ▶

MEDIUM– Fast ▶

MEDIUM ▶

MEDIUM– Slow ▶

SLOW– Fast ▶

SLOW– Medium ▶

SLOW ▶

FAST

MEDIUM

SLOW

10

9

8

7

6

5

4

3

2

1

Hair textures can be charted to show their rate of progression, or **tempo**. Tempo can vary along the length of the hair shaft. It can be accelerated, as in very curly hair, or decelerated, as in very straight hair.

Charting assigns a numerical value to the tempo; with higher numbers indicative of a faster tempo and lower numbers indicative of a slower tempo.

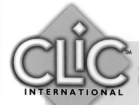

Biological Powers REVIEW QUESTIONS

TRUE OR FALSE

_____ 1. We use four of our five senses to assist us in designing hair.

_____ 2. An inverted triangle face shape has a wide forehead and a narrow chin line.

_____ 3. The client's profile view is not important to the hairdesign.

_____ 4. Only a client's eyes determine the placement of a part.

_____ 5. When designing hair, knowing your client's body type does not matter.

_____ 6. A client's lifestyle should be considered in planning a hairdesign.

_____ 7. A person can have only one fashion personality.

_____ 8. A client's posture has no effect on the hairdesign plan.

_____ 9. Too many textures overwhelm the hairdesign.

_____ 10. A hairdesigner should recommend the length of children's hair.

MULTIPLE CHOICE

1. How many face shapes are there?
   A. Three
   B. Five
   C. Seven
   D. Ten

2. Facial features are important to hairdesigning because we want to:
   A. Enhance desirable attributes
   B. Emphasize weak features
   C. De-emphasize strong features
   D. Ignore all features

3. Body type of a person with an athletic build.
   A. Mesomorph
   B. Endomorph
   C. Ectomorph
   D. Anthropomorph

4. The ideal profile is approximately this sloping angle at the nose.
   A. 30-degree
   B. 20-degree
   C. 10-degree
   D. 180-degree

5. A well-balanced hairdesign is in proportion to the:
   A. Number of accessories
   B. Client's ego
   C. Hair's texture
   D. Face and body

6. A person who prefers unstructured clothing tends to have what fashion personality?
   A. Romantic
   B. Sporty
   C. Classic
   D. Dramatic

7. A round hair follicle produces:
   A. Wavy hair
   B. Straight hair
   C. Curly hair
   D. Coarse hair

8. The tempo of curly hair is considered:
   A. Accelerated
   B. Decelerated
   C. Accentuated
   D. Varied

9. The head is divided vertically into:
   A. One division
   B. Three zones
   C. Three hemispheres
   D. Three divisions

10. It is helpful to have this at your workstation for visually-impaired clients.
    A. A paper and pen
    B. An extra chair
    C. A magnifying mirror
    D. An interpreter

shape
line
sequence
angles
space
proportion
components

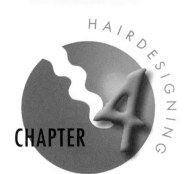

Mathematics

MATHEMATICS

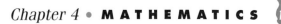

"Mathematics, rightly viewed, possesses not only truth, but supreme beauty..." Bertrand Russell
(1872-1970) British Philosopher

Mathematics *is the common thread that runs throughout the fabric of the biological factors we discussed in Chapter 3 that affect hairdesign, such as our senses and the clients' physical characteristics. This chapter explores how hairdesigns resemble elements of nature in form, and uses mathematics to discuss the structured organization found within the art and practice of hairdesign.*

Mathematics is merely a formalized attempt to find order in what appears to be chaos in the natural world. **Counting, measuring,** finding **proportions** and **patterns** and describing the **shapes** of objects are some of the ways that we apply mathematics to everyday life.

"View the patterns in the world around you. What do you SEE?"

Mathematicians throughout the ages have attempted to find the key to understanding patterns in nature and why we as humans respond positively to those patterns.

The Mathematics of Design...

Setting the Stage

In the 12th century, *Leonardo Fibonacci (fi-be-nä'-chE) identified a method for explaining naturally occurring sequential patterns (for example, the markings on a seashell). Fibonacci believed that connections and predictions could be made regarding man and his environment by studying the natural order of our surroundings.*

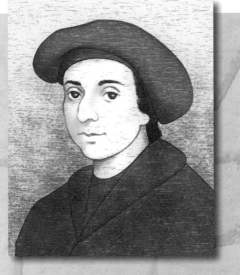

Fibonacci's Sequence can ultimately help professional hairstylists understand how to apply mathematical design elements such as **space, color, texture, line** and **form** into a creative and aesthetically pleasing hairdesign.

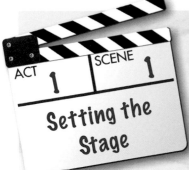

1

Visually stimulating hairdesigns resemble elements of nature in form.

2

Fibonacci's Sequence is the relationship among numbers in which to get a third number, one adds the preceding two. It begins with 0, 1, 1, 2, 3, 5, 8, and continues infinitely. Can you identify the next number in the sequence? That is right; it is 13. In looking at the natural examples of a conch shell or a sunflower, you will find Fibonacci's Sequence.

The credit card's basic pattern shows evidence of a graphic designer's innate understanding of Fibonacci's Sequence. The eye naturally flows easily over a well-designed image, since harmonious balance and graceful proportion are both stimulating and pleasing to the eye.

2408 7018 6225 4289

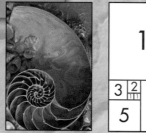
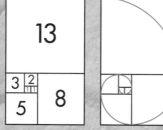
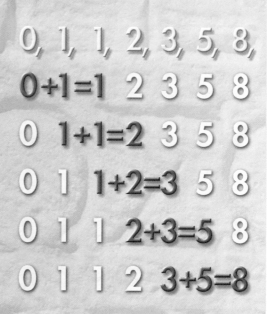

Notice the beautiful spiral pattern created by nature in this seashell. The design begins in the center, and as each section increases according to Fibonacci's Sequence, it gradually forms a spiral rotation.

0, 1, 1, 2, 3, 5, 8,

0+1=1 2 3 5 8

0 1+1=2 3 5 8

0 1 1+2=3 5 8

0 1 1 2+3=5 8

0 1 1 2 3+5=8

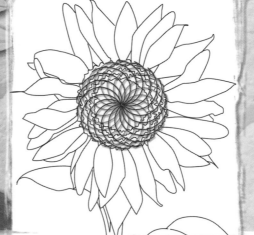

"Notice the sequential spirals in the sunflower."

The Mathematics of Design...

Numbers create phi

Mathematicians took Fibonacci's ideas further and realized that adjacent numbers in the sequence can be used to create a ratio (a proportional relationship between two quantities); 1/2, 2/3, 3/5, 5/8, and so on. The ratio 2/3 is known as the **Golden Ratio** or **phi** (fI). Mathematicians believe this divine proportion is demonstrated as beauty and organization in the cosmos.

phi=0.618
(roughly two-thirds)

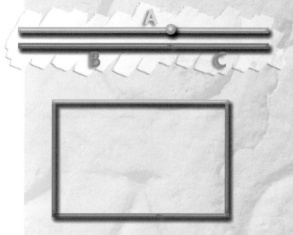

phi creates lines

Look at more examples of the Golden Ratio. It is shown in segments of a line that is 2/3 larger than another line, and a line that is again 2/3 larger than the first line, mimicking Fibonacci's Sequence. Applying these proportions to the lengths of a rectangle's sides results in a well-balanced figure.

Lines create art

The Greeks used phi's proportional relationship of lines in their architecture. The Egyptians adopted the Golden Ratio to design the pyramids. Artists used it in the creation of paintings and sculptures during the Renaissance.

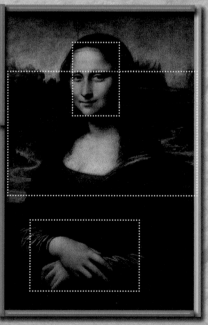

Positioning objects about one-third of the way across a picture rather than centering them makes the composition more pleasing to the eye.

The Mathematics of Design...

To the professional of hairdesign, *the Golden Ratio is the key to a well-designed hairstyle.*

Look at the ratio or proportion of face to hair in this example.

The Golden Ratio demonstrates that beauty comes from graceful proportion, the relationship of a part to the whole. Instead of a sculptor's block of marble, hair is your medium in which to create the illusion of perfect proportion. The Golden Ratio is what the hairdesigner uses, if even unconsciously, when they attempt to correct imbalance in the facial structure by using the hair to create visual harmony.

This model's face is approximately 1/3 of the total design area. Her hair equals 2/3 of that area, creating the perfect balance for her features. The Golden Ratio of 2:3 or 3:2 is straight from Fibonacci's Sequence.

"Think in thirds, just like the Egyptians, the Greeks, and all artists through the centuries."

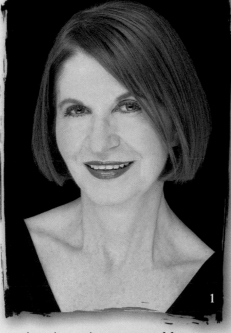

In this photo, the amount of face showing is similar to the amount of hair. **1** plus **1** equals **2** ... another ratio from Fibonacci's Sequence.

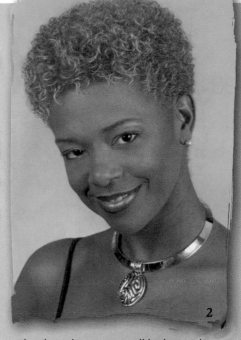

This hairdesign is well-balanced because the face is about two-thirds and the hair is one-third of the total area.

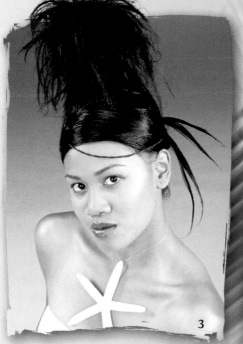

In this example, the face area is about 3/4 as large as the hair area. These numbers do not follow the Golden Ratio, making this design's proportions appear unbalanced. The hairdesign is too large for the model's relatively small body size.

Here again, the model's face is 3/4 of the total area, but her hair equals only 1/4, leaving the hairdesign out of proportion. A hairstyle with a larger form would have corrected the overall appearance by counterbalancing the larger upper body.

Consider the client's entire image when choosing elements and components to enhance the hairdesign; adjust for proportion, personality and physical characteristics. Master stylists who create illusions of balance are in high demand.

RETAIL • RE-BOOK • REFERRAL

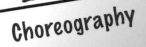

ACT **2** SCENE **1**

Choreography

4

The applications of hairdesign

involve two distinctly different aspects – theoretical and practical.

Theoretical applications of hairdesign involve ideas or **concepts**. Inspiration can come from anywhere ... art, music, nature.

The next step is to plan the concept based on your inspiration. A **design plan** is a guide that outlines the elements and components involved in creating the hairdesign's composition.

The artistic or creative part of the hairdesign is known as an **element**. An element is the smallest component into which something can be divided. Because of their mathematical foundation, elements are discussed throughout this chapter as essential building blocks in the creation of beautiful and artistic hairdesigns.

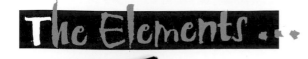

1

As in any art form, there are some basic principles of design that need to be understood before you begin. Applying two or more elements creates a scientific **principle** of hairdesign, which is covered in Chapter 5.

The **practical** application of hairdesign implements the principle idea to achieve a **composition** or finished style by arranging **component** parts.

A single component is like an individual musical note to be arranged toward the creation of a melodic masterpiece. The resulting hairstyle is like fine **choreography**, the artistic arrangement of a composition in a hairdesign performance.

DESIGN PLAN

COMPONENT

2

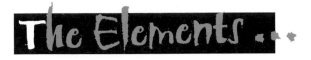

The Elements ...

The elements of hairdesign along with the principles and concepts (which are addressed in the science chapter) are the instruments employed to create beautiful and artistic hairdesigns.

The basic styling elements utilized in hairdesigning are **space**, **color**, **texture**, **line** and **form**. As we introduce these elements one by one, look for ways to creatively combine and apply them to fit your client perfectly.

One of the **most important aspects of design** is visualizing the entire image before you choose the individual elements.

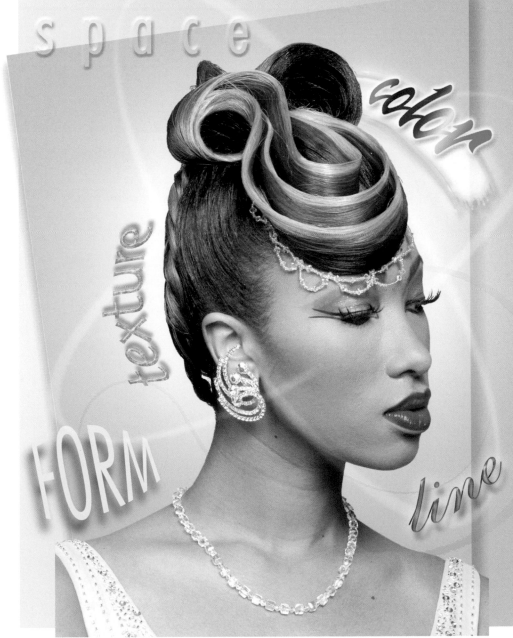

Each element of hairdesign **adds** to the total effect, but **cannot stand alone** and must work together with other elements to achieve total **harmony** in the finished look.

An example of this would be to presume that all people with square faces and short body stature must wear long hair to create the **illusion** of length in a vertical line. Only the element of length **(Line)** is given consideration. We have ignored the identification of other possible elements necessary to achieve the best hairdesign **balance** for our client's features. In this example, we also need to round out or soften the angular features of the square face.

All design elements must be considered before selecting one to dominate a design plan.

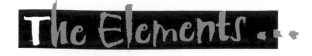

ELEMENT 1

Space is a three-dimensional area in which the hairdesign can move or be formed. Space can be in or around your hairdesign, distinguishing the design from the background.

Without adequate space considerations, hairstyles can become too busy and overwhelm the eye. Less is more.

When a style is open and airy, there is space showing through the hairdesign. This is called **negative space**, while the space that is occupied by the hair is called **positive space**. When a hairstyle has a lot of negative space, it appears to have less mobility and volume (mass) than a similar size hairstyle without negative space. The scientific principle relating physical mass to hairdesign space is explored in more detail within the Theory of Motion section of Chapter 5.

POSITIVE

NEGATIVE

POSITIVE

NEGATIVE

POSITIVE

POSITIVE

POSITIVE

NEGATIVE

NEGATIVE

The Elements...

Dimension

In planning a hairdesign we work in all three forms of dimension, with each dimension taking up a different amount of space.

The design plan is where we pre-plan and first view our hairdesigns as a one-dimensional image, either by sketching on paper or molding on the head. We work on the two-dimensional form when we wet set or airform the hair into the desired pattern. It is during the three-dimensional form where we see all of the elements in the composition of design coming together by working on the hair after it is dry to create the finished design.

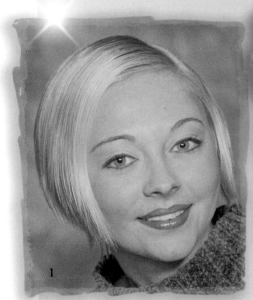

1

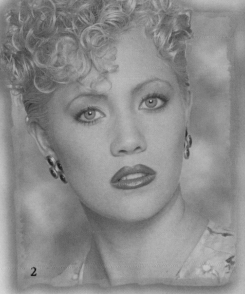

2

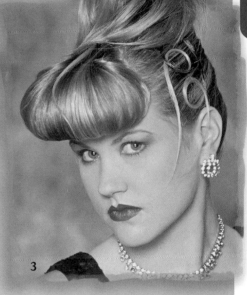

3

One-dimensional designs have only the single spatial measurement of length without depth or width.

Two-dimensional measures space in two directions, producing designs with length and width, but no depth.

Three-dimensional is the measurement of space in three directions: length, width and depth.

4

Not all hairdesigns will include the third dimension. Some only contain two dimensions in their finished form, but the most interesting will contain at least a component of the third dimension. For example, a style finished with a flip on the ends.

ELEMENT 2

Color is a visual sensation experienced when light of varying wave lengths reaches the eye. Color helps invoke an emotional response to a hairdesign. Using the element of color enhances your design by reinforcing other design principles.

Color can create value, contrast, illusion, mood, emphasis and dimension. It is used to emphasize line, texture, rhythm, repetition, balance and patterns within a hairdesign.

1

Value is the amount of light or darkness in the tone of a particular color.

Contrast occurs when two or more opposing colors are placed close to each other within a hairdesign.

3

Illusion is a visual perception created by the strategic placement of color. Lighter shades accentuate hairdesign components while darker colors help them recede.

2

Mood is created from the tonal value of colors. Blue-based colors invoke feelings of coolness and depth. Yellow-based colors add visual lift using lightness and brightness. Red-based colors create warmth or vibrancy.

Emphasis of color is used to give prominence to a component or area of a hairdesign.

5

4

Dimension is created by the use and placement of contrasting elements within the hairdesign. Lighter colors give the overall design the appearance of being larger, closer, brighter and more airy. Darker colors give the effect of being smaller, recessed, denser and more compact.

"For more information on color, consult the CLiC Haircoloring module."

6

The Elements ...

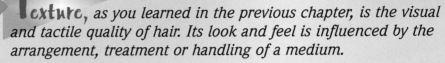

ELEMENT 3 *Texture*, as you learned in the previous chapter, is the visual and tactile quality of hair. Its look and feel is influenced by the arrangement, treatment or handling of a medium.

We know that biological or **natural textures** occur in hair when it assumes the shape of the follicle from which it grows. When planning a hairdesign, a stylist either allows the natural texture to take center stage or chooses to choreograph its arrangement into a command performance, altering the hair's natural texture permanently (chemically) or temporarily (physically).

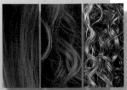

4

In a **permanent change of texture**, when the hair is shampooed it will retain its altered form.

PERMANENT WAVING

1

COLORING

CHEMICALLY RELAXING

2

3

SETTING

4

AIRFORMING

5

6

BRAIDING

In a **temporary change of texture**, when the hair is shampooed it will revert to its natural form.

Artificial textures occur when adding ornamentation to the hair, such as a hairpiece (natural or synthetic), man-made fibers (like ribbon) or natural fibers (like a feather).

7

ARTIFICIAL TEXTURES

"Combining natural and artificial textures provides you with an array of styling options limited only by your imagination!"

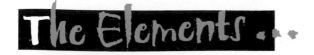

ELEMENT 4

Lines are everywhere. Look around and you will see lines that are curved, straight, diagonal, zigzagged! Whether perpendicular, circular, ovaloid, geometric or parallel, all the lines you see are made up of points in space.

Points, lines, shapes, forms, spaces and proportions make up our world. Our goal is to understand how to apply the naturally occurring lines of our world to create beautiful hairdesigns.

4

A **point** in space

A **line** is comprised of points in space.

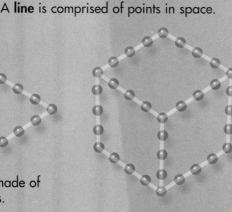

A **shape** is made of multiple lines.

A **form** is made of multiple shapes.

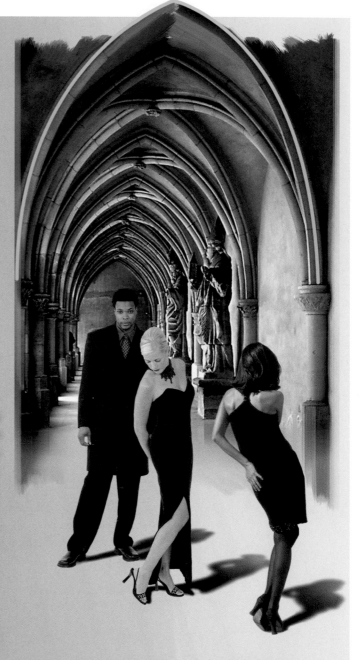

When we think of classically beautiful forms like pyramids, Grecian temples, swans, even cars – we think of lines.

It is the lines within the design that create motion and mood.

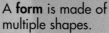

The Elements ...

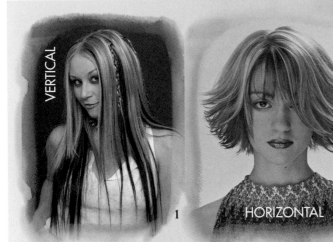

VERTICAL

HORIZONTAL

DIAGONAL

CURVED

1

2

3

4

Lines are created by the shifting points in a straight or curved direction. When constructing lines within a hairstyle, be aware of the directions and illusions they create.

- **Vertical** lines create the illusion of length or height.
- **Horizontal** lines create the illusion of width.
- **Diagonal** lines create depth or dimension.
- **Curved** lines create movement and waves.

Theatrical set designers and costume designers know that straight lines appear masculine, adding strength to soft, childlike features. Curved lines repeat the rounded female silhouette, softening the appearance of hard or angular features. Throughout history great artists drew, painted and sculpted the simplest but most elegant art line, the "S."

Even today, the smooth flow of the "S" line element is considered the most regal of all designs. Two "C's" connected together produces a variation of the "S" curve: the back-to-back or bell-to-bell "C."

Color, cut, texture or wet and dry styling create these lines within a hair design.

► EXERCISE

Identify the curved lines present within these illustrated hairdesigns.

ELEMENT 5 Form

The form of a hairdesign is the structural outline of the hair that makes it identifiable from all angles.

By darkening an image and following the contours of a figure's detailed shape, you create a **silhouette** (si-le-wet). The silhouette of a client with fine, straight hair is small and narrow, and a very wide silhouette may appear on wavy, coarse hair that has not been properly shaped.

► EXERCISE

Look at the outline of each form identified on the images of these two pages. Develop a collection of similar forms and shapes to use when designing hair by looking through magazines or making notes as you observe various hairstyles in everyday life. How does the form or shape chosen add to or detract from the person's physical characteristics?

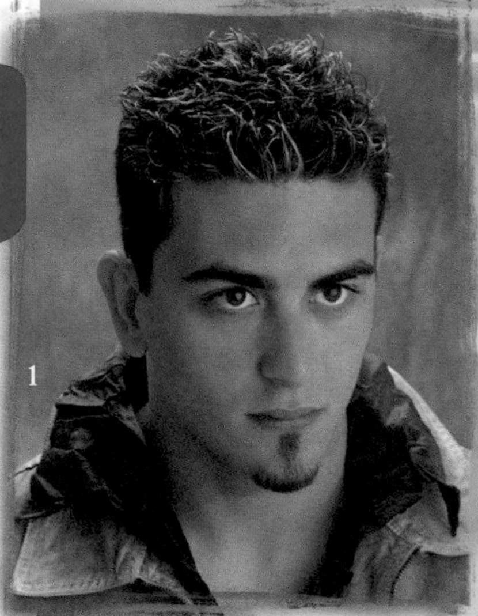

TRIANGLE FORM

1

SQUARE FORM

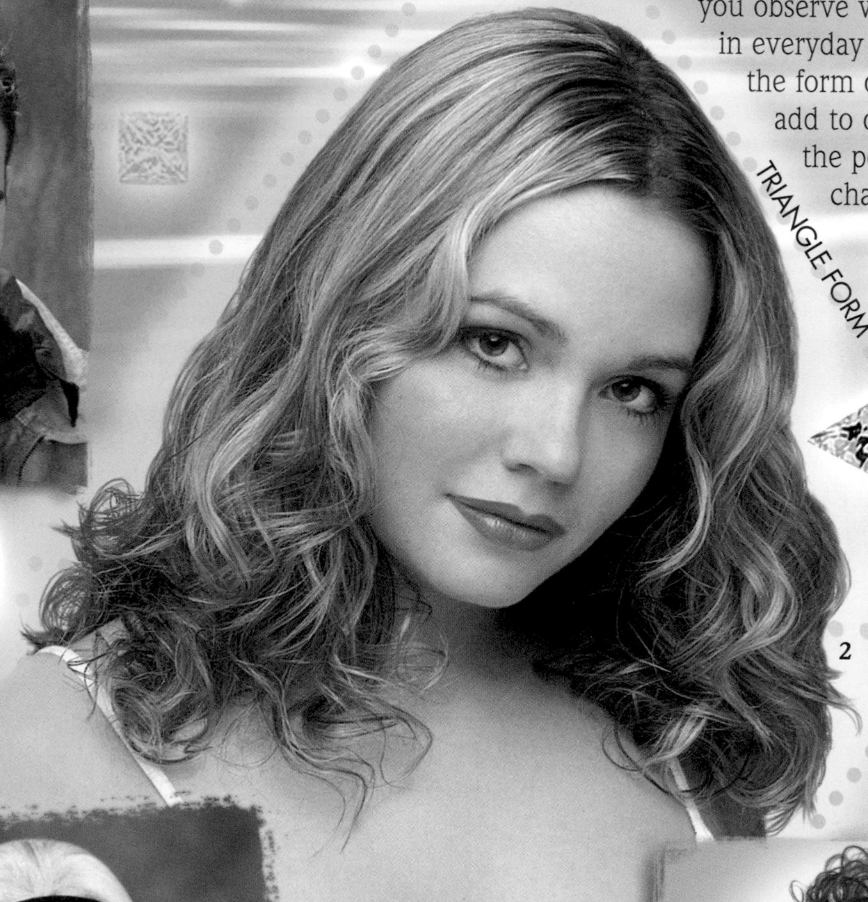

2

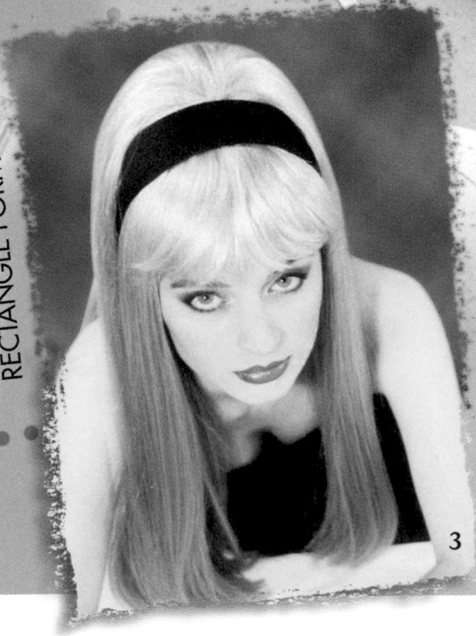

RECTANGLE FORM

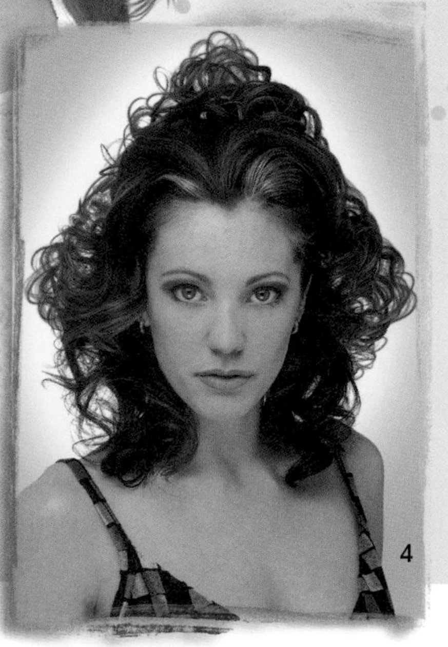

3

DIAMOND FORM

4

The Elements ...

Shapes *are made up of connecting lines of straight or curved geometric figures (square, rectangle, triangle, round, oval and ovaloid).*

Hairdesigns are like a puzzle. The sequential patterns are the pieces that compose the final picture of the puzzle. Design elements such as colors, textures or shapes are used as **blending lines** to connect one traveling motion to another. This will produce a continuous flowing motion in the hairdesign, which your eye will naturally follow. Extending or breaking lines within a hairdesign will produce an **interruption of motion.**

Our study of biology and the human form in the previous chapter led to identification of **seven facial shapes.** Now we can use these shapes to identify how **design forms** are created.

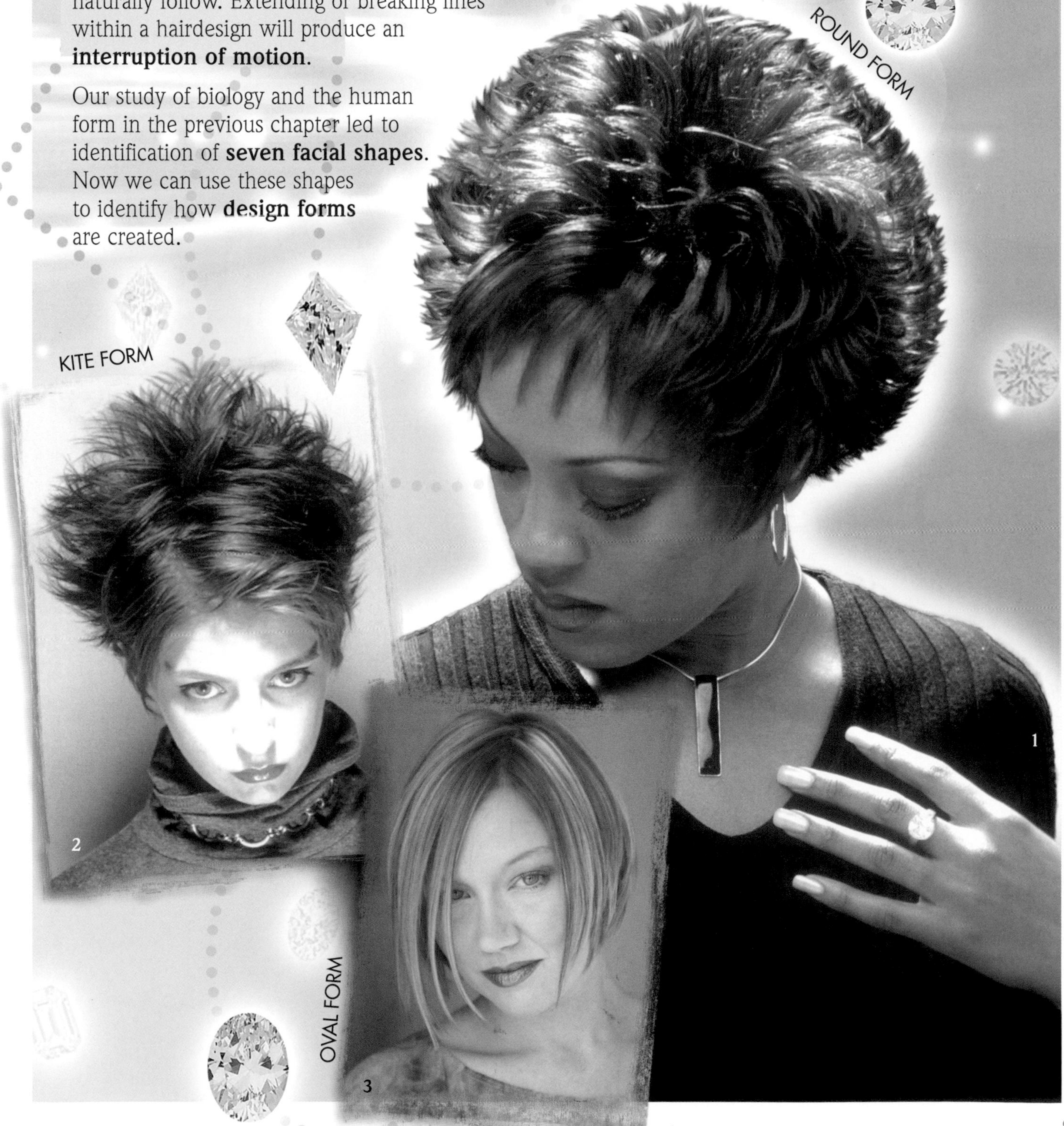

ROUND FORM

KITE FORM

OVAL FORM

1

2

3

4

SIDE   SIDE

VERTEX   ANGLE

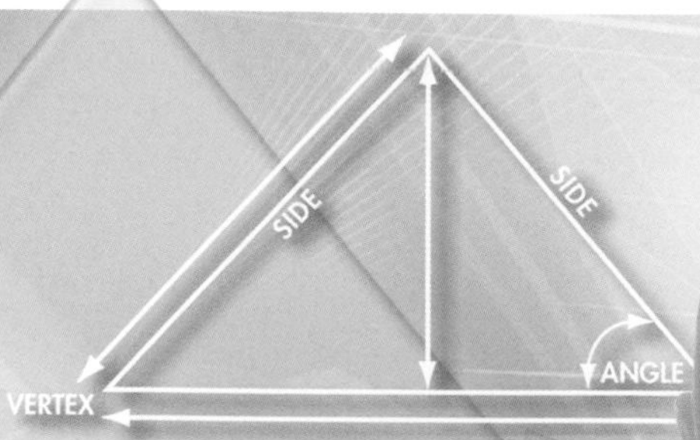

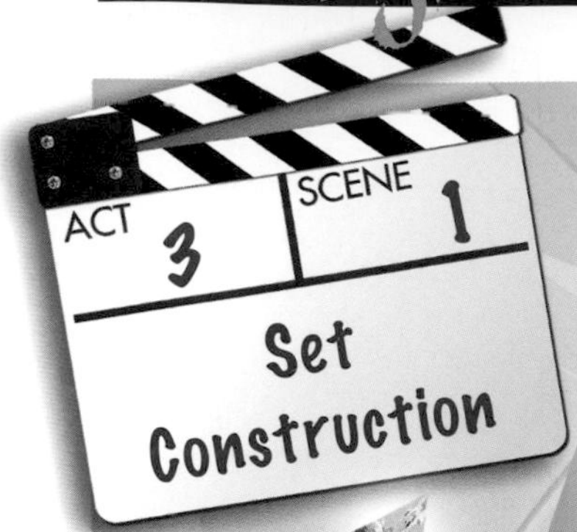

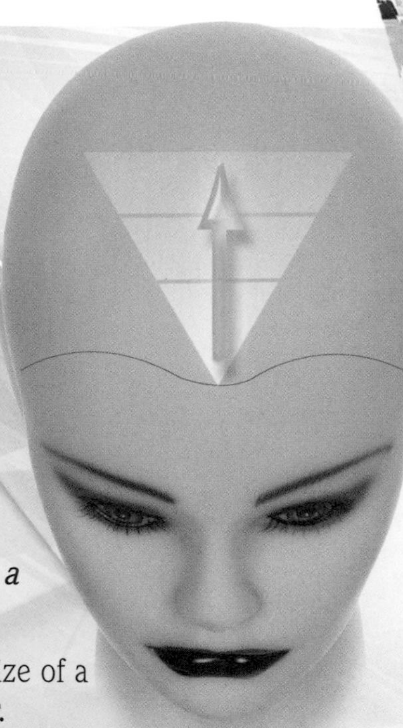

The most perfect shape
in hairdesign is the triangle. It has a naturally strong design since the base is broad and supportive of its top. Of all the straight shapes, the triangle has the fewest number of sides and points. Hairstylists can use triangles to construct a variety of straight and curved shapes.

The degree or sharpness of the angles determines the shape and size of a triangle. The **vertex** is the point where the two sides come together.

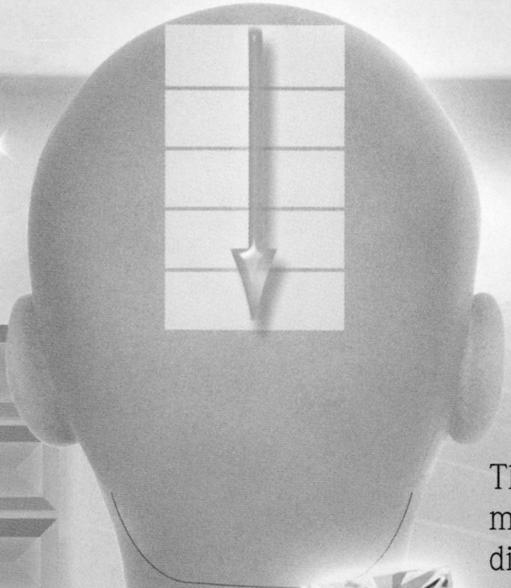

"The same mathematical shapes previously used to identify facial contours in Chapter 3 can be used to FORM COMPONENTS in hairdesigns."

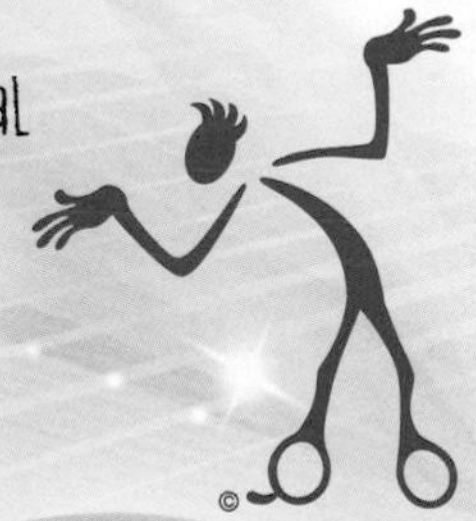

The ancient Greek mathematician Pythagoras discovered that combining two right triangles together formed a **square**.

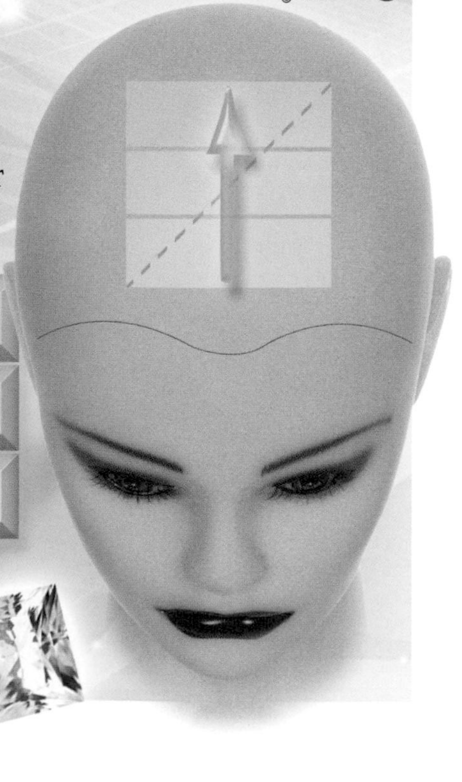

Mathematicians later established that four right triangles formed a **rectangle**. In a rectangle, all four sides must be 90-degree angles. A square shape becomes a rectangle when elongated to the point where its sides are no longer considered even in length.

Therefore, the **straight shapes** consist of a square, a triangle, and combinations of these to form a rectangle.

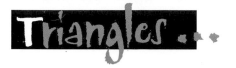
Triangles

"Now apply the same mathematical reasoning that led to the creation of these straight shapes. Use them to create hair art!"

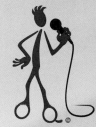

EXERCISE

The **straight shapes** consist of the square, triangle, and combinations. Each component in your style's design plan is directly related to the facial shapes and precious gem stone shapes we studied in Chapter 3. Practice setting the geometric shapes below. Remember, straight shapes are set into the hair using **cylinder** rollers. Cylinder rollers are always fastened in the direction hair is rolled onto the roller.

4

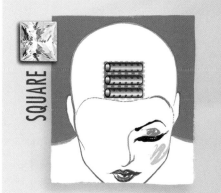

SQUARE

RECTANGLE

TRIANGLE

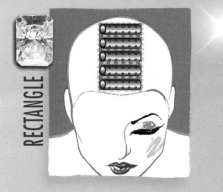

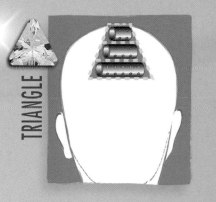

1. In order to create a **square** setting formation, set the hair with three rollers of the same length. The hair is directed in a straight line from the front hairline to the crown.

2. To produce the **rectangle** setting formation, combine the same length rollers in an elongated pattern, placed from the front hairline toward the nape or other control point identified in the design plan.

3. To imitate a **triangle's** equality of proportion, set the hair formation using a half-length roller followed by one three-quarter length roller and one full length roller. The hair in the triangle setting formation travels in a straight direction from one location.

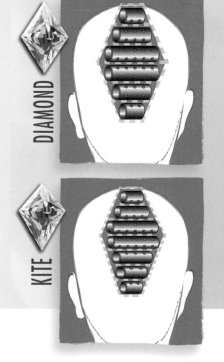

DIAMOND

KITE

4. Develop the **diamond** setting formation (with two equal triangles) by using a half-length roller followed by one three-quarter length roller and one full length roller. Reverse this pattern (creating a back-to-back effect with these triangles) by placing another full length roller next, followed by one three-quarter length roller and a half-length roller.

5. To form a **kite** shape setting formation, put two triangles with different side lengths (one equal and one unequal triangle) together at their bases. Set the hair using a half-length roller first, followed by a three-quarter length roller and one full-length roller. Continue setting this pattern by placing a three-quarter length roller next, followed by two half-length rollers.

Curved shapes consist of circles, ovals, and ovaloids (also known as oblongs). Ovaloid shapes in alternating directions produce wave formations. These three curved shapes can travel in clockwise or counter-clockwise directions. Each component in your style's design plan is directly related to the facial shapes and precious gem stone shapes we studied in Chapter 3.

▶ EXERCISE

To create the curved shapes of a circle, oval and ovaloid, set the hair using **conical** rollers. Conical rollers were designed for setting curved shapes and are fastened at the small end of the roller in the direction that the hair has been rolled. Practice setting these shapes in clockwise and counter-clockwise directions.

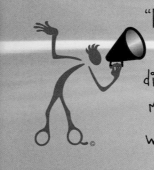

"First, use the width from the small end of a conical roller to measure diameter. Next, lay the roller flat to measure length. Diameter plus length will determine the width of a circle or oval shape."

CIRCLE

CIRCLE
(Eight equal length conical rollers)

1/2 CIRCLE

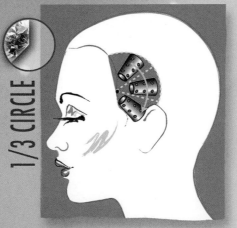

1/3 CIRCLE

1/4 CIRCLE

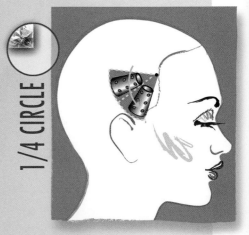

1/2 CIRCLE
(Four equal length conical rollers)

1/3 CIRCLE
(Three equal length conical rollers)

1/4 CIRCLE
(Two equal length conical rollers)

Triangles...

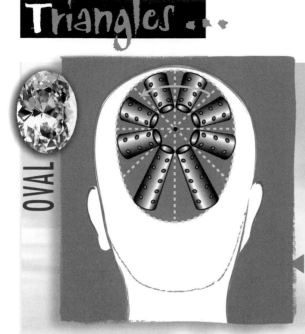

OVAL
(Eight unequal length conical rollers)

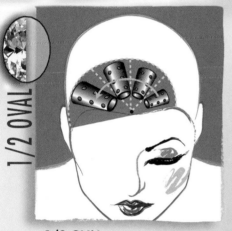

1/2 OVAL
(Four unequal length conical rollers)

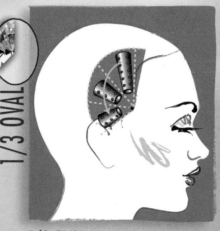

1/3 OVAL
(Three unequal length conical rollers)

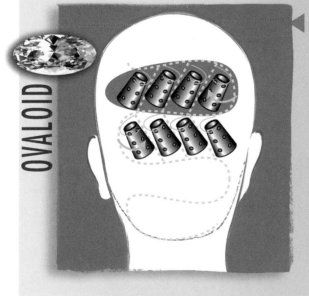

OVALOID (Two ovaloids (oblongs) set with four short, equal length conical rollers in each oblong) Partings are zig-zag to each other.

"Remember, a circle is set with equal length rollers. An oval is set with unequal length rollers. An ovaloid (oblong) is also set with equal length rollers, but on 45 degree partings and in alternating directions. The diameter of these rollers may vary within the same shape depending on the hair's length and the amount of curl desired."

ACT **4** SCENE **1**

Arrangements

4

Elevation in hairdesign is equal to height or how much the hairdesign is lifted off of the scalp.

A term frequently used in haircutting, elevation refers to the angle created when the hair is lifted before being cut. The same principle is used for hairdesigning. Although the hair is not cut, it is styled in such a way as that it produces **lift** from the surface.

Styling the hair using **positive** elevation increases the **mobility** of the design and also the convexity **(volume or mass)** it fills in space, whereas **negative** elevation is used when styling hair **closer** to the scalp area of the head form.

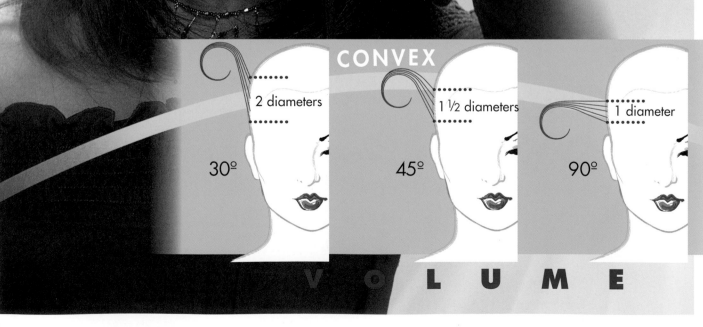

CONVEX

2 diameters

1 ½ diameters

1 diameter

30º

45º

90º

VOLUME

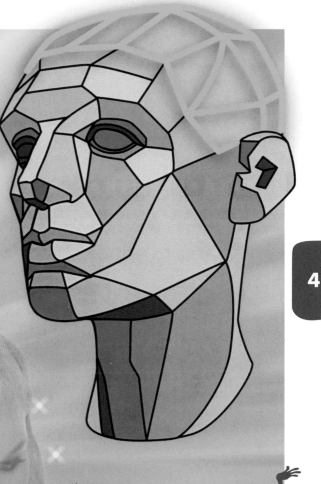

Planes are identified as straight areas on the head's relatively spherical surface. For simplicity, the **360 degrees of a circle** are reduced to vertical and horizontal planes, each from 0-90 degrees in area. Combining the planes of the head will produce **lines, shapes and directional movement** within a hairstyle. Our eye will perceive these **connecting lines** as a curved surface following the form of the head.

We use the planes of the head to create convexity (volume) and concavity (indentation) within a hairdesign. This can be accomplished using liquid tools, pin curls, rollers, an airformer and/or irons to create the appropriate volume or indentation established when creating your design plan. **To create convexity (volume), turn the ends under** in your design plan. **For concavity (indentation), turn ends up.**

4

"To create indentation in a hairdesign, you must first have a hill before a valley!"

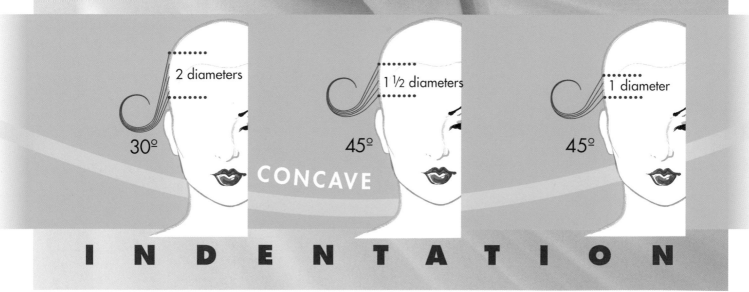

2 diameters

30°

CONCAVE

1 ½ diameters

45°

1 diameter

45°

I N D E N T A T I O N

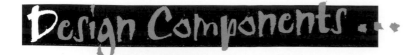

RA

Finger waves are ovaloid shapes placed into the hair in alternating directions using the fingers and a comb. They can be created on horizontal, vertical or diagonal planes (positions) of the head form.

Finger waving helps develop the finger strength and manual dexterity necessary to perform more complex hairdesign skills. This art of molding hair to the curved surface of the head is seen frequently on Hollywood's red carpet, where retro styles show history's influence on today's hairdesign.

Structure

The shaping is the section of hair that is molded prior to the formation of a wave. Shapings give the **hair direction** for the ridge to be formed. Traditional waving lotion is made from plant sources, but commercially-prepared gels may also be used. Its thick viscosity is combed in before shaping to control coarse hair and can be diluted for use on very fine hair. To keep hair pliable and avoid overuse of styling product, apply waving lotion or gel to one section at a time while molding.

Caution: Applying too much waving lotion may cause the material to flake when the finger waved hair is dried. Using a high quality liquid styling tool will prevent flaking when dry.

SHAPING

HOLLOW

RIDGE

The ridge is the raised convex (volume) section of hair created in the shaping of a finger wave when the alternating ovaloids connect. **Do not overdirect** the hair or pinch fingers together to increase the height of the ridge; this will create an unstable and uneven hair placement.

The hollow is the concave (indentation) ovaloid section directly under the ridge that **determines the wave's depth and tempo.** The hollow will have the opposite direction of the ridge and always follow the plane of the ridge.

"If the finger wave's ridge is on a horizontal plane, then the hollow must be on a horizontal plane."

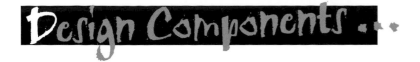

The design plan

Prior to creating a finger wave, a design plan is needed to determine the starting direction for the wave and on what plane the wave is going to travel. Complete directions for each type of finger wave formation are within the art chapters of this manual. Chapter 8, the Art of Design Sculpting.

▶ EXERCISE

Basic finger wave formation

Practice shaping the hair into a basic finger wave pattern by creating alternating oblongs (ovaloids) with two ridge formations on the side of the head.

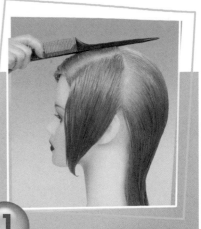

1 Shampoo the hair and apply the liquid tool of choice. Create a side part.

2 Mold a 'C' shaping on the heavy side of the part line.

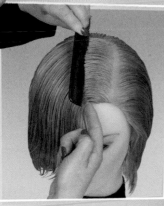

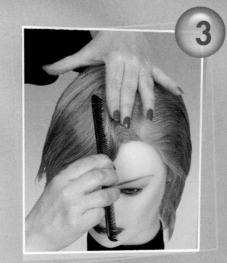

3 Place your index finger on the open end of the 'C' shaping at the front hairline two finger widths from the part. The first section of the ridge is created by inserting the comb parallel to the part and directly under your index finger. Draw the comb forward along your index finger, working in 1 to 1.5 inch (2.5-3.8 cm) panels as measured with the second knuckle of your index finger to the tip.

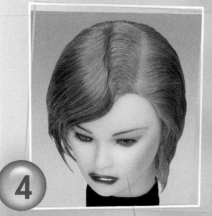

4 Lay the comb flat to the scalp. Place your middle finger into the index finger position, with your index finger on top of the comb. Apply pressure by closing the two fingers together, which will produce the ridge of the wave. **Caution:** Do not push the hair up to form the ridge.

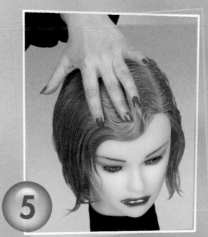

5 Without lifting your fingers, remove the comb while rotating the teeth toward the scalp. Reinsert the fine teeth of the comb and smooth the ridge by retracing the movement. Redirect the hair in the reverse direction to create the hollow.

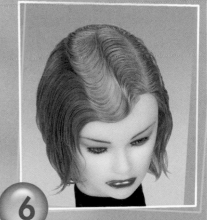

6 Slide your hand back with the tip of your index finger resting on the back side of the ridge and repeat the steps above to join the panels.

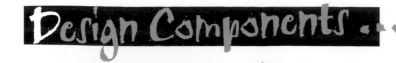

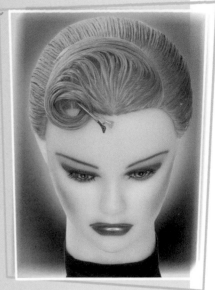

SCALING

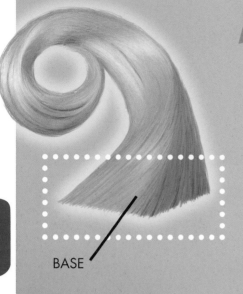

BASE

Pin curls

Structure

Scalings are panel subsections created prior to pin curl placements from which the bases of pin curls are selected. Scalings are geometric, may be straight or curved, and can be placed in forward, reverse, horizontal, vertical or diagonal planes.

The **base** is the portion of hair that is attached to the scalp. The geometric shapes used in hairdesign are present in bases, shapings, waves and curls.

The **straight** shaped bases used for pin curl designs consist of the square, rectangle and triangle.

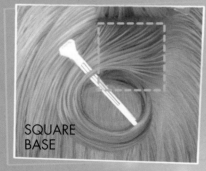

SQUARE BASE

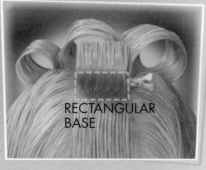

RECTANGULAR BASE

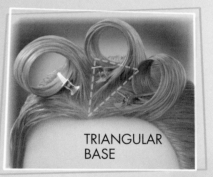

TRIANGULAR BASE

- **Square** based pin curls can be flat or convex (volume). **Flat** square bases are used for areas that require curl but no lift, such as the side of the front hairline or the nape. **Convex** square pin curls are used to add lift or volume.

- **Rectangle** based pin curls which stand up are known as **barrel curls,** and are used to create convexity (volume) anywhere on the head.

- **Triangle** bases are used for flat as well as convex (volume) pin curls, primarily along the front hairline to **prevent breaks** in the finished design.

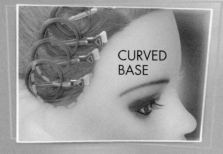

CURVED BASE

The **curved** bases for pin curl placements (circles, ovals and ovaloids) are shaped like the letter "c" and are also referred to as arc or half moon shapes. Arc-based pin curls are most commonly used and recommended for use in the side hairline or nape area.

"Another name for a curl that is sliced from a scaling and formed without elevation is a carved curl. A pin curl that creates height is also known as a cascade curl."

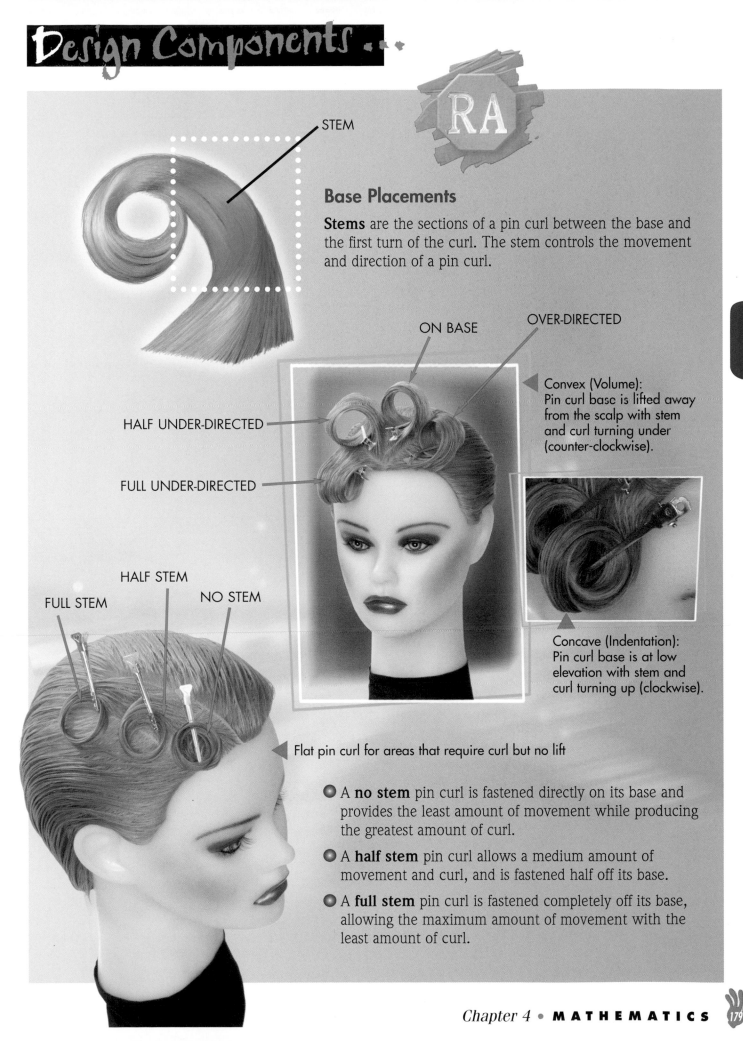

Design Components...

RA

STEM

Base Placements

Stems are the sections of a pin curl between the base and the first turn of the curl. The stem controls the movement and direction of a pin curl.

ON BASE

OVER-DIRECTED

HALF UNDER-DIRECTED

FULL UNDER-DIRECTED

Convex (Volume):
Pin curl base is lifted away from the scalp with stem and curl turning under (counter-clockwise).

Concave (Indentation):
Pin curl base is at low elevation with stem and curl turning up (clockwise).

FULL STEM

HALF STEM

NO STEM

Flat pin curl for areas that require curl but no lift

- A **no stem** pin curl is fastened directly on its base and provides the least amount of movement while producing the greatest amount of curl.

- A **half stem** pin curl allows a medium amount of movement and curl, and is fastened half off its base.

- A **full stem** pin curl is fastened completely off its base, allowing the maximum amount of movement with the least amount of curl.

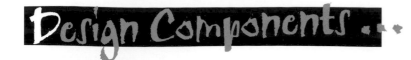

RA

A circle at the ends of the hair that produces the wave pattern is known as a **curl**. The center of the curl can be open or closed, but the ends of the pin curl should be contained **within the circle**.

A **closed** center will produce maximum curl with less definition and may be used to help hold a style in fine hair. An **open** center will produce curls that are more uniform, but not as tight. The larger the circle or curl the wider the finished wave pattern.

CURL

Pin curl direction is either clockwise or counter-clockwise.

- Pin curls formed in the same direction as the hands move on a clock (to the right) produce a **clockwise** direction.

- Pin curls formed in the opposite direction from which clock hands move (to the left) produce a **counter-clockwise** direction.

CLOCKWISE

COUNTER-CLOCKWISE

12

9   3

6

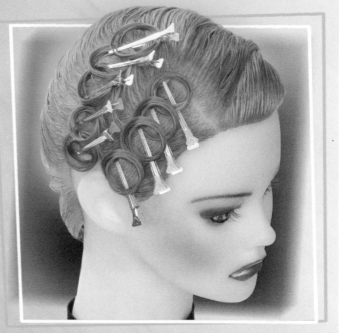

PIN CURL WAVE FORMATION

- Alternating rows of pin curls will produce a **complete wave pattern.**

- **Ridge curls** form a strong wave pattern by following the finger wave's ridge with a row of pin curls. Pin curls placed behind a ridge and followed by another ridge produce a **skip wave.**

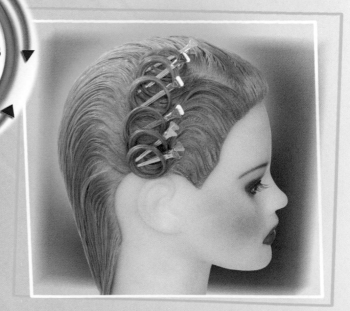

RIDGE CURL PATTERN; TWO ROWS FORM A SKIP WAVE

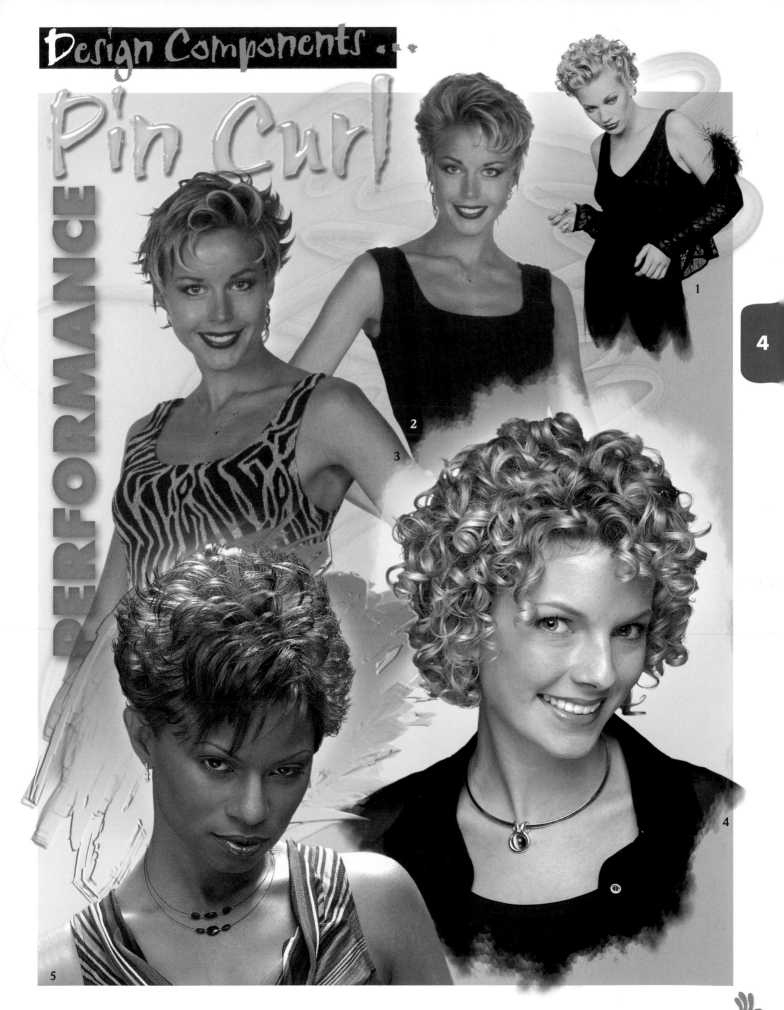

Design Components

Pin Curl

PERFORMANCE

The design plan

The pin curl design plan should include the geometric shape bases and curl placements that are needed to achieve the desired look. For example, rectangular bases and convex (volume) pin curls create barrel curls similar to roller curls.

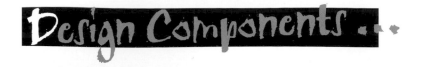

▶ EXERCISE

Pin Curl Technique

Practice pin curl design on all bases and shapings in recommended areas of the head form. Pin curls can be placed in tight areas too small for rollers.

PREPARATION: Shampoo the hair and evenly apply the liquid tool of choice. Identify the bases and controls to achieve the final hairstyle.

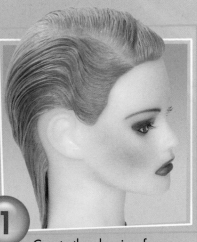

1 Create the shaping for the pin curls.

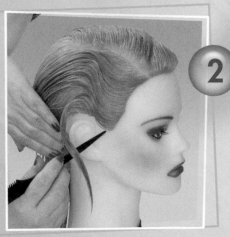

2 Select the strand for the first pin curl from the open end of the shaping. Smooth the strand with the comb. Pinch the strand and **ribbon** until smooth by running it between the index finger and thumb.

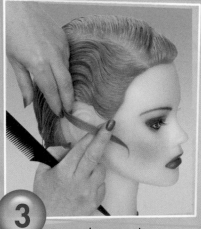

3 Grasp the strand at the end and begin to form the curl.

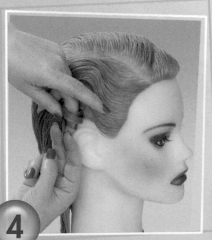

4 Roll the curl around one finger, either center or index finger, keeping the ends enclosed within the circle or curl.

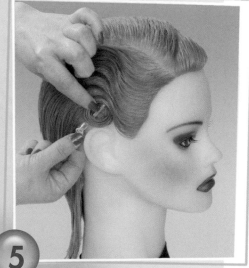

5 When the desired placement has been reached, slide the curl off of the finger and pin it with a clip. Clips should be secured in the direction in which the curl has been formed.

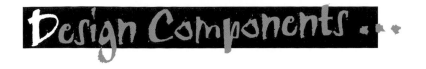
Alternate Pin Curl Techniques:

Ends to Base – Grasp the ends of the hair strand and turn them to form a circle. Making sure the ends remain inside the circle, roll the ends into the stem of the curl, and continue winding until the curl has reached the desired base placement. Secure the curl with a clip.

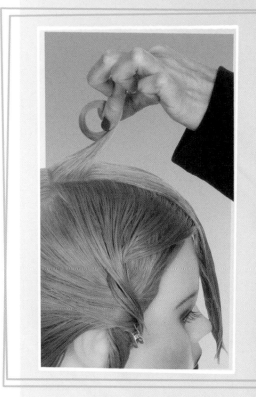

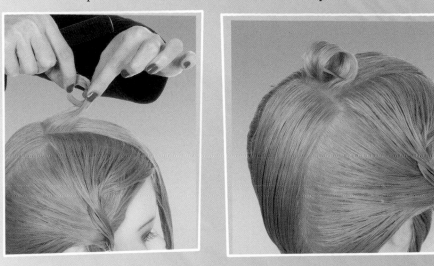

Winding Clipped Ends – Grasp the ends of the hair strand to smooth and secure them with a clip. Turn the clipped end of the strand to form a circle. Making sure the ends remain inside the circle, roll the clipped ends into the stem of the curl, and continue winding until the curl has reached the desired base placement. Hold the curl securely while removing and fastening the clip at the base to secure the curl.

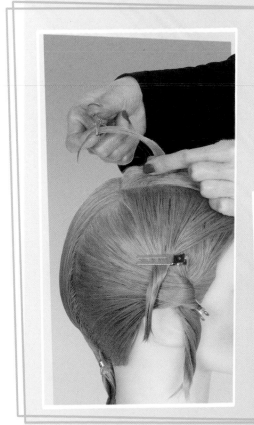

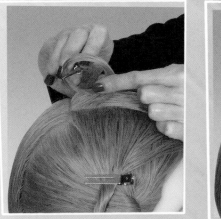

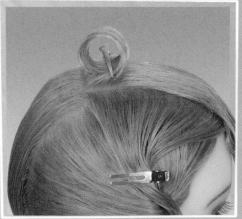

Design Components...

Roller Curls

The roller design plan should include the geometric shape components necessary to achieve the finished look. Curved shapes are generally used around the perimeter of a hairdesign and straight shapes are most frequently found within the interior of a hairdesign plan. Rollers sets are firmer than airformed or pin curled styles. An area set with rollers covers a surface equal to using two to four pin curls.

BASE

The **base** is the section of hair that is attached to the scalp. When making the base selection, use the diameter and length of the roller as a measuring device. Design decisions will also be influenced by the length of the hair, diameter of the roller and how it is placed on the base to achieve the desired finish. The smaller the diameter of the roller, the tighter the curl formation.

STEM

Roller **stems** are the section of hair between the base and the first turn of the roller. Stems are held at an angle as the hair is wrapped onto the roller. It is the stem or control that determines the placement of the roller in relation to the base. The controls for roller placement are on base, over-directed and under-directed for both convexity (volume) and concavity (indentation).

CURL

The **curl** or **circle** is the end of the hair that is wrapped completely around the roller. The size of the circle along with the length of the hair determines the amount of the curl produced in the pattern.

▶ Convex (Volume) – Creates fullness or lift in the hairdesign

- **Full over-directed:** Rolled at a 10-degree angle above the base and secured above the top parting; produces minimal volume with maximum stem mobility.

- **Half over-directed:** Rolled at a 30-degree angle above the base and secured on the top parting; creates moderate volume and stem mobility.

- **On base:** Rolled above the top parting at a 45-degree angle and secured within base partings; creates maximum volume with no stem mobility.

- **Half under-directed:** Rolled at a 90-degree angle from the base's center and secured directly on the bottom parting; creates minimal volume and moderate stem mobility.

- **Full under-directed:** Rolled at a 45-degree angle below the bottom parting and secured below the base; creates minimal volume and maximum stem mobility.

▶ Concave (Indentation) – Creates a hollow or flat area in the hairdesign

- **On base:** Rolled at a 45-degree angle below the bottom parting and secured within base partings; creates minimal hollowness or indentation.

- **Half under-directed:** Rolled at a 45-degree angle below the bottom parting and secured directly on its bottom base parting; creates moderate hollowness or indentation.

- **Full under-directed:** Rolled at a 30-degree angle or lower and secured below the bottom base parting; creates maximum closeness or indentation.

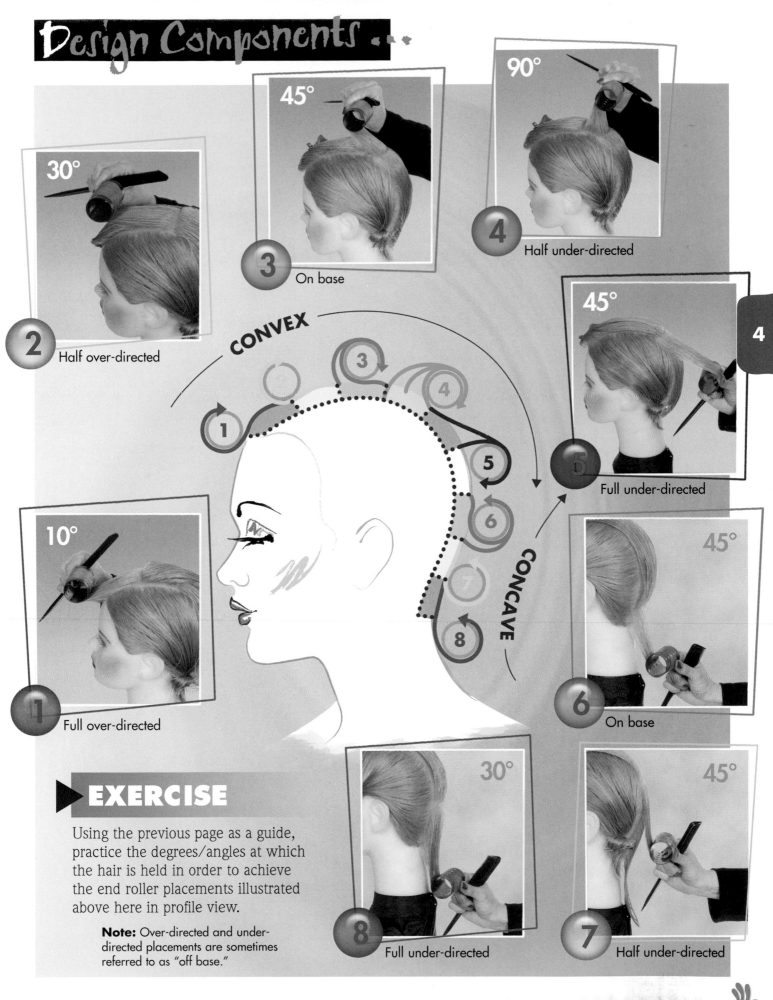

Design Components...

30° — 2 — Half over-directed

45° — 3 — On base

90° — 4 — Half under-directed

45° — 5 — Full under-directed

10° — 1 — Full over-directed

45° — 6 — On base

CONVEX

CONCAVE

45° — 7 — Half under-directed

30° — 8 — Full under-directed

▶ EXERCISE

Using the previous page as a guide, practice the degrees/angles at which the hair is held in order to achieve the end roller placements illustrated above here in profile view.

Note: Over-directed and under-directed placements are sometimes referred to as "off base."

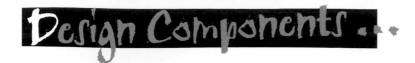

► EXERCISE

Cylinder Roller Technique
PREPARATION:
Shampoo the hair; evenly apply the liquid tool of choice.

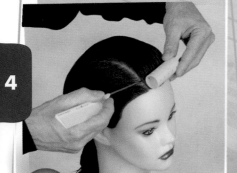

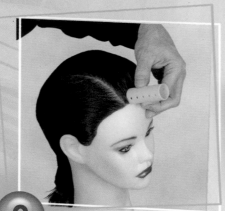

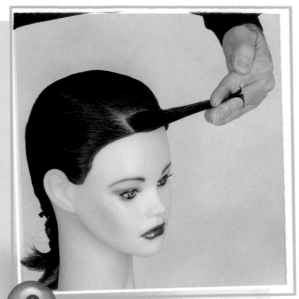

1 Identify the bases needed to create the desired look. Use the length of the roller to create the panel section for roller placement.

2 Use the diameter of the roller to measure for the subsection or base selection. Diameters of 1, 1 1/2, or 2 times the roller size may be used. This will vary the amount of hair placed in each roller, which influences the movement and strength of the curl produced.

3 Insert the tail comb at the scalp, and comb through the hair strand to create the subsection. Comb the strand twice on the underside and once on the outer side to smooth the subsection while holding the hair with tension at the desired angle for proper roller placement.

Finished convex (volume) roller placement   Finished concave (indentation) roller placement

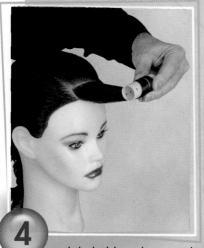

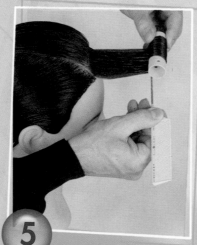

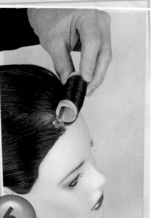

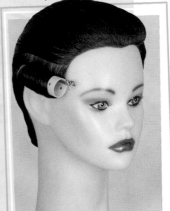

4 While holding the strand in position, insert the roller. Use your thumbs to adhere the hair to the roller. Do not pinch the strand together; keep it evenly distributed across the roller.

5 If necessary, use the tail of the comb to smooth any irregular ends. Wind the roller with the hair toward the scalp.

6 Holding the roller firmly in place, fasten the clip in the center of the roller to maintain tension to provide the proper curl formation.

Note: The hair must be long enough to wrap around the roller's diameter 1 1/2 times to produce a wave pattern, although one complete turn will result in the formation of a "C" shape.

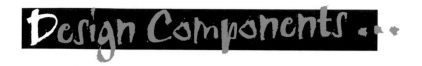

▶ EXERCISE

Conical Roller Techniques

PREPARATION: Shampoo the hair; evenly apply the liquid tool of choice.

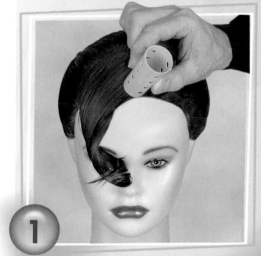

1 Use a control point from which the hair is distributed for the individual conical roller selections. The roller will sit one diameter (small end of the roller) away from the control point.

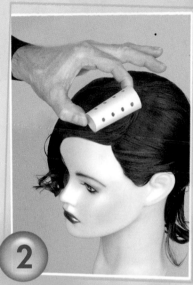

2 The diameter of the small end plus the roller's length determines the size of the scaling.

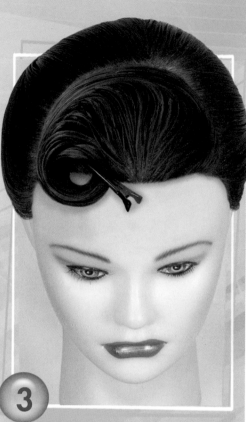

3 Create the scaling in which the conical rollers will be placed.

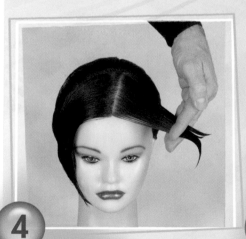

4 Insert the tail of the comb at the control point and create the subsection within the scaling. Comb through the strand to smooth.

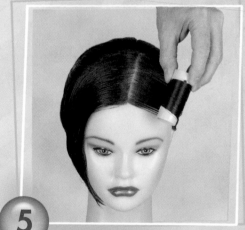

5 Hold the strand in position. Insert the roller, following the hair with your thumbs to smooth the ends around the roller. Maintain tension and roll toward the scalp.

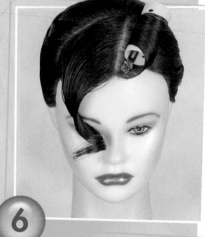

6 Secure the roller with a fastener in the direction the hair has been rolled.

"Many factors determine the end result: base size, roller diameter, placement and tension."

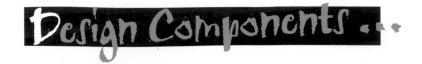

Design Components...

Airforming

Proper airforming technique is quickly becoming a lost art. As technology advances, emphasis is placed more on the speed in which the hair is dried rather than focusing on performing the technique correctly. To eliminate fatigue and work more efficiently, stylists must first learn the proper airformer, body and brush positions.

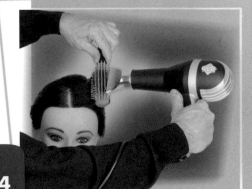

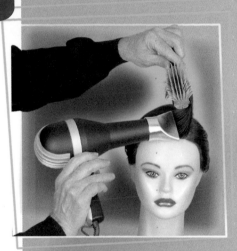

Airformer Positions

The proper position is achieved by holding the airformer by the handle with the cord placed over the arm for maximum mobility and control. This technique will keep the electric cord out of the stylist's way and prevent it from hanging in the client's face. The stylist's elbows are extended outward with the flow of air directed inward. Keep the air flow directed at the stylist to prevent the air from accidentally hitting the client. Feel and adjust the temperature of the propelled air if it becomes excessive in order to protect the client's skin and hair.

The concentrator attachment should be on the airformer at all times to **keep the air flow focused.** It must be positioned next to the brush to eliminate any space between the two tools, which should travel through the hair as one unit. The placement of the brush along with the airformer creates curl formations when rotated with hair.

To properly form the curl the hair should be 50 percent dry. Trying to form the curls without the hair being dried sufficiently will delay the hydrogen bonds' reformation into their new positions. To create straightness in the hair, keep good tension. To produce curl, relax the hair by creating a loose bend when airforming.

Continually rotating the brush while drying the hair in the direction of the cuticle will smooth and polish the hair strands. **To maximize the curl formation,** first heat and then cool the base with the airformer prior to removing the brush. **Hot air forms the pattern, and cool air sets the pattern.** Pin the hair at the base after removing the brush to allow the hair to stay in the curl formation until cool.

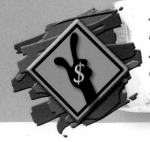

Stand out from your competition by making sure your clients can maintain their new hairdesigns at home. Recommend appropriate styling tools and finishing products for their hair type and the desired look to be achieved. Instruct them on the proper use of these tools to build their confidence and loyalty.

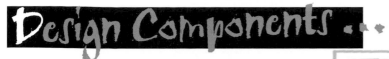

Design Components...

To perform the proper airforming techniques, you must learn the components of curls and how to achieve them. As in roller curls, each airformed curl contains a base to determine its placement, a stem for direction and a circle that defines the diameter of the curl. Instead of rollers, the stylist uses an airformer and a styling brush.

Stems are created in airforming by the angle of the hair strand while the curl is rolled and placed on, above or below the base.

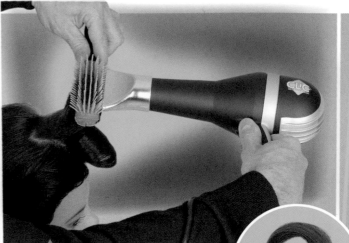

4

An **on** base curl placement creates maximum volume. The strand is held at a 45-degree angle above the base. The curl is fastened directly within the base partings.

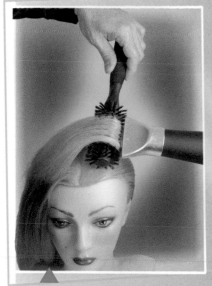

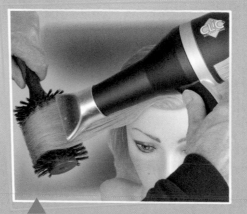

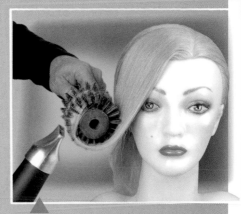

An **over-directed** volume base placement is held at a 10- to 30-degree angle. The curl is fastened either above (full over-directed) or on the top parting (half over-directed) to create moderate volume.

An **under-directed** volume base placement is held at a 90-degree angle or lower. The curl is fastened on or below the bottom parting (half or full under-directed), creating minimal volume.

An **indentation** curl is held at a 45-degree angle or lower. The curl is fastened on or below the bottom parting, according to base placements.

"To produce convex volume and lift, always over-direct the hair. To produce concave indentation and closeness, keep hair close to the scalp."

▶ EXERCISE

1. Help the hair reach the proper degree of moisture for airforming.

2. Make the curl formations using the proper airforming techniques.

3. Use the proper techniques within geometric shapings.

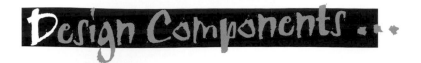
Iron Curls

The component parts of iron curls are the same as with roller and airformed curls. They include a base, a stem and a curl or circle. Other names for iron curls include thermal curling or Marcel waving.

Electric and conventional irons produce the same curl formations; therefore, the techniques are identical for both types of irons. The only difference between the irons involves their heat source (self-heating/electrical or conventional/stove-heated).

In iron styling it is important to establish the base on which the curl will be formed. Use a comb to select and carve the desired geometric base shape from the head. The diameter of the tool used will determine the size of the base.

To prepare the base you must warm the strand close to the scalp. Insert the hair between the groove and barrel of the curling iron, hold in place for a few seconds and then slide the iron down the length of the hair strand.

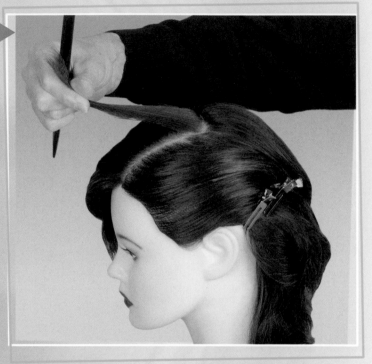

Selecting Base Size

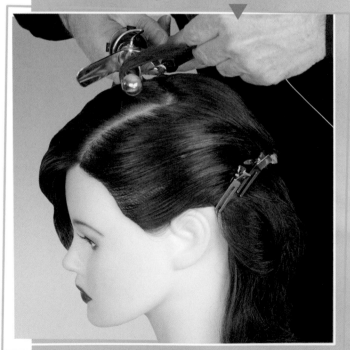

Warming the Strand

Curls are formed by rotating the iron with hair using the correct techniques. **The curl techniques consist of neutral, base to ends and ends to base.** See Chapter 2 iron dynamics for conventional iron ends to base volume curl technique and electric iron base to ends spiral curl technique.

Placement of the hair to be curled is identified by its relation to the base of the curl. **On base** placement assures maximum lift and convexity (volume) from the head form. **Half under-directed** placement allows the stem more freedom of movement. **Full under-directed** base placements produce minimal volume but maximum direction of the curl's movement.

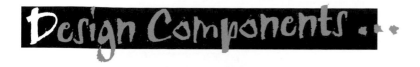

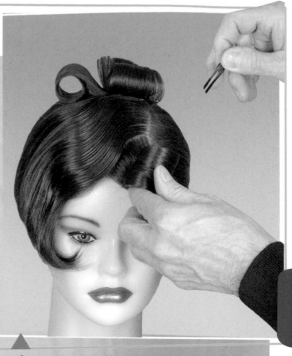

Volume Curl Direction

The direction in which the hair is placed onto its base will also help determine the strength of the curl. To produce convexity (volume) and lift, always overdirect the hair.

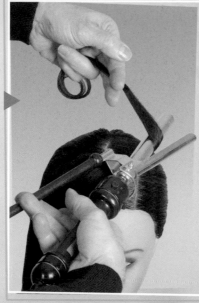

Indentation Curl Direction

To produce concavity (indentation) or closeness, keep hair close to the scalp (under-directed).

Spiral Base Position

Curls positioned vertically are referred to as spiral curls.

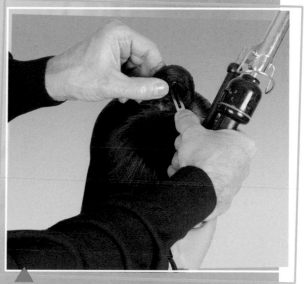

The amount of curl or movement within the finished hairdesign is determined in part by the **diameter** of the curling iron chosen along with the **hair's length** and by the **wrapping technique** at the stem area. The weight of longer hair will pull down a curl, whereas shorter hair wrapped with the same diameter iron will produce a stronger curl with more volume or lift.

Clip Curl until Cool

To increase the strength of the curl, iron curls may clipped after the iron has been removed. The pins should remain in place during the cooling process for maximum strength and durability of the curl.

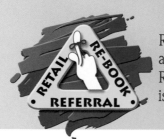

Remember to book the next appointment and ask your clients for referrals. Rewarding loyal, satisfied customers is the best way to build your clientele.

Proper Iron Techniques

▶ EXERCISE

Neutral Curls

Neutral curls can move in any direction and are created by directing the hair into the iron in a neutral or straight position.

PREPARATION: The hair must be clean and dry to ensure a good thermal curl. Create the individual geometric shapes from which the partings for individual curls will occur.

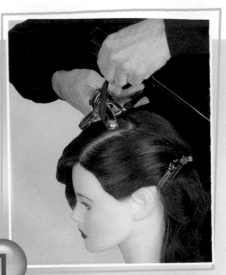

1 Establish a base and warm the strand.

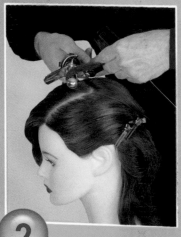

2 Insert the iron at the base of the curl while supporting the ends of the hair.

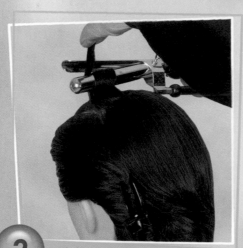

3 While maintaining tension, rotate the iron using the fingers to manipulate the movement. Continually open and close the groove of the iron while supporting the ends until they have been enclosed within the curl.

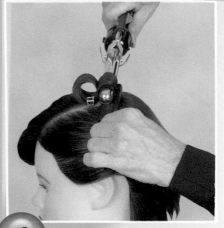

4 Once the ends have been enclosed within the center rotate the iron one complete turn to refine the curl. Place a hard rubber comb under the iron to form a protective barrier for the scalp.

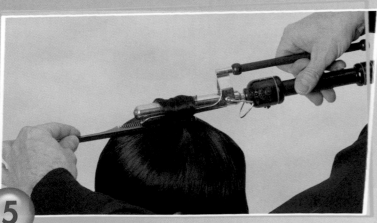

5 Slide the iron along the comb while opening the groove to remove the iron.

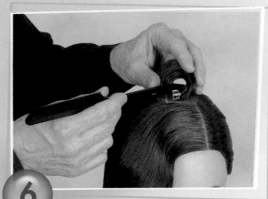

6 Secure the curl with a clip and allow to cool.

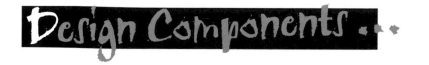

Figure Eight Base to Ends Double-Looped Curls

PREPARATION: Create the individual geometric shapes from which the partings for individual curls will occur.

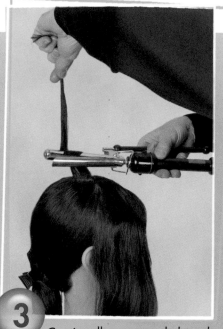

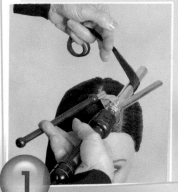

1 Establish a base and warm the strand.

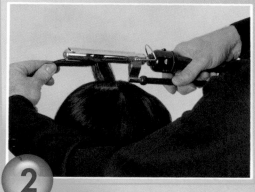

2 Insert the iron at the base of the curl. Rotate the iron's shell one half turn while opening and closing the groove. Direct the hair toward one side of the iron to form the first loop of the curl.

3 Continually open and close the iron while rotating the iron's shell. Direct the hair strand toward the opposite end of the iron as the previous loop and form the second loop.

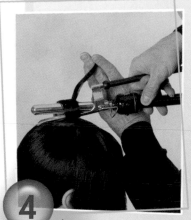

4 Alternate creation of each loop until hair ends have been enclosed within the curl. Remember to open and close the shell continually throughout the rotations.

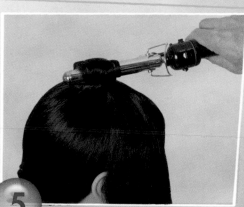

5 After the ends have been enclosed within the curl, complete one final rotation of the iron to smooth and define the curl formation. Avoid "fishhooks" caused by crimping ends not properly rolled into the iron.

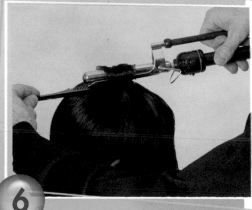

6 Place a heat-resistant comb between the iron and the scalp for protection, and hold the iron in place for a few seconds.

7 Remove the iron from the curl by opening the clamp and sliding the iron along the comb. Pin the curl and allow it to cool for maximum curl strength.

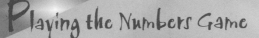

Design Components ...

Playing the Numbers Game

► EXERCISE

Here's a game that will help you quickly analyze pleasing proportions in a hairdesign. Study the examples shown here and then try it yourself on the next page.

As a general rule, the most pleasing and dynamic hairstyles will have three main components; when it has more than three, it may become too busy. Less than three could result in a lack of excitement.

Each component will make up a certain percentage in the design. This game uses only odd numbered hairdesign components, because our goal is to create styles which stimulate and capture our interest. Since we are viewing only flat, one-dimensional images in these photographs, you will need to make allowances for the unseen portion; therefore, the percentages will not add up to 100 percent.

HOW TO PLAY:

STEP A: Find and outline the main components in the hairdesign. (Our sample outlines are in color so you can see them clearly.)

STEP B: List the design components according to their size – the smallest to the largest. Add them to the COMPONENT column, using a simple name to easily identify them.

STEP C: Using only odd numbers (1, 3, 5, 7 and 9), determine the percentage of each component's total area and write the corresponding number in the # column as shown below.

Note: Not all numbers from 1 to 9 apply in every hairdesign. Your figure should show only a relationship of one component to another, not the percentage each component contributes in relation to the whole design. The total will not equal 100%.

STEP A   STEP B   STEP C

EXAMPLE 1

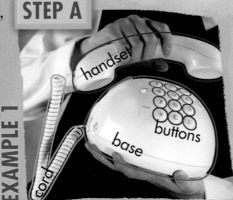

COMPONENT	#
buttons	1
cord	3
handset	5
base	7

STEP A   STEP B   STEP C

EXAMPLE 2

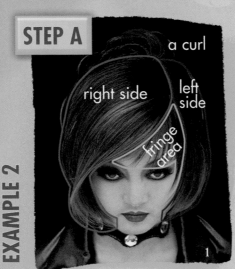

COMPONENT	#
a curl	1
fringe area	3
left side	5
right side	7

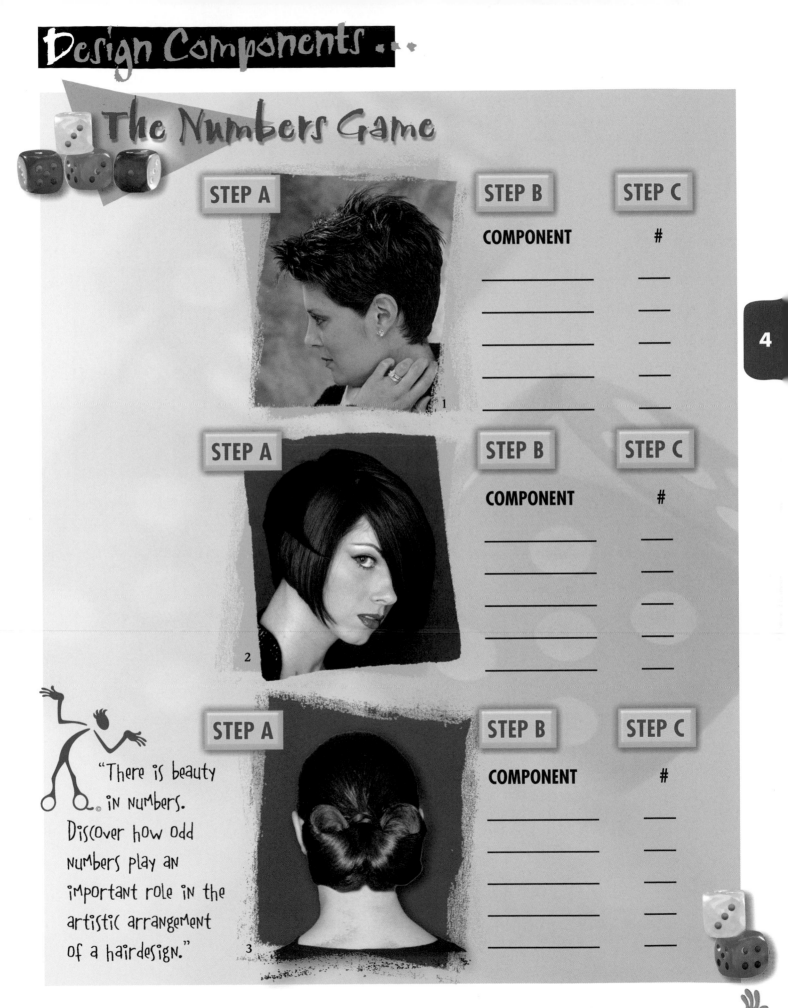

Design Components...

The Numbers Game

STEP A **STEP B** **STEP C**

COMPONENT #

_____ ____

_____ ____

_____ ____

_____ ____

_____ ____

STEP A **STEP B** **STEP C**

COMPONENT #

_____ ____

_____ ____

_____ ____

_____ ____

_____ ____

STEP A **STEP B** **STEP C**

COMPONENT #

_____ ____

_____ ____

_____ ____

_____ ____

"There is beauty in numbers. Discover how odd numbers play an important role in the artistic arrangement of a hairdesign."

FIBONACCI'S SEQUENCE

The relationship among numbers in which, to get a third number, one adds the preceding two. This sequence mimics the natural patterns found in nature that are pleasing to the eye.

$$0+1=1 \quad 2 \quad 3 \quad 5 \quad 8$$
$$0 \quad 1+1=2 \quad 3 \quad 5 \quad 8$$
$$0 \quad 1 \quad 1+2=3 \quad 5 \quad 8$$

Numbers create phi: Adjacent numbers in Fibonacci's Sequence create the Golden Ratio (2/3 is also known as phi).

13
3 2
5 8

phi creates lines: Applying 2/3 proportion in creating lines results in a well-balanced figure.

Lines create art: Positioning objects in thirds (2:3 or 3:2) adds visual stimulation.

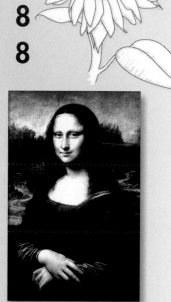

APPLICATIONS OF HAIRDESIGN

Plan designs based on a **concept**, which can be inspired anywhere (nature, art, music).

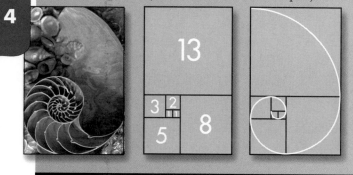

1

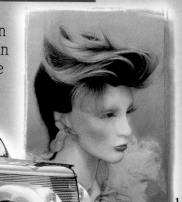

FORM or SHAPE

DIMENSION

LINES

COLOR

SPACE

TEXTURE

Elements are essential building blocks in the creation of artistic hairdesigns. Two or more elements combined create a **principle** theory behind how elements are applied to create a hairdesign.

A style is achieved by arranging **component** parts into a **composition**. Hairdesigns using odd numbers of components are more aesthetically pleasing.

2

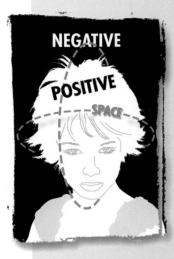

SPACE

A three-dimensional area in which a hairdesign can move or be formed.

When looking at a hairdesign, the space hair occupies is called **positive** space. When a style is open and airy, **negative** space shows through the hairdesign. Without adequate space considerations, hairstyles can become too busy.

DIMENSION

One-dimensional designs have only a single spatial measurement of length without depth or width.

Two-dimensional designs produce length and width but no depth.

Three-dimensional designs include length, width, and depth.

4

COLOR creates:

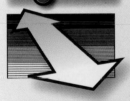

Mood (base tones; blue adds depth, yellow adds brightness, red adds warmth)

Emphasis (gives prominence to a component or area)

Dimension (placing contrasting elements; light colors look larger or less dense than dark ones)

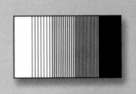

Value (the amount of lightness or darkness)

Contrast (placing opposing colors to add interest)

Illusion (a visual perception; light colors accentuate, dark colors recede)

TEXTURE changes

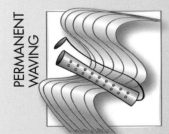

PERMANENT WAVING

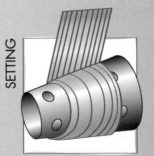

SETTING

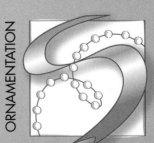

ORNAMENTATION

Permanent: When hair is shampooed it retains its altered form (relaxing, coloring).

Temporary: When hair is shampooed it reverts to its natural form (setting, braiding).

Artificial textures are created by adding ornamentation, such as hairpieces, ribbon or jewels.

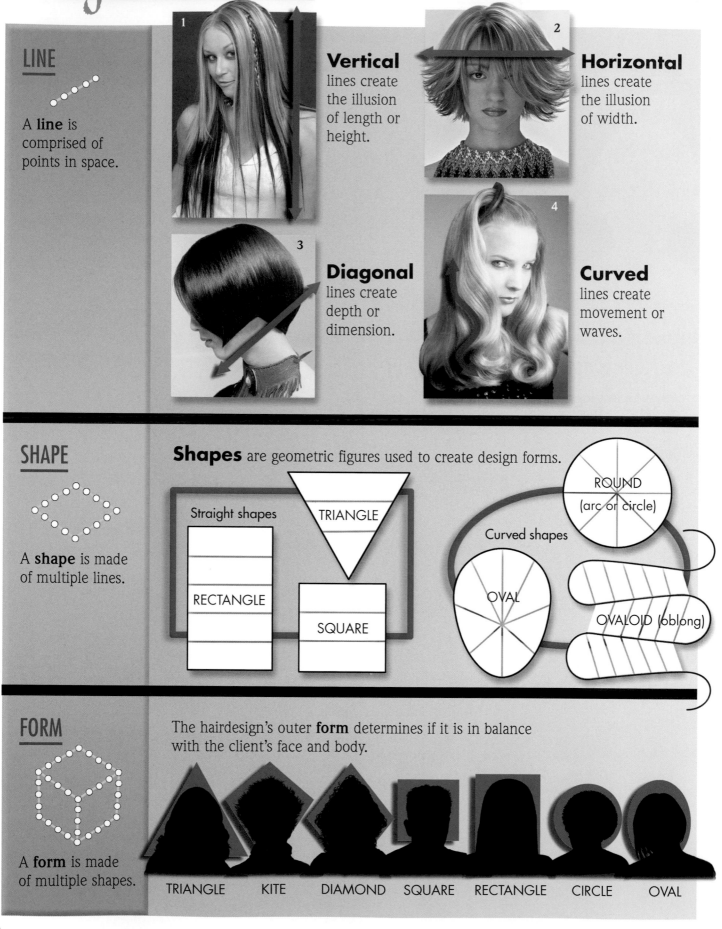

LINE

A **line** is comprised of points in space.

Vertical lines create the illusion of length or height.

Horizontal lines create the illusion of width.

Diagonal lines create depth or dimension.

Curved lines create movement or waves.

SHAPE

A **shape** is made of multiple lines.

Shapes are geometric figures used to create design forms.

Straight shapes

TRIANGLE

RECTANGLE

SQUARE

Curved shapes

ROUND (arc or circle)

OVAL

OVALOID (oblong)

FORM

A **form** is made of multiple shapes.

The hairdesign's outer **form** determines if it is in balance with the client's face and body.

TRIANGLE KITE DIAMOND SQUARE RECTANGLE CIRCLE OVAL

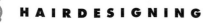

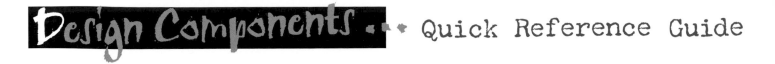

ROLLER CONTROLS Applications and Base Placements:

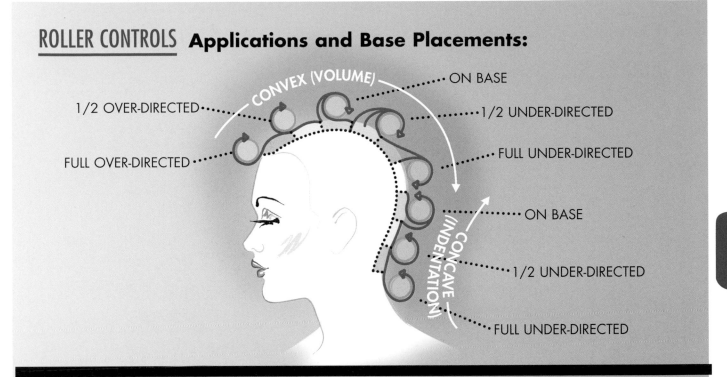

- 1/2 OVER-DIRECTED
- FULL OVER-DIRECTED
- CONVEX (VOLUME)
- ON BASE
- 1/2 UNDER-DIRECTED
- FULL UNDER-DIRECTED
- ON BASE
- CONCAVE (INDENTATION)
- 1/2 UNDER-DIRECTED
- FULL UNDER-DIRECTED

4

PIN CURLS

The **base** is the section attached to the scalp. Various base shapes are used throughout the head: square (when flat, produces curl with no lift), rectangle (for barrel curls), triangle (avoids splits in hairline), arc-shaped (side hairline, used for wave formations).

Stems are between the base and the first turn of the curl. Stems control movement and direction.

The **curl** is the circle at the end of the hair that produces the wave pattern. The larger the circle, the wider the finished wave pattern. Pin curl direction is either clockwise or counter-clockwise.

STEM
CURL
BASE
CLOCKWISE
COUNTER-CLOCKWISE
12
9
3
6

FINGER WAVES

Ovaloid shapes placed into the hair in alternating directions using the fingers and a comb.

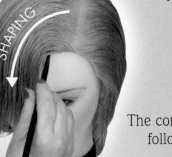

SHAPING

Shaping: Molding a section of hair prior to the wave formation.

Ridge: The raised section of hair created when the alternating ovaloids connect.

Hollow: The concave ovaloid section directly following a ridge that determines the wave's depth and tempo.

MULTIPLE CHOICE

1. One of the ways that we apply mathematics to everyday life is in:
   A. Reading literature   B. Finding proportions   C. Chaos   D. Using a dictionary

2. Determines if the hairdesign will be in the most balanced proportion for the client's face and body.
   A. Line   B. Texture   C. Form   D. Profile

3. Used to emphasize line, texture, rhythm, repetition, balance and patterns within a hairdesign.
   A. Dimension   B. Elevation   C. Color   D. Partings

4. Adds to the total hairdesign effect, but cannot stand alone.
   A. Element   B. Design plan   C. Concept   D. Ornamentation

5. Hairstyles can become too busy and overwhelm the eye without adequate considerations for:
   A. Contrast   B. Space   C. Elasticity   D. Divisions

6. The key to a well-designed hairstyle.
   A. Golden Ratio   B. Code of Conduct   C. Golden Rule   D. Theory of Motion

7. An example of artificial texture would be adding this to the hair.
   A. Ornamentation   B. Cornrows   C. Highlights   D. Finger waves

8. To properly airform a curl, the hair should be dried to what percentage?
   A. 20   B. 50   C. 75   D. 90

9. To produce volume and lift, always do this to the hair.
   A. Wet Style   B. Airform   C. Condition   D. Over-direct

10. This type of roller was designed for use with curved shapes.
    A. Conical   B. Cylinder   C. Steam   D. Electric

TRUE OR FALSE

1. _____ An under-directed placement creates maximum volume.

2. _____ A convex placement creates indentation.

3. _____ Pin curls placed behind a ridge and followed by another ridge produce a skip wave.

4. _____ The triangle can be used to create both curved and straight shapes.

5. _____ Ovaloid shapes in alternating directions produce wave formations.

6. _____ In a temporary change of texture, shampooed hair retains its altered form.

7. _____ Horizontal lines create the illusion of width.

8. _____ The center point of a circle is called the axis.

9. _____ Neutral curls cannot move in any direction.

10. _____ The artistic or creative part of the hairdesign is known as an element.

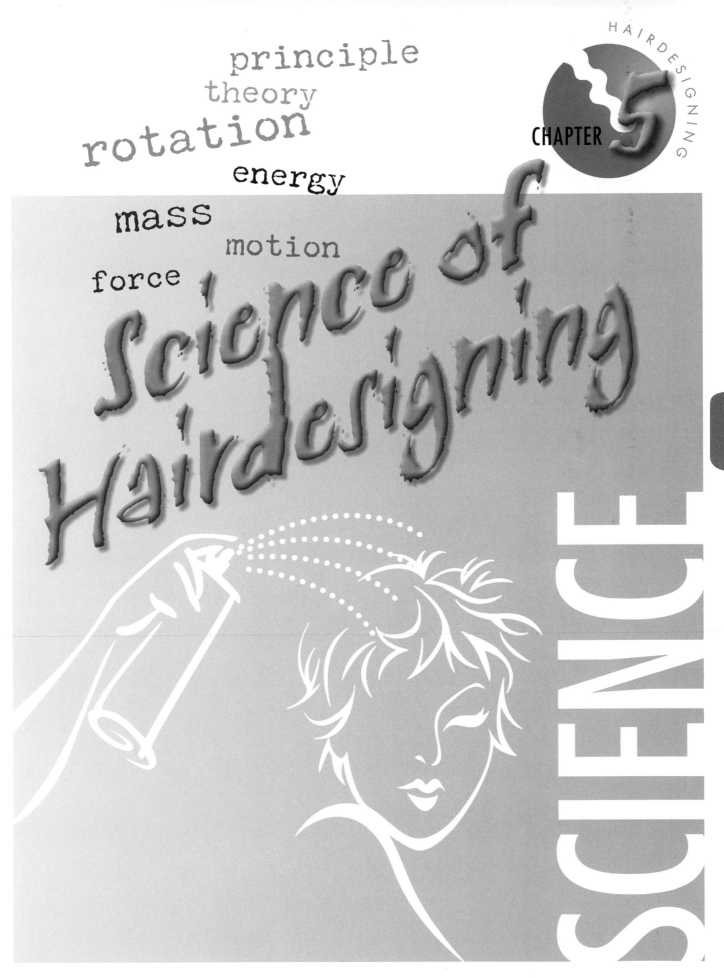

principle
theory
rotation
energy
mass
motion
force

Science of
Hairdesigning

SCIENCE

Principles of Design ...

A Principle is a law in nature as formulated and accepted by the mind. A principle of hairdesign is a theory behind how elements are applied to create a hairdesign. Once a hairdesigner is trained and experienced in the principles and elements of design, educated and calculated risks may be taken to build on this strong art foundation.

Scientific influences, theories and laws demonstrate how the hair will react when various combinations of **principles** and **elements** are applied. Principles move hairdesign from the theoretical **concept (design plan)** to the practical actions necessary for creation of the finished style. By recognizing, practicing and applying these principles, the hairdesigner will master the art of hairdesign.

ACT 1 **SCENE** 1

Principle Characters

Concept

THEORETICAL

DESIGN PLAN

Action

PRACTICAL

ARRANGING COMPONENTS

FINISHED COMPOSITION

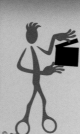

"A CONCEPT is an idea that combines the theoretical and practical applications of hairdesigning. Inspiration can come from anywhere... art, music, nature."

5

Principles of Design

Applications of Hairdesign

Theoretical

● **Element**
An artistic part of a hairdesign. Two or more elements combined create a principle of hairdesign.

● **Principle**
A theory behind how elements are applied to create a hairdesign.

Practical

● **Component**
One part of the whole design.

● **Composition**
The arrangement of components to create a finished hairstyle.

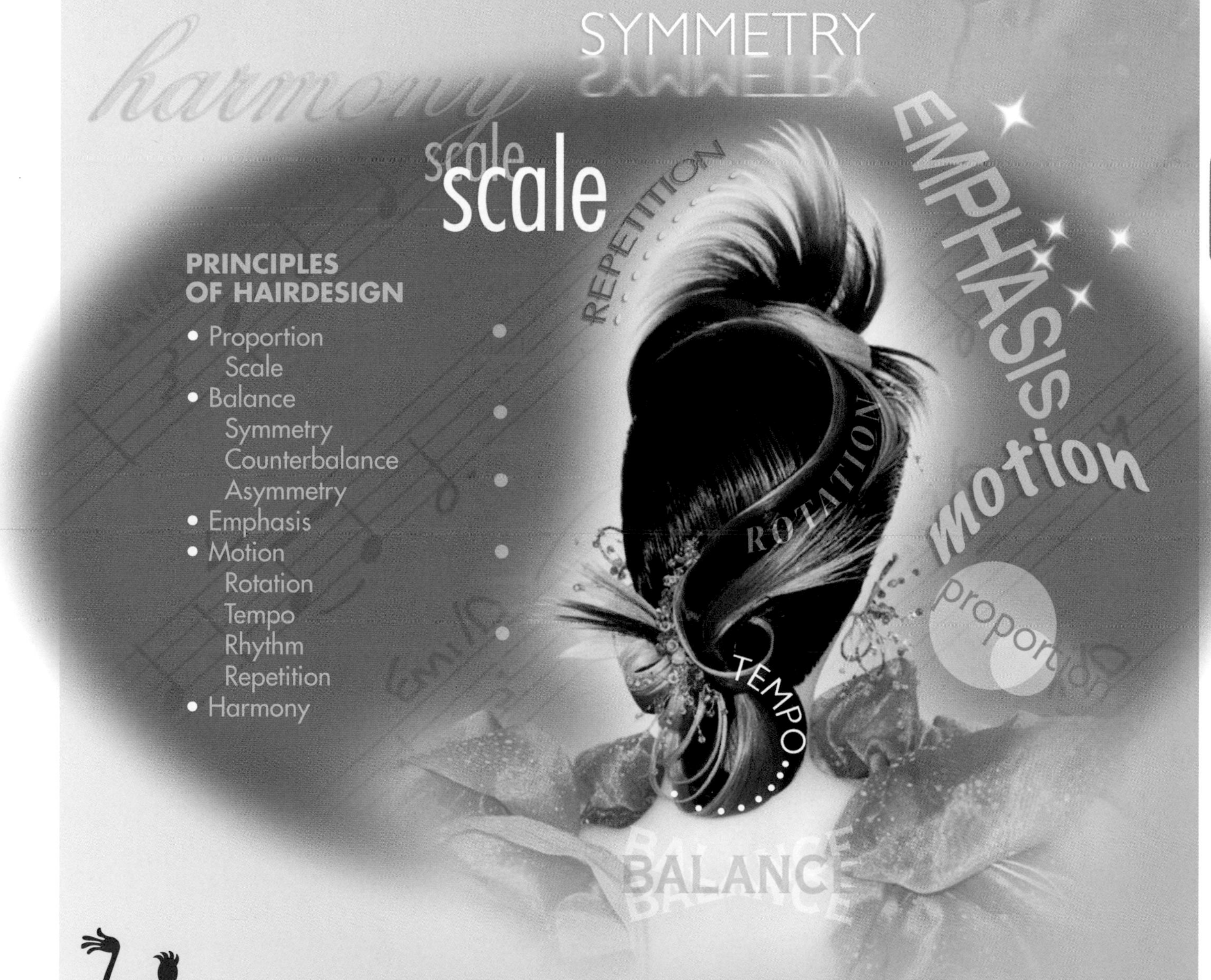

PRINCIPLES OF HAIRDESIGN

- Proportion
    Scale
- Balance
    Symmetry
    Counterbalance
    Asymmetry
- Emphasis
- Motion
    Rotation
    Tempo
    Rhythm
    Repetition
- Harmony

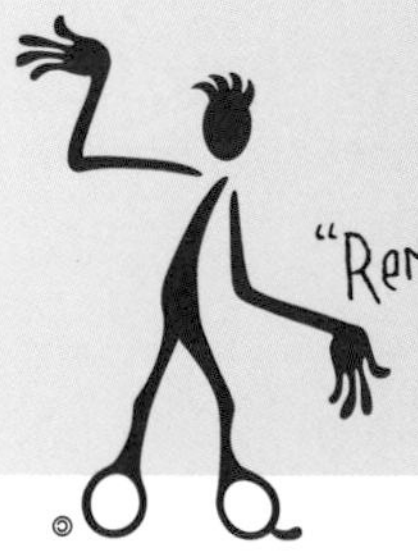

"Remember your design plan! It lays out how you will use these principles to combine elements and components into a unique hairdesign composition."

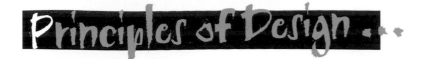
PRINCIPLE 1

Proportion *is the direct correlation of size, distance, amount and ratio between the individual characteristics when compared with the whole. A design with proper proportion is arranged to be harmonious or graceful.*

Dividing components into thirds using the Golden Ratio of divine proportion (3 to 2, or 2 to 3) balances the hairdesign in relation to the entire image (not just the head) and reinforces the artistic principle of proportion.

This principle will help you in these areas of design:

The comparison of hair to face (Example: 1/3 face to 2/3 hair; always following the 2:3 or 3:2 ratio – 2 parts face, 3 parts hair, or vice versa)

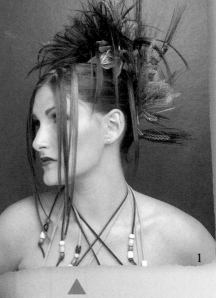

The comparison of designs within the form (Example: too many textures will produce a 'busy' hairstyle)

1

3

The comparison of the body to the hair (Example: large body/small hairdesign would be out of proportion)

3:2 ratio

2

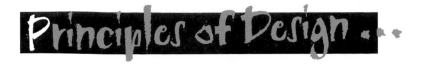

Principles of Design . . .

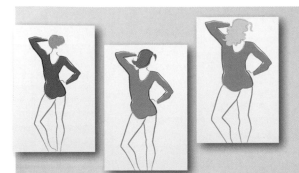

Scale *refers to the proportion of size or mass to the total volume of a hairdesign.*

A **design plan** for a hairstyle can be adjusted either up or down in volume or length to accommodate clients of different sizes. It is from this word that the term **scaling** was developed, meaning to sketch shapes, sizes and proportions of a hairdesign.

The principles of hairdesign include a chronological work order with four stages:

1 SKETCH

Sketch (mold) the design into the desired shape (one-dimensional).

2 SCALE

Scale (proportion) the design into distinct areas or sections (one-dimensional).

3 SET

Set the design (two-dimensional).

4 SCULPT

Sculpt/comb the design (three-dimensional).

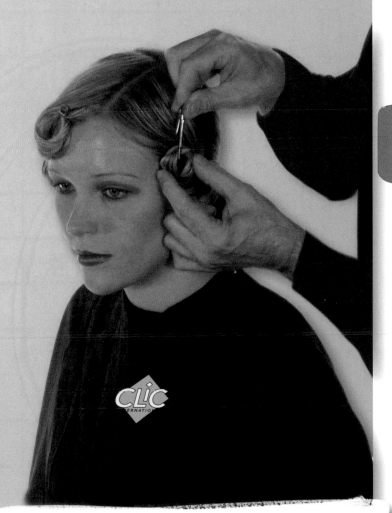

Scaling is used to create the general movement of geometric shapings by distributing wet hair around the head form. This **one-dimensional** design has only length and little to no elevation, and becomes **two-dimensional** by setting the hair into the desired pattern, which now exhibits both length and width. When the design is combed or finished into its **three-dimensional** form (with length, width and depth), the style should reflect the scale of the individual's body and facial proportions.

Balance *is the visual comparison of weight used to offset or equalize proportion. By arranging the elements of a hairdesign with nothing emphasized or out of proportion, balance is achieved.*

We develop a sense of balance at an early age by observing the world around us on a daily basis. Lack of balance is disturbing, while visual weights or attractions that have symmetry give a **feeling of order.**

Develop your personal sense of balance in design by observing the arts, floral design and fashion. Then round out your skills by studying the principle of balance in order to possess the ability to create a hairdesign with style and symmetry.

The principle of balance will help in these areas of design:

◉ Symmetrical/Asymmetrical balance within the hairdesign

◉ Symmetrical/Asymmetrical balance of hair with the body

Hairdesigners use a center or **axis** point of reference to view balance within the hairdesign and in relationship to the body. This axis point of the head occurs by dividing the face horizontally and vertically with an imaginary line.

On the straight (front) view, the axis point of reference on the head occurs where the lines intersect around the nose. The axis point of reference on the head in the profile view occurs where the lines intersect around the top of the ear.

The axis point of reference on the body will fall at the area approximately around the navel or hip area, depending upon the person's body type as referenced in Chapter 3.

Principles of Design...

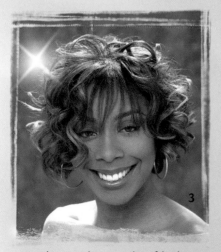

The Theory of Balance in Hairdesign

We have already discussed how to find the axis point of reference on the head during the principle of balance. Once the axis is identified, you can then decide how to balance a hairdesign – symmetrically or asymmetrically.

Symmetry: Each visual weight is the exact same distance from the axis and is equally important in all symmetrical balances. The imaginary design line on which these **balances** are located will emphasize whatever features are also present on this line. Symmetrical balances can occur on a horizontal, diagonal or vertical line.

SYMMETRICAL HAIRDESIGNS

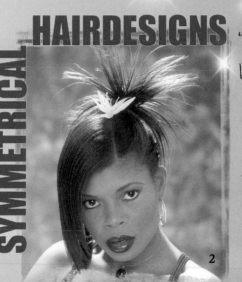

"Diagonal balance at less than 45 degrees but greater than 15 degrees is the most pleasing to the eye."

Identical balance
The visual weight and/or movement of a hairdesign is the same on opposite sides of the axis point.

Calculated balance
The weight of the hairdesign is equally distributed on both sides of the axis point, but the movement or shape is different.

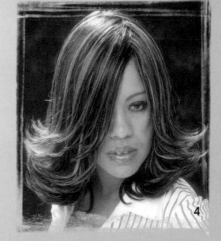

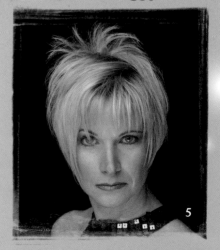

By placing the weight of balance toward the front of the head on a horizontal design line you create the appearance of adding width to the overall design.

By placing the weight of balance on the diagonal design line you create the appearance of length and/or width.

By placing the weight of balance on the vertical line you create the appearance of adding height to the overall design.

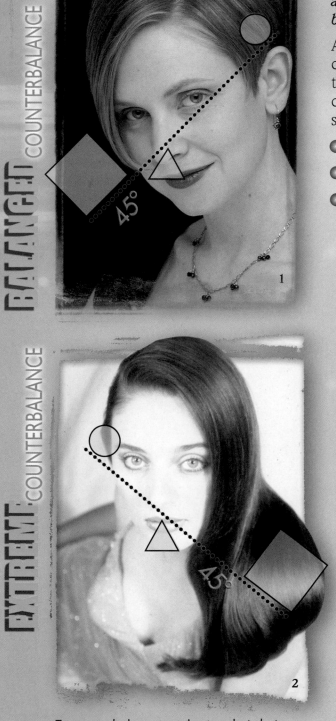

BALANCED COUNTERBALANCE

1

EXTREME COUNTERBALANCE

2

To counterbalance weights in a hairdesign, draw an imaginary line. If the counterbalance is more than 45 degrees from point to point, the hairstyle is out of balance.

Counterbalance is the use of different weights and lengths in opposite areas that offset each other to create a balanced overall form.

As we explored in Chapter 3, planning for counterbalance begins with an evaluation of the overall body shape and size. Analyze the curves and features of the face, head, neck, shoulders and body to determine:

- Where to create either closeness or fullness
- The optimal length of the hair
- The direction of the hairdesign

After analyzing the body, evaluate your client's facial features and proportions. Consider each feature both individually and also as part of the entire body. A **good design plan** will counterbalance facial and body irregularities to **create symmetry** and also fit your client's lifestyle and personality. Is it easy to manage at home? Does it fit his/her lifestyle? Hairdesign examples used to counterbalance facial and body feature flaws were included in our study of biology in Chapter 3.

3

EXERCISE

Create a scrapbook from magazine clippings of balance and counterbalance techniques you find in everyday life.

5

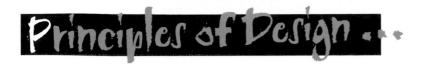

Principles of Design

ASYMMETRICAL HAIRDESIGNS

Asymmetry: *The visual weights in the hairdesign are unequal and/or placed at different distances from the axis' central point of reference.*

- The **heavier** visual weight, fullness, or attraction should be placed **closer** to the axis, and the **lighter** visual weight, fullness, or attraction is placed **farther** away from the axis.

- As the **heavier** weight moves **away** from the axis point, the **lighter** weight will move **closer** to the axis to counterbalance the hairdesign.

The weight should remain on the same design line, whether horizontal or diagonal, and maintain proportion (3:2, 2:3).

In either case, positioning the weight correctly will produce eye-pleasing hairdesigns, whether symmetrical or asymmetrical.

1

Typical Asymmetry

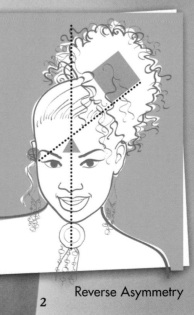

Reverse Asymmetry

2

Principles of Design...

PRINCIPLE 3

Emphasis *may also be called a focal point or the heart of interest. It is the main excitement, attraction or action whether it is in a work of art, on stage or in a hairdesign. The professional hairdesigner creates a focal point first through form or shape, which is then emphasized over the rest of the design through color, texture, height or ornamentation. As you become more skilled in the art of hairdesign, you will recognize infinite ways to create focal points.*

5

Zone 1

1

By placing the focal point or emphasis in the proper division or zone, you **counterbalance undesirable features** such as close-set eyes, a large nose or a receding chin. The following examples show how focal points **emphasize or divert interest** to or from different **facial zones** or **cranial divisions**.

2

An imaginary line drawn through the widest portion becomes a hairdesign's focal point. By placing the widest point in Zone 1 **on or around the forehead** (and drawing the eye upward), a wide chin can be **minimized**.

3

On stage, the director sets the focal point – the place where everyone in the audience looks – by the arrangement of performers, scenery and lighting. Artists may use color, contrast, framing, texture or all four to create a focal point.

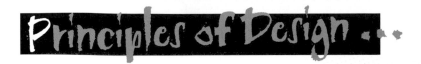

Principles of Design . . .

In the photograph to the right, the widest part of the hairdesign is **in line with the eyes**. Emphasis on this area of Zone 2 is effective for triangle-shaped faces since it creates the **illusion of width** in the temple area.

1

Zone 2

2

The widest part of the hairdesign in the photos above and to the right falls directly **across the bridge of the nose**. Emphasizing this area creates the **illusion of width** across the cheekbone area. This style is effective for long, narrow faces.

3

The widest portion of the hairdesign emphasizes **the mouth** in the photo to the right. This helps camouflage the wide forehead of an inverted triangle (heart) shaped face.

Zones

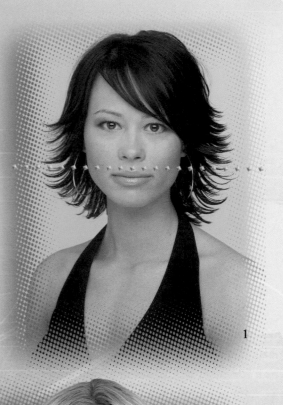

1

The focal point falls at **the chin** in Zone 3 to shorten an elongated face.

2

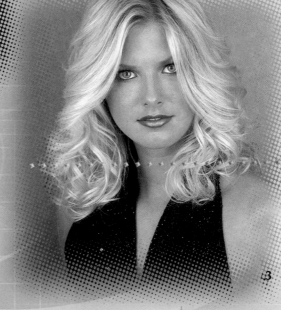

3

Gateway to the Body

Placing the widest portion of the hairdesign in the **neck and shoulder area** can shorten an elongated face while narrowing and elongating the neck.

4

5

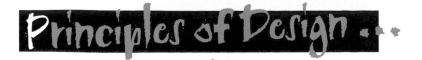

Principles of Design

When placing the emphasis in a hairdesign, stylists must consider all views of the head. Some focal points in hairdesigns cannot be seen from the front. In this instance, try placing emphasis in relation to cranial divisions instead of facial zones.

While looking at a client in profile, determine the best division in which to place the focal point to **balance the head form and features** for the hairdesign you have created. Then, view the head from the front and back to ensure that placement of the focal point enhances the overall view. Hairdesigns that are the most flattering counterbalance head form anomalies or facial flaws.

◀ Facial Division

Many focal points seen from the front are placed in the facial division. However, some focal points placed in the facial division may not be seen clearly from the front. In the photograph on the left, the hairdesign's focal point is seen most clearly from a profile view.

Forward movement in facial division creates a focal point in the profile view.

1

Parietal Division ▶

The central division allows the most options to make the head form more balanced. Make focal points above the ears in this division to give the appearance of width when viewed from the front, or by adding height to create the illusion of length in hairdesigns.

Height in parietal division creates a focal point.

2

Occipital Division ▼

The updo is most common type of hairdesign that places the main focal point in the occipital division. The focal point is best viewed from the profile or back views for hairdesigns in this division.

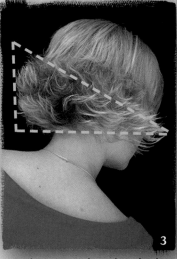

3

Focal point is placed in the lower section of the occipital division.

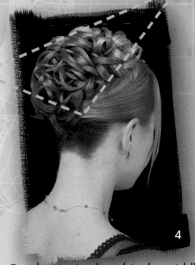

4

Focal point is placed in the middle section of the occipital division.

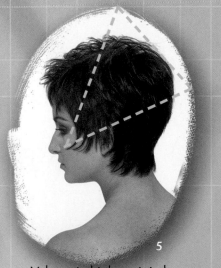

5

Volume in high occipital division creates a focal point.

Principles of Design ...

The Theory of Emphasis is used to create a primary or secondary focal point. When the design's focal point is strategically placed, it will accent or give prominence to the most important element or component feature.

If a hairdesign only contains one focal point, it is the primary emphasis. Secondary emphasis draws the eye toward the focal point within a hairdesign. It does not always become the focal point, but can be used to direct the hair to a focal point or to counterbalance one.

PRIMARY

There should only be one dominant focal point and a limited number of secondary focal points. Too many points of emphasis within the design will create confusion, as the eye does not know what to view first.

SECONDARY

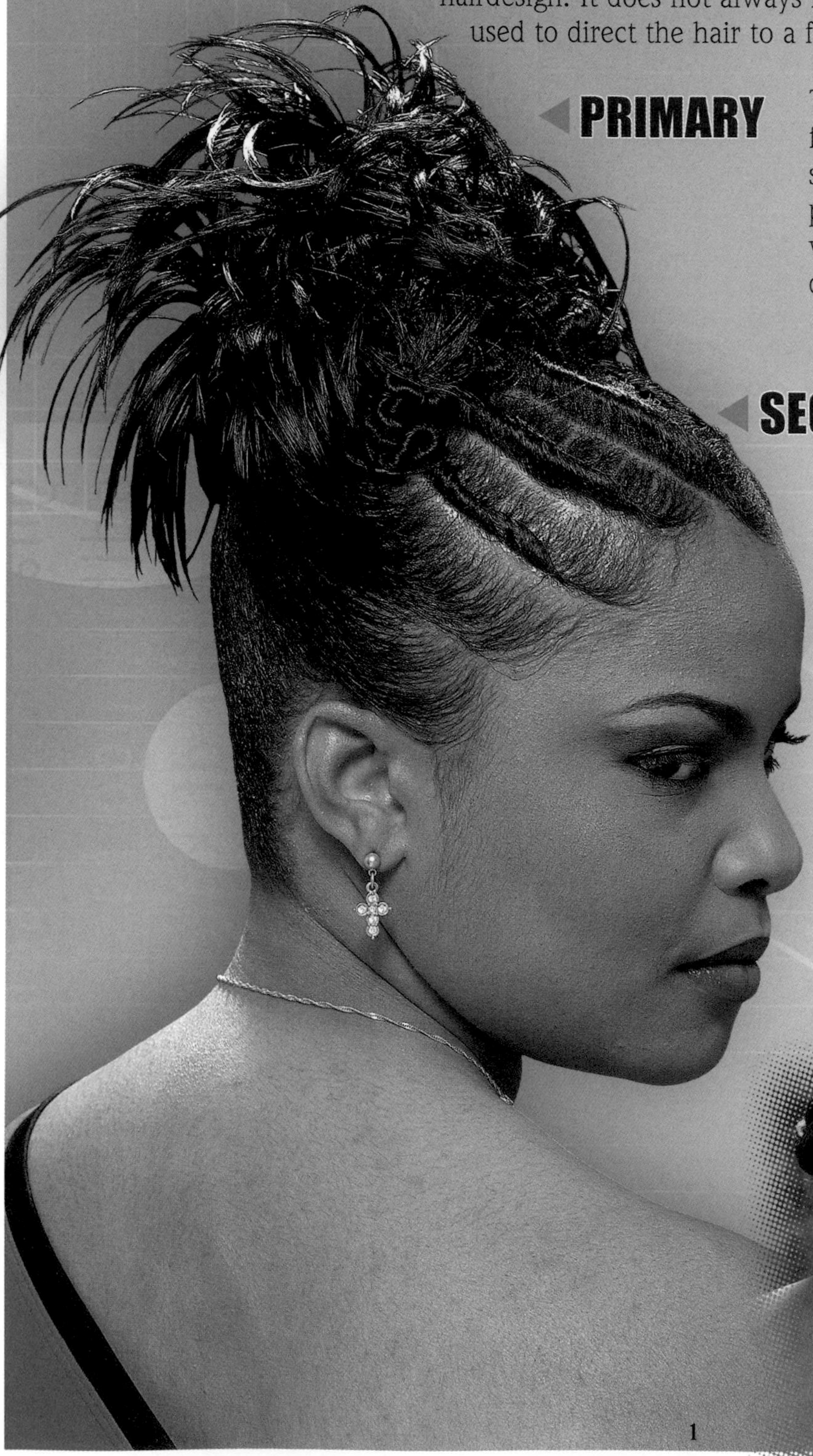

COLOR
Focal Point

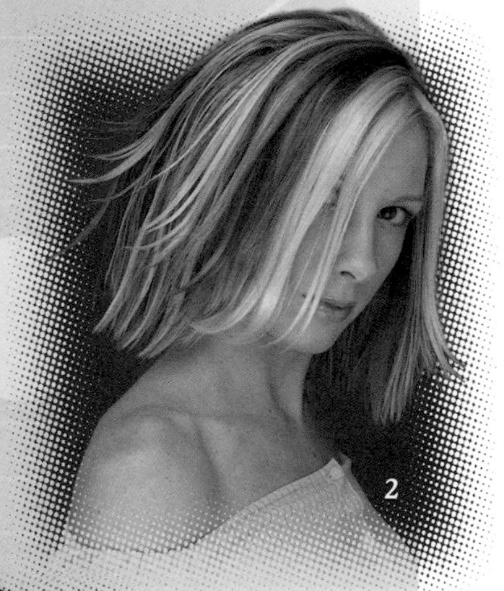

TEXTURE
Focal Point

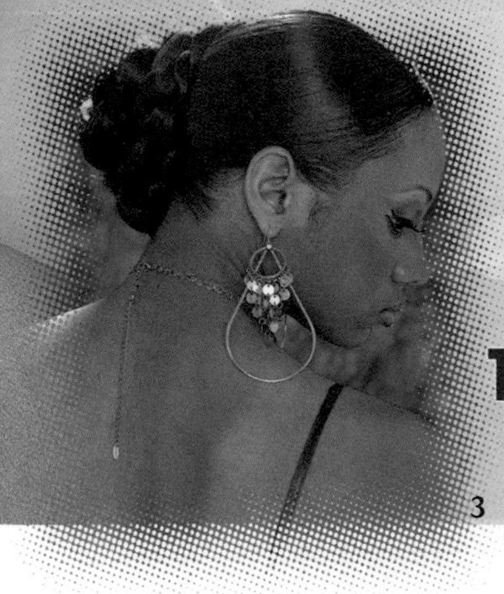

5

1

2

3

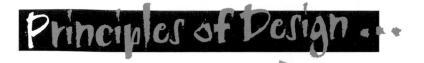
Principles of Design...

Ornamentation

Music adds strong emotional elements to the visual experience of a theatrical performance. At times the music becomes the focal point. Ornamentation in hairdesign and fashion adds to the visual experience of a client's hairdesign or outfit. It can either embellish or become the main focal point.

Hairdesign ornamentation may include decorative hairpins, barrettes, hair bands or other material to attract the eye and establish the "theme" or **main emphasis** of the hairdesign. The size and amount of the ornamentation must be reasonable in order to create interest in the design without overpowering it.

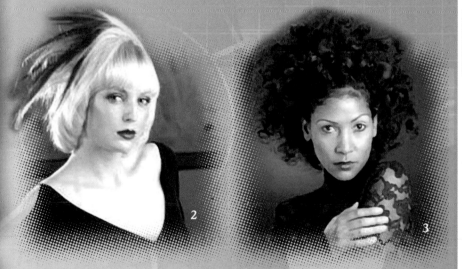

Fashion ornamentation, like jewelry, colorful pins or other accessories, embellishes or becomes the **focal point** of a client's outfit. Hairdesign and fashion ornamentation should collaborate to complete your client's overall appearance.

"Remember the RULE OF 13."

RULE OF 13: Never wear more than thirteen pieces of ornamental attire. Add up all flowers, bows, or hair accessories, belt buckles, jewelry, shiny buttons and metal decor on shoes. Less is more!

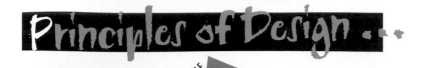

Principles of Design ...

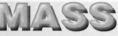

PRINCIPLE 4 — Theory of Motion

The principle of motion involves the action of movement, direction or force. Hairdesign is controlled by basic art principles, although scientific influence controls the physical properties of the hair.

The first influence is **Energy**. Gravity holds the hair and all objects down. The force of **gravity** on the hair keeps hair from rising upward. When the hair falls downward, we refer to this gravitational energy as the **natural directional motion** of the hair.

The second influence is **Mass,** the amount of space matter takes up. Hair takes up space; therefore the size, bulk or magnitude of a hairdesign will determine the amount of mass created. Mass can be deceptive, like an optical illusion. A fuller or wider hairstyle with space within its design may appear to be greater in mass than a solid design that takes up less space but more total mass.

The third influence is **Tempo**. When creating design movements, the rate of motion in the hair will produce a decelerated (slow), moderate (medium), or accelerated (fast) tempo, or any combination of tempo rates.

Energy

1

MASS

2

3

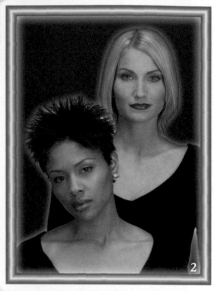

▶ EXERCISE

View the images on this page and label the following:

A. Identify anti-gravity areas (energy).

B. Locate the largest and the smallest mass (size).

C. Find a slow, moderate and fast tempo (acceleration or speed).

Tempo

4

5

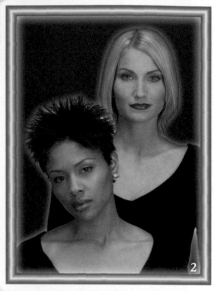

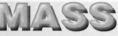

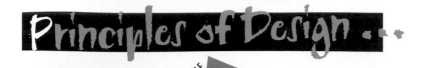

5

Principles of Design …

Sir Isaac Newton, the famed English physicist, developed the laws of motion. He explained how objects of nature moved on earth as well as through the heavens, converting the laws of science into mathematical theories.

Sir Isaac Newton
1642-1727

Newton created three laws of motion:

● Law One
"Every object in a state of motion tends to remain in that state unless an external force is applied to it."

● Law Two
"The relationship between an object's mass, its acceleration and the applied force is F = ma." (**force** equals **mass** times **acceleration**)

● Law Three
"For every action there is an equal and opposite reaction."

Now that we have **introduced** Newton's laws, let us **simplify** and **adapt** them to the field of cosmetology. Here are a few examples to help **relate** these laws to our art.

Law 1 states that an object (hair) remains **in motion until a force is applied** to stop it (hairspray) or to divert its direction.

Law 2 shows a direct relationship between mass (size), speed (acceleration) and force (energy). This law simply says that **the larger an object is the more force and speed** it takes to move it. Therefore, when working with large amounts of hair, more speed and force are needed.

Law 3 states that in every movement there is a **second opposite movement**. This law applies in making a wave in hairdesign; when one arc goes forward, the second arc must travel backwards.

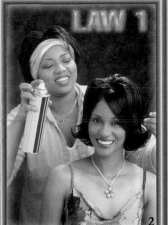

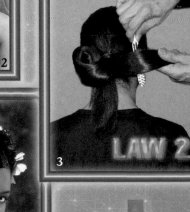

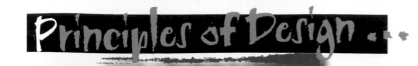
Principles of Design . . .

Diversion or Interruption of Motion

creates a visual break in the continuity of a design by changing the direction of a line or movement after it traveled too far in one direction.

The theory of diversion or the **interruption of motion** is present when the emphasis or motion directs the attention away from an undesirable area and shifts it to a more pleasing area of the finished design. The eye will focus on the emphasized part of the design, distracting it from the problem area.

5

1

2

3

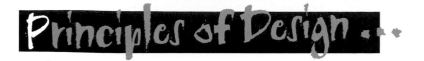

Principles of Design

The Theory of Rotation

*By first understanding how the laws of motion work, we can then start to evaluate rotation. **Rotation** is the act of turning a solid body on an axis. An **axis** is a fixed point of reference from which a body or geometric shape rotates.*

Hairdesigners turn hair on an axis to create different looks. One axis that we use is a base in the head form. A **base** is the stationary area of hair attached to the scalp from which directional controls or stems rotate.

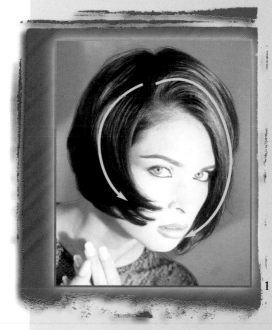

CLOCKWISE

COUNTER-CLOCKWISE

1

2

5

Rotational Direction

Direction is the path in which the hair flows. The directional movement or aim of the hair within a hairdesign is created by joining straight or curved lines.

In hairdesign, we use the terms clockwise and counter-clockwise to describe curved directional motions.

The term **clockwise** describes curls which are formed in the same direction as the hands move on an analog-type clock or timepiece (to the right). The term **counter-clockwise** describes curls formed in the opposite direction from which clock hands move (to the left). The directions are constant; however, the line on which they sit can change.

▶ EXERCISE

Practice creating different directions (clockwise and counter-clockwise) using the following skill factors:

Simple Skill - mold hair with alternating wave patterns

Intermediate Skill - mold hair with alternating wave patterns using pincurls

Complex Skill - mold hair with alternating wave patterns using rollers and pincurls

Applying Rotational Force

In making design decisions, you must account for the force needed to move the hair into the desired style.

Remember that when rotating a circle you need more force to close the outer loop at the same time as you close the inner loop. For example, when ice skaters in a line begin to rotate, the first (inner) ice skater in line barely changes her position while the last (outer) skater uses all of her strength and force to get into the line.

In hairdesign, concentric shapes have a common axis or starting point and repeat in different sizes from smaller to larger.

"I believe at the heart of science are the words 'I think, I wonder and I understand.'"

– Physician Mae Jemison, first female African American astronaut

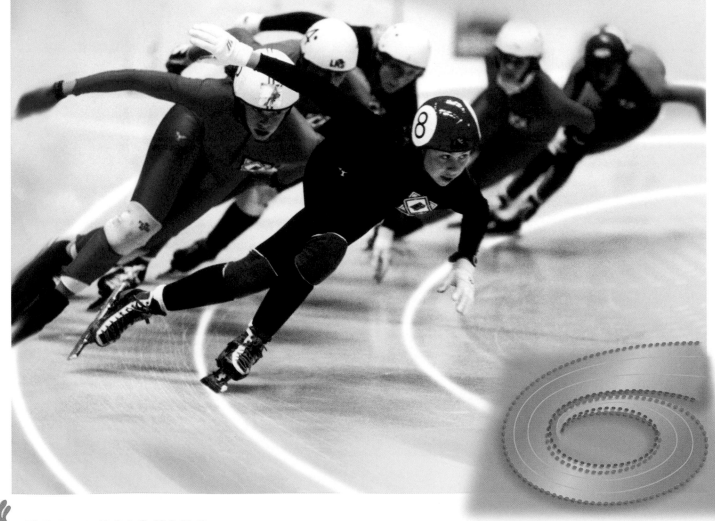

Principles of Design...

Rotational Tempo (speed)

***The pace or tempo of direction** relates directly to how far the hair must travel.*

Previously, we showed how the outer circle must travel faster than the inner circle. However, the inner circle will make more rotations than the outer circle, creating a more accelerated tempo. Therefore, pin curls, rollers or iron curls with a smaller diameter will produce tighter wave or curl formations with a more accelerated tempo than those with a larger diameter.

1

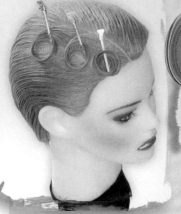

Examples:

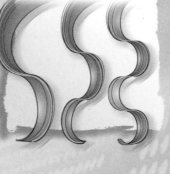

● A pin curl with no stem produces a curl with an accelerated tempo or wave pattern with the least amount of movement. A half stem pin curl allows moderate movement or tempo. A full stem pin curl will produce a decelerated tempo, but the greatest amount of movement from the base.

● An on base placement using a smaller diameter roller creates more lift and an accelerated tempo compared to a larger under-directed roller's closeness to the scalp and decelerated wave pattern.

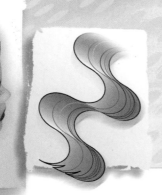

● Ovaloid patterns in finger waving produce a tempo which starts in the narrower open end as accelerated and travels toward the wider closed end, becoming more decelerated in tempo. By alternating the ovaloids you can produce balanced wave formations.

Rotational Force

*How far the hair must travel and the momentum that it takes to get there is **force**.*

The hair will react to **gravitational force** by falling downward. In order to get the hair to react against gravity when styling, an external force must be applied.

From a point of reference called an **axis**, the hair moves in a specific curved direction (clockwise or counter-clockwise). The placement of the axis in combination with the amount of gravitational force applied will determine the amount of movement (lift or fall) the hairdesign pattern will have.

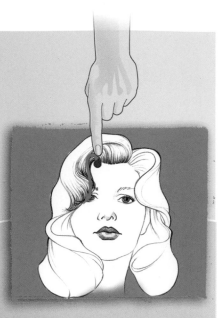

▲ 1/4 Fringe

To place a minimal amount of hair falling into the fringe area and expose most of the forehead, create the axis point on the client's right side of hairline, using the client's right eyebrow as a reference area.

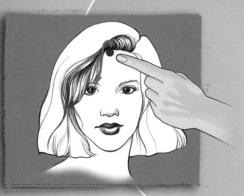

1/2 Fringe ▶

To place a moderate amount of hair falling into the fringe area, create the axis point at the center hairline, directly above the nose.

3/4 Fringe ▶

To place a maximum amount of hair into the front hairline's fringe area and cover most of the forehead, place the axis point on the client's left side of hairline, using the client's left eyebrow as a reference area.

▶ EXERCISE

Finding the Axis of Rotation

Practice placing the axis point at various areas along the hairline and placing a design tool (round brush, pin curls, rollers, etc.) to finish the fringe.

- Use your index finger to place the axis at the desired area for lift or fall in the hair's design flow.

- All hair to one side of the axis placement will have lift, and all hair to the other side will fall into the fringe.

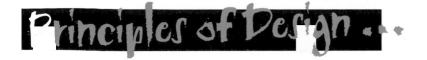

This rotational theory can be applied anywhere on the head. Another design plan example shows how to place the axis at the side hairline.

For less lift/more fall, place the axis point at the upper portion of side hairline.

For moderate lift/fall, place the axis point at center of the side hairline.

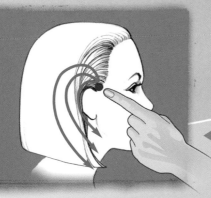

For more lift/less fall, place the axis point at lower portion of the side hairline.

"What goes up must come down! To develop a successful design plan, a stylist must consider how design elements create different patterns when affected by scientific forces and influences."

International Combing Concepts

Perfecting the skills necessary to give hair lift, direction and form requires practice, attention to detail and knowledge of the following international combing concepts.

The Three Memories of Hair Formation:

○ **Wet memory** is achieved when the hair has been formed onto rollers, set in pin curls or molded into a specific design.

○ **Dry memory** is achieved when heat has been applied to a wet style. This can be accomplished by using a hood dryer, airformer or curling iron.

○ **Directional memory** is achieved when you relax the dry form with a brush.

"When applying directional memory, the term LACING means to compress hair together with a comb or brush for height and control."

Applying Directional Memory

When the hair has been dried and cooled thoroughly, remove all setting tools. Relax the set by brushing, starting at the ends of the hair and working toward the scalp. Follow the brush with the palm of your hand to ensure the hair is smooth.

Place the palm of your hand on the client's head and gently push the hair forward. This will direct the hair into the general style in which it was set. Apply the desired lacing (backcombing) technique from the next page. Always follow the direction in which the style was set.

Using the end of a rattail comb, lift areas of your hairdesign where necessary and smooth with your palm to achieve the form of your finished hairdesign.

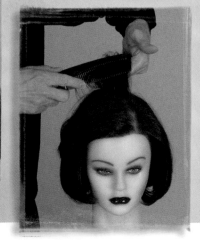

Being careful not to remove the cushioning, gently smooth the laced hair with a comb to finish the style.

Principles of Design...

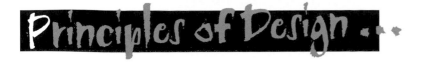

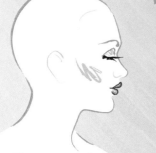

French Lacing Techniques
(also called cushioning, interlocking, backbrushing or backcombing)

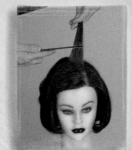
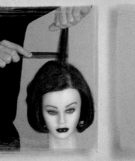
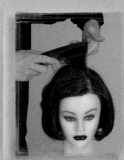

Compact Lacing
is used to create the most volume (convexity) in a hairdesign.

Hold a smoothed section of hair firmly between your middle and index fingers at 90 degrees from the scalp.

Compact the hair by inserting a comb 1-2" (2.5-5 cm) from the scalp and pushing the hair downward, repeating until a firm cushion has been achieved.

Smooth the surface of the cushioned hair while retaining the lift built into the design's form.

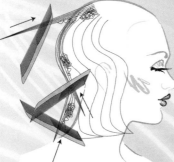

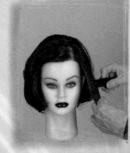
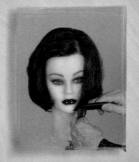
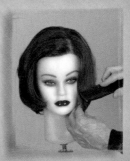

Directional Lacing is used to follow a particular line in a set or to create moderate volume (convexity) in a hairstyle. Larger sections of hair are used than when compact lacing.

The hair is held at less than 90 degrees to achieve the desired amount of lift and direction.

Always lace in the direction the hair will travel. Lacing the underside of the hair strand produces volume; lacing on top of the hair creates closeness.

Smooth the surface of the cushioned hairdesign's form while maintaining the direction established during the lacing technique.

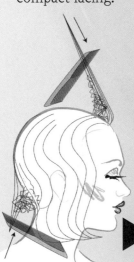

Interlocked Lacing is used to create little to no volume (convexity) in the hair. This technique joins hair from one section into the next, creating one fluid movement or design.

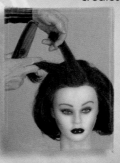
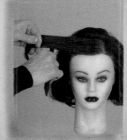
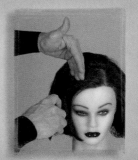

Divide the hair into sections and lace each one separately.

Picking up two sections, lace sections together.

Smooth the surface of the joined sections to finish the style.

▶ **EXERCISE** Practice all three lacing techniques to finish a hairdesign.

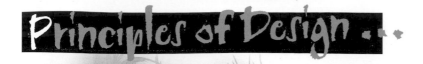
Rhythm *creates the relationship between movement or motion and the lines of a pattern; one part to another that harmoniously flows as one.*

Hairdesigning is like a symphony. Singular movements (and shapes) blend to create a fluid line of notes (design) with form and function. The movement's tempo can be fast or slow, repeated or conflicted. Rhythm can be progressive and either decrease or build to a crescendo.

The principle of rhythm will help decide:

- How often shapes, textures, or colors are repeated within the design

- The size of the elements or components

- The interruption of motion within the design

- The rhythm of texture (tempo) as accelerating (increasing), staying the same, or decelerating (decreasing) throughout the hairdesign

▶ **EXERCISE**
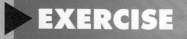

Find the rhythmic components in each hairdesign.

5

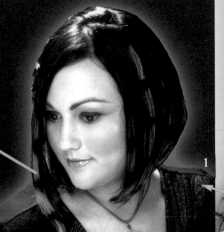

Rhythm can have activity, described in terms like recurring, sequential or radiating.

Recurring rhythm is defined as even distributions within the hairdesign. Evenly distributed patterns can be considered beautiful, but if no interruption or point of interest is included, they tend to be very boring.

RECURRING RHYTHM
WITH COLOR

FAST

SLOW

Sequential rhythm is defined as increasing or decreasing the various patterns in a predetermined order within the hairdesign.

Radiating rhythm patterns are dispersed evenly from a common center.

5

Principles of Design ...

Repetition is how often the lines, angles, colors, textures or patterns are repeated in sequence within a design.

The principle of repetition is used within hairdesigns to:

- Help create the outer silhouette or form

- Emphasize a shape or other component by repeating it

- Relate the other elements of a total look to the hairstyle, such as clothing and makeup choices

The theory of repetition is the act of repeating patterns, colors, shapes, textures and other designs. Repetition can be created on vertical, horizontal or diagonal directions in clothing, makeup and hairdesign, individually or combined.

Repetition creates the unity used within the design to link common features together. However, hairdesigns can become boring if elements or components are repeated too often. When considering odd and even patterns in design, think in terms of **repetition versus randomness.**

1

REPETITION IN WAVE PATTERN

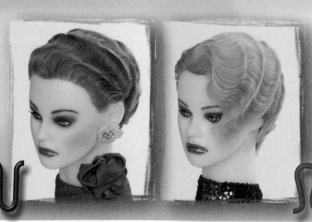

The hollow between ridges in this finger wave pattern is repetitively-spaced or uniform and therefore considered even-looking and predictable.

Ovaloid spacing between finger wave ridges (where the open end is smaller than the closed end) is considered random or odd, producing a more varied and stimulating visual pattern.

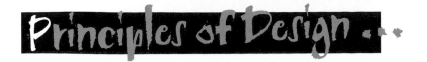
In art, as in nature, *creations are artistically arranged in uneven components (numbers or size). The common factor is that all things in nature are not equally balanced (proportioned). Each is designed by nature to attract and keep your interest by having odd proportions in their design elements.*

The human brain tries to find order in chaos. Examine what happens when people attempt to insert the perfect shape into nature's art. The shape may become too evenly organized in its proportioned elements, creating a design that is repetitious and uninteresting to our brain.

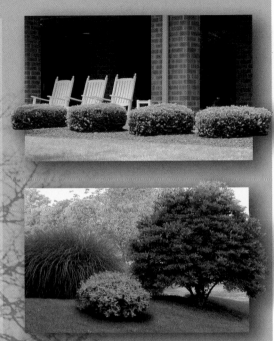

When you take the time to examine a tree, a mountain range or a field of flowers, notice the odd proportions and numbers appearing everywhere in nature are what makes them so interesting.

Even numbers create repetition. Our brain quickly learns what to expect next and loses our interest.

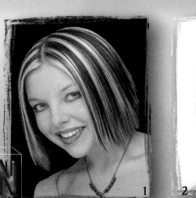

1

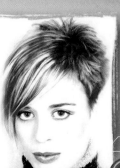

2

Odd numbers and sizes create contrast and excitement, capturing and holding our interest.

EVEN

odd

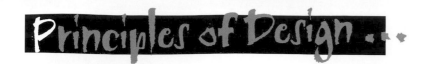

PRINCIPLE 5

Harmony *is the aesthetic placement of shapes and lines. It creates a flow or sense of consistency throughout the entire hairdesign.*

The principle of harmony is used to create a predictable pattern either within a hairdesign or on its surface. The design can be either **contrasting** or **similar**. Abrupt changes in rhythm will disrupt the harmony.

Harmony in Makeup

1

Harmony in the Total Look

2

Harmony in Clothing

3

5

4

The theory of harmony is when one or more components are synchronized. Harmony exists if the design is pleasing to the eye. The makeup, hair and clothing all **complement** the client's personality, lifestyle and features.

In competition hairdesign, fashion and hair ornamentation must coordinate.

Examine the competition hairdesign below. There are multiple design patterns, colors, textures and ornamentation all working together **harmoniously**. Even the choice of clothing, makeup and accessories are **coordinated** to produce an award-winning hairdesign.

▶ EXERCISE

Create a design plan listing each principle, element and component utilized to produce harmony in the finished style.

"An excellent design has both form and function, as they work harmoniously together."

History of Hair

Stone Age 4500BC - 2500BC

Natural Discovery
In the beginning, mankind evolved and adapted to his environment in order to survive. Hair served only as protection. As humans became civilized during the Stone Age, grooming or controlling the hair became a concern.

Our ancestors used the backbones of fish in order to comb lice and nits from their hair.

Cave paintings show mud, feathers and animal skins used as hair adornment as much as for protection. Twine wrapped around a stick, stone or bone helped them arrange their hair to look more attractive, a key factor in perpetuating the species. As they discovered another utilitarian purpose for everyday objects, styling tools were born!

Bronze Age 900BC - 600BC

Heat and Metal
During the Bronze Age (3000-600 BC), people created tools out of metal—knives, razors and tweezers—to cut and style their hair. Early in the third century, single prong hair pins made out of silver or gold were designed as hair ornamentation; some even included jewels. Technological advancements continually produced machinery to control, shape and style the hair. The Greeks developed the calamistrum, a hollow bronze stick with a row of bristles used to reshape hair. The result may be seen in many antique statues and busts.

Middle Ages to the Age of Enlightenment
500BC - 1500CE

Plants and Herbs

Natural dyes from plant leaves, like Egyptian henna and indigo, influenced hairdesign. Greeks would color their hair with saffron, a dried purple-flowered crocus.

Roman women copied the Germans and bleached their hair with Hessian soap, which contained a strong base, ashes and fats. Wigs made of organic materials first served as protection from the sun. Feathers, ivory, pearls, leaves, flowers or precious stones were added as adornments to create an elaborate hairdesign.

Primitive styling products developed from beeswax, oils, clays or mud caused wigs or hair to become stiff or sticky. This allowed the hair to be molded into almost any shape desired.

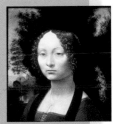

Cultural Influences

Through the centuries, fashions in hairdesign have reflected many facets of economic, social and political standing. Hairstyles symbolized civilization (cornrows represented cultivation), marital status (veils for women) and religious beliefs (requiring shaved heads, long side locks or beards).

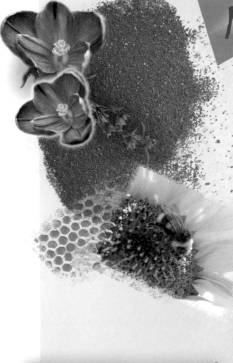

It was fashionable in fifteenth century Europe to create a higher and broader hairline by removing eyebrows and fringe hair and exposing more forehead.

In sixteenth century England, ladies turned their hair up and over pads to give the hair added fullness. Cultured ladies embraced haircolor inspired by Queen Elizabeth's red hair. A type of hairnet called a snood became very popular, along with headbands decorated with jewels and pearls.

In Asia, the wealthy class set themselves apart from the working class through elaborate styles, expensive ornaments and wigs.

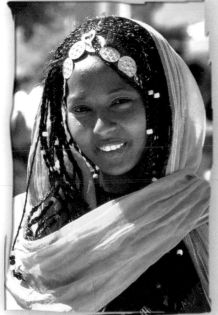

In the seventeenth century, a long singular lock of hair worn over one shoulder was called a Lovelock. In the eighteenth century, France became the center for fashion. Men and women had styles indicative of their class within the society. Men wore a long bob, or followed the king's example by covering their thinning hair with elaborate wigs. Women formed their hair into braids, twists, chignons or curls.

Technological Innovation:

19th—20th Century

Electricity

Electricity

Electricity transformed the world! Inventors were harnessing these newfound abilities into electrical designing tools. The nineteenth century brought the invention of the Marcel curling iron (named after Marcel Grateau, who developed the technique), solid and soft hood-type hair dryer, airformer (blow dryer), curling brush, flat irons and clippers.

In the Victorian age, hair was pulled over a hot iron resulting in a wave known as crimping.

Children wore long drop curls called barley curls. Nineteenth century barbers, formerly frequented for dental extractions, were now seen in a new light and viewed as necessary. Salons were booming with the introduction of the first permanent waving machine, requiring operation by a skilled professional.

The first electric hair dryer was invented in 1890, adapted from a vacuum cleaner. As this century closed, the Gibson Girl, Pompadour and French Twist were seen.

Chemical Revolution

Chemical Revolution

The early 20th century produced the first chemical haircolor formula, permanent wave (1905) and hair straightening solutions. Hair texture changed dramatically throughout the century, from tighter croquinole curls to softer airformed styles, from harsh or solid matte coloring to subtle form-enhancing highlights. Present-day hair conditioner was created in the 1950's, with chemists taking a cue from fabric softeners.

The aerosol spray can was perfected with the development of a clog-free nozzle in 1953, and ozone-friendly pump alternatives were introduced due to consumer demand twenty years later.

From the mid to late 20th century, hair dressing products like pomade, gel, and mousse rose in popularity and started a retail boom, as people styled their hair more at home in an attempt to duplicate more polished or finished-looking salon hairdesigns.

Nestle
COLOR'nTONE
Adds new color!
BLACK
6 Week
Hair Color Rinse

5

History of Hairdesign...

1900's-1920's

Madame C.J. Walker develops a method to soften and smooth black women's hair. Entertainer Cab Calloway initiates a trend known as the conk in which curly hair is relaxed with lye, and fabric called a do-rag is worn on the head to prevent reversion of the hair back to its natural curly state due to humidity.

Sammons patents the straightening comb.

As the war ends, a few women with newfound independence are bravely starting to bob their hair. Since stylists in beauty salons up to this point in time are trained primarily in dressing hair and not cutting, women invade traditional male barber shops for this service.

The invention of the bobbie pin is named after its use on bobbed hair.

1930's

With movies in their infancy, the ladies and gentlemen of this decade start to get their fashions and hairdesigns from their favorite stage and screen stars. Taking note of changing style demands, hairdressing schools begin to include training in the art of hair cutting.

"Enjoy hair fashion... see how history and technological advances have influenced fashionable styles. Everything old is new again!"

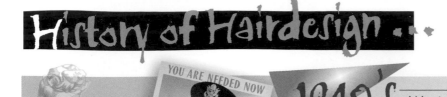

1940's

People style their hair after various World War II pin-up girls.

Wartime work in radar is developed into laser and imaging systems. The development of a scanning electron microscope makes it possible to analyze the internal structure of the hair to detect damage, and a smaller modified version is utilized decades later by manufacturers as a tool to promote retail conditioner sales in salons. Velcro® hook and loop fasteners are patented in 1948, and the technology is later adapted to rollers, requiring no clips.

1950's

Heavily-sprayed sets for women and dove-tailed haircuts for men mimic the conflict between propriety and rebellion of this time period.

Nuclear age hair is backcombed and sprayed at the salon every week into a helmet of perfectly-formed curls, waves and bouffants. Wiglets and switches of false hair called falls are often used to create the illusion of more volume. Full wigs regain popularity as women enjoy the ability to change their hairstyle or haircolor at whim. Starlet Marilyn Monroe's blonde and Lucille Ball's red hair prompts women to try both home and salon chemical services as permanent hair dyes and cold waves are improved.

1

1960's

The conk style fades out, as a return to pride in black heritage leads to the revival of the natural Afro look.

Hairspray is the best-selling beauty product. Many favor the **flip hairstyle** as Jacqueline Kennedy sets the pace for both hair and clothing fashion. Teenagers roll their hair onto large rollers or even cans to control curl, with some using ironing boards with irons to completely smooth tresses.

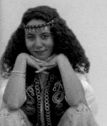

The musical "Hair" debuts, and the hippie look of the flower generation leaves its mark.

History of Hairdesign...

The first unisex salons are opened. Wash and wear hair and precision cutting impact hairdesign choices. The shag, wedge, and pageboy styles for both men and women create an androgynous blurring of gender lines. Terms like wings or feathers are used to describe layered fringe area hair.

Spiked, punk styles in fluorescent colors appear in London along with the tightly-cropped pixie look the model Twiggy sports.

Henna regains popularity as a naturally based pigment alternative, and milder heat-activated acid waves are introduced.

1980's

Reggae dreadlock styles hit the mainstream population.

Big hair is the fad, and mousse is in demand for both men and women. The modern curling iron is patented. Spiral perm and reverse curl techniques jumpstart a permanent wave revolution.

Bo Derek takes cornrows across racial barriers.

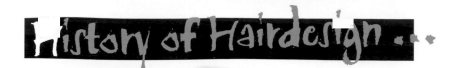

1990's

Straighter hairstyles with fewer perms or curls are accompanied by finger-drying techniques and smoothing liquid tools. Stylists make more use of haircolor to define design lines.

1

2

3

21st Century

The creative art of hair styling returns. Short, messy, multi-textured designs with more dimension emerge beside graceful, flowing, retro hairdesigns. Emphasis in hairdesigning is on the condition, shine and texture of the hair.

4

"Now it's your turn to influence the future by creating new hairdesign trends or tools for the 21st Century."

5

6

FUTURISTIC Forecasters

In store for the FUTURE?

Science and technology continue to advance the formulation of styling tools, haircoloring or permanent waving/straightening methods, hair additions and replacement systems. The salon industry grosses in excess of $50 billion annually. As the world grows smaller through digital communications, we are witnessing medical laser and imaging advancements. Researchers are currently working to adapt biological triggering devices for natural haircolor recall, which would make hair dye obsolete. Fashion trends will embrace cross-cultural integration through hairdesign.

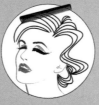
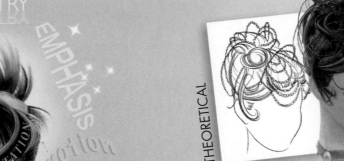
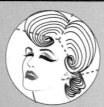
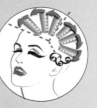
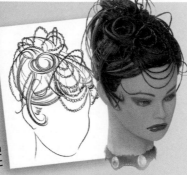
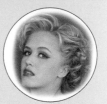
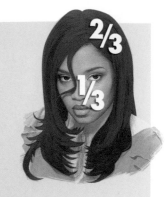

THEORETICAL

PRACTICAL

2/3

1/3

PRINCIPLE

A theory behind how elements are applied to create a hairdesign.

DESIGN PLAN

A guide outlining how stylists use principles to combine elements and components into hairdesign compositions.

PROPORTION

To arrange to be harmonious or graceful. Use the Golden Ratio of 3:2 or 2:3 when comparing individual characteristics to the whole.

CHRONOLOGICAL WORK ORDER OF A DESIGN

1. SKETCH

Mold the design into the desired one-dimensional shape.

2. SCALE

To proportion geometric shapes and sizes into distinct one-dimensional sections of a hairdesign.

3. SET

The practical application and placement of tools to create a two-dimensional design.

4. SCULPT

Comb the design into its three-dimensional form.

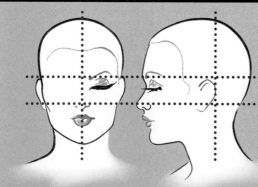

SYMMETRICAL – Each visual weight is the same distance from the axis.

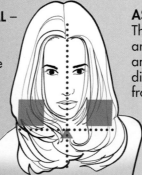

ASYMMETRICAL – The visual weights are unequal and/or placed at different distances from the axis.

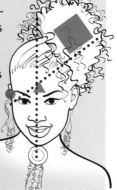

BALANCE

The visual comparison of weight used to offset or equalize proportion.

COUNTERBALANCE

The use of different weights and lengths in opposite areas to create a balanced form. If the counterbalance is more than 45 degrees from point to point, the hairstyle is out of balance.

5

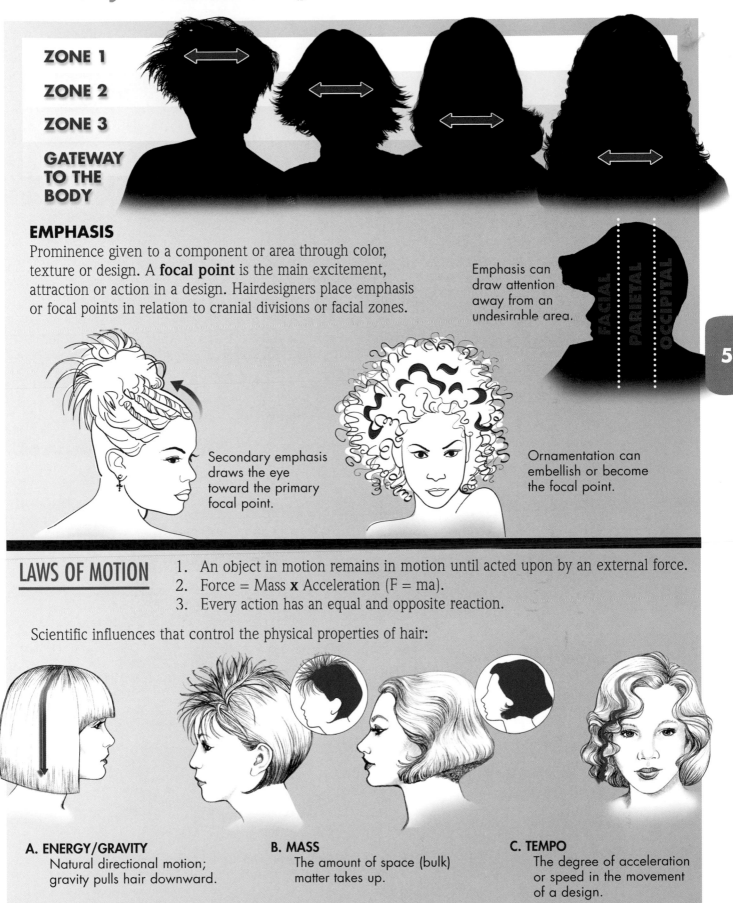

ZONE 1

ZONE 2

ZONE 3

GATEWAY
TO THE
BODY

EMPHASIS

Prominence given to a component or area through color,
texture or design. A **focal point** is the main excitement,
attraction or action in a design. Hairdesigners place emphasis
or focal points in relation to cranial divisions or facial zones.

Emphasis can
draw attention
away from an
undesirable area.

FACIAL   PARIETAL   OCCIPITAL

Secondary emphasis
draws the eye
toward the primary
focal point.

Ornamentation can
embellish or become
the focal point.

LAWS OF MOTION

1. An object in motion remains in motion until acted upon by an external force.
2. Force = Mass **x** Acceleration (F = ma).
3. Every action has an equal and opposite reaction.

Scientific influences that control the physical properties of hair:

A. ENERGY/GRAVITY
Natural directional motion;
gravity pulls hair downward.

B. MASS
The amount of space (bulk)
matter takes up.

C. TEMPO
The degree of acceleration
or speed in the movement
of a design.

5

DIVERSION OR INTERRUPTION OF MOTION creates a visual break in the continuity of a design. Direction or movement is created by joining straight or curved lines within a hairdesign.

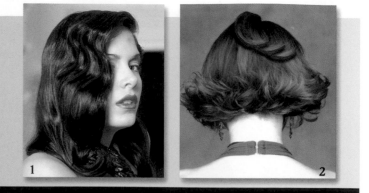

ROTATION is the act of turning a solid body on an axis. The terms **clockwise** and **counter-clockwise** describe curved directional motions.

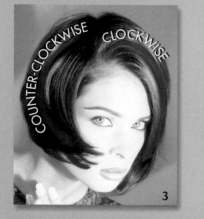

When rotating a circle you need more **rotational force** to close the outer loop at the same time as the inner loop. However, the inner circle will make more rotations than the outer circle, creating more **rotational tempo** (acceleration or speed); therefore, smaller diameters produce tighter curl formations than those made with larger diameter tools.

THREE MEMORIES OF HAIR FORMATION

WET MEMORY
Hair is molded into a specific design while damp.

DIRECTIONAL MEMORY
Relaxing the dry form with a brush and/or applying the desired lacing technique in the direction the style was set.

DRY MEMORY
Heat is applied to a wet style to set the curl pattern.

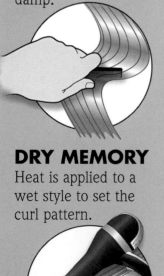

Compact lacing creates a cushion to achieve the most volume.

Directional lacing follows a particular line in a set.

Interlocked lacing joins hair from one section to the next.

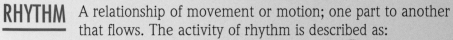

RHYTHM A relationship of movement or motion; one part to another that flows. The activity of rhythm is described as:

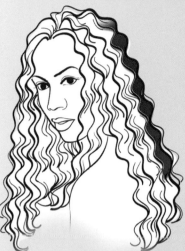

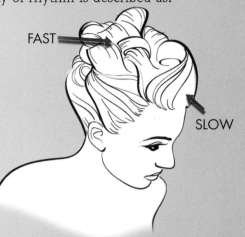

FAST

SLOW

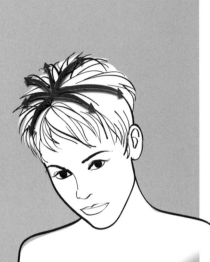

RECURRING RHYTHM
Even distributions within a hairdesign.

SEQUENTIAL RHYTHM
Patterns increase/decrease in a predetermined order.

RADIATING RHYTHM
Patterns are evenly dispersed from a common center.

5

2468 13579

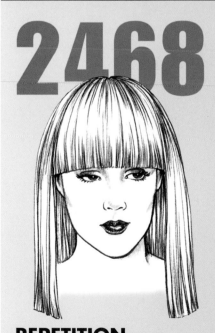

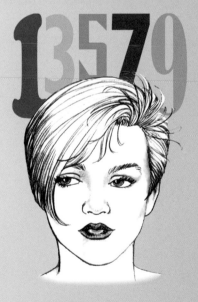

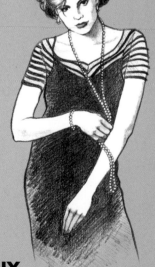

REPETITION
How often elements or components are repeated within a design. Work in odd numbers, not even. Repetition (even) is unappealing to the eye.

CONTRAST
Contrast (odd) is exciting and appealing to the eye.

HARMONY
The aesthetic placement of shapes and lines. The clothing, makeup, hairdesign and accessory choices complement each other and the client's personality, lifestyle and physical features.

MULTIPLE CHOICE

1. Refers to the force of gravity on the hair.
   A. Mass   B. Tempo   C. Energy   D. Weight

2. The amount of space matter takes up is called:
   A. Mass   B. Volume   C. Texture   D. Gravity

3. Occurs when each visual weight is the exact same distance from the axis.
   A. Emphasis   B. Symmetry   C. Illusion   D. Counterbalance

4. The proportion of mass to the total hairdesign.
   A. Motion   B. Component   C. Harmony   D. Scale

5. The ideal comparative ratio in design of size to the whole is:
   A. half and half   B. 2:3 or 3:2   C. 1/4 to 3/4   D. 3:1

6. A theory behind how elements are applied to create a design.
   A. Principle   B. Ratio   C. Composition   D. Sequence

7. The use of different weights and lengths in opposite areas to offset each other.
   A. Disturbance   B. Proportion   C. Counterbalance   D. Neutralizing

8. Created by placing the weight of balance on the vertical line.
   A. Width   B. Height   C. Asymmetry   D. Sections

9. Diagonal balance at less than this degree is most pleasing to the eye.
   A. 90   B. 10   C. 45   D. 60

10. Turning on an axis is called:
    A. Repetition   B. Rhythm   C. Force   D. Rotation

TRUE OR FALSE

1. _____ Curved directional motions always travel clockwise.

2. _____ A two-dimensional design has length and width.

3. _____ Shifting attention away from a problem area is called division.

4. _____ Patterns with radiating rhythm are dispersed evenly from a common center.

5. _____ More force is needed to close the inner loop of a circle at the same time as the outer loop.

6. _____ The smaller the circle, the slower the tempo or motion it will have.

7. _____ Harmony is the aesthetic placement of shapes and lines.

8. _____ Repetition in hairdesign is used to de-emphasize individual components.

9. _____ Ornamentation was the original purpose for hair.

10. _____ Social status, religious beliefs, and civilization affect hairdesigns.

STUDENT'S NAME   DATE   GRADE

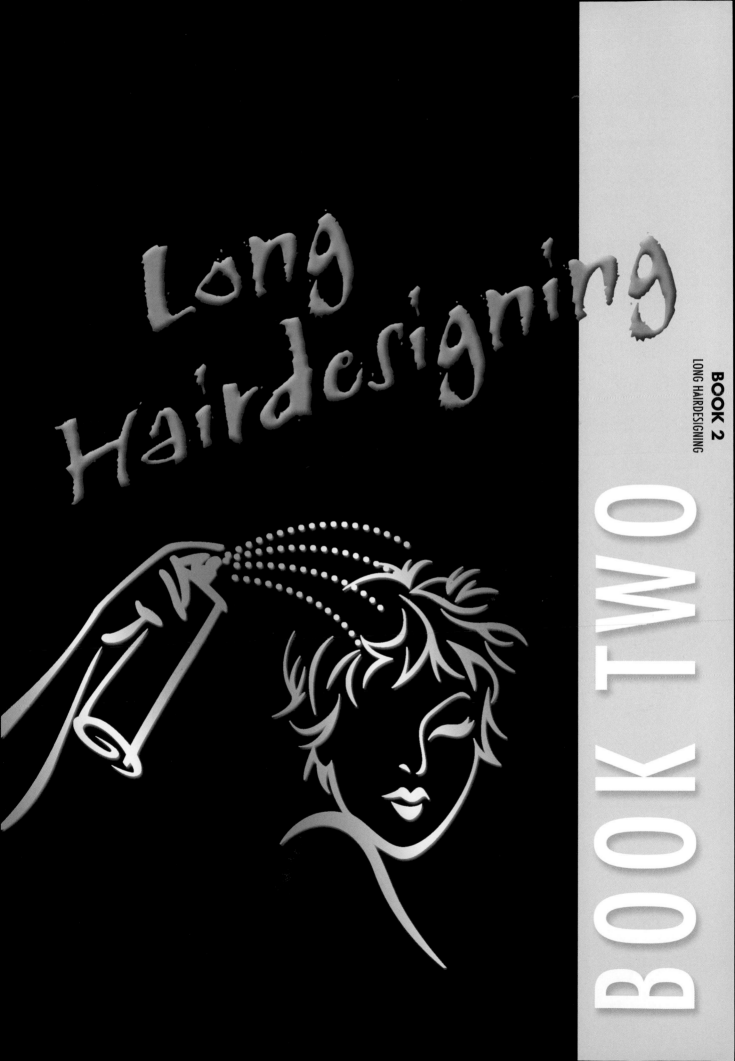

Long Hairdesigning

BOOK 2
LONG HAIRDESIGNING

BOOK TWO

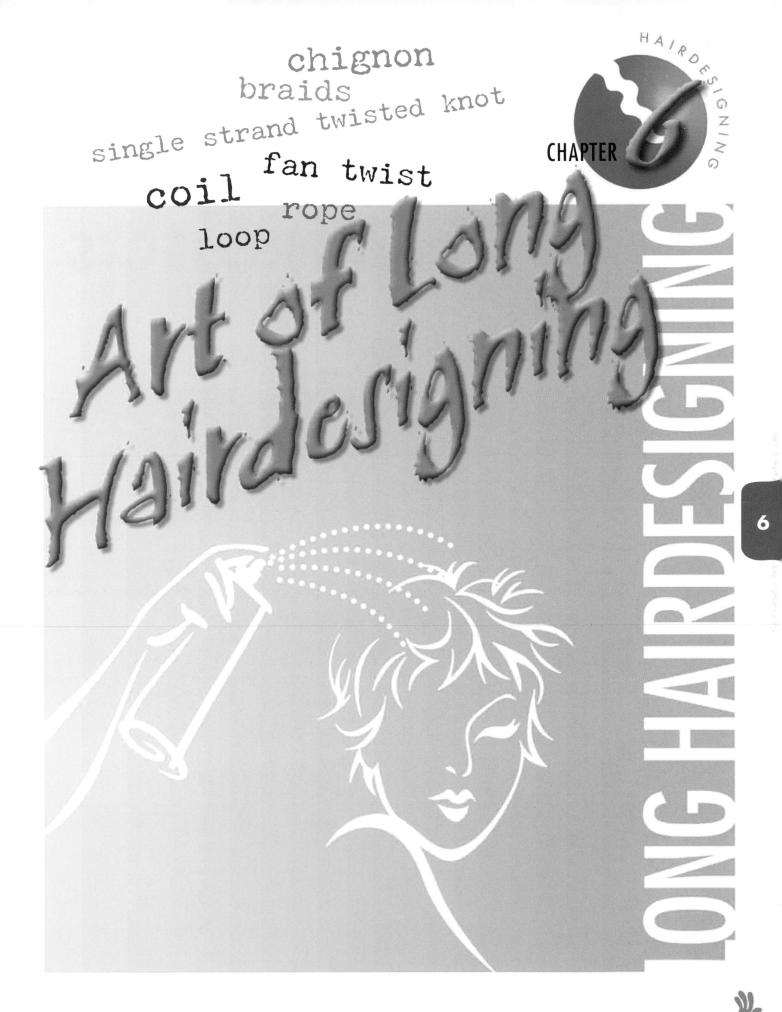

chignon
braids
single strand twisted knot
coil fan twist
rope
loop

Art of Long Hairdesigning

Long Hairdesign
LAB PROJECTS

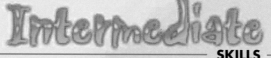

Simple SKILLS

Intermediate SKILLS

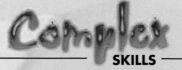

Complex SKILLS

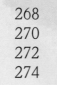

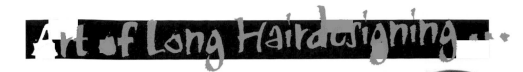

The concept of designing and finishing hair is truly an art form. This chapter and those that follow will help you to develop professional perception, manual dexterity, and tactile sensitivity using basic art elements and principles.

1

6

2

3

4

Each lab project is part of our competency-based learning system, progressing from simple to complex skill levels.

These pages were established to allow freedom of innovation and adaptation to current trends.

Long Hairdesign

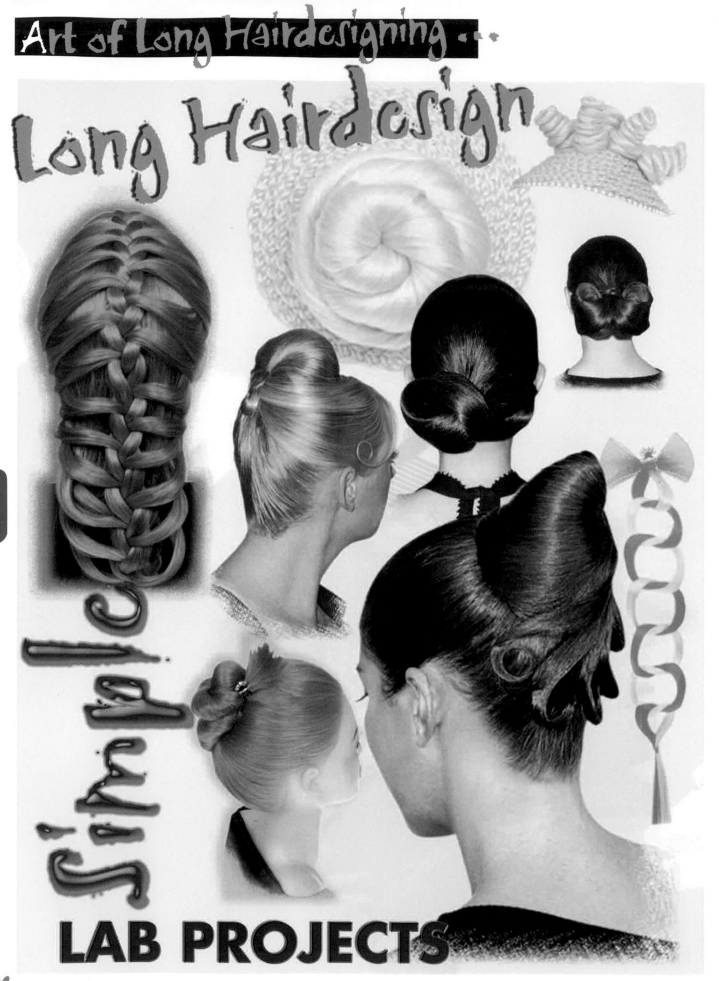

6

Simplicity

LAB PROJECTS

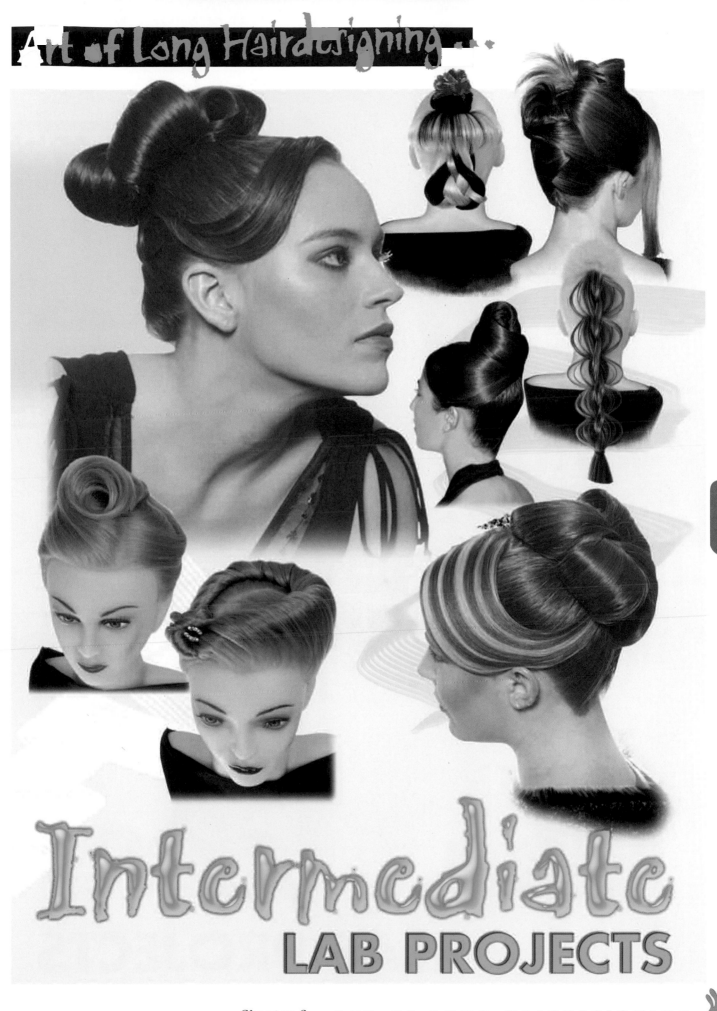

Intermediate
LAB PROJECTS

6

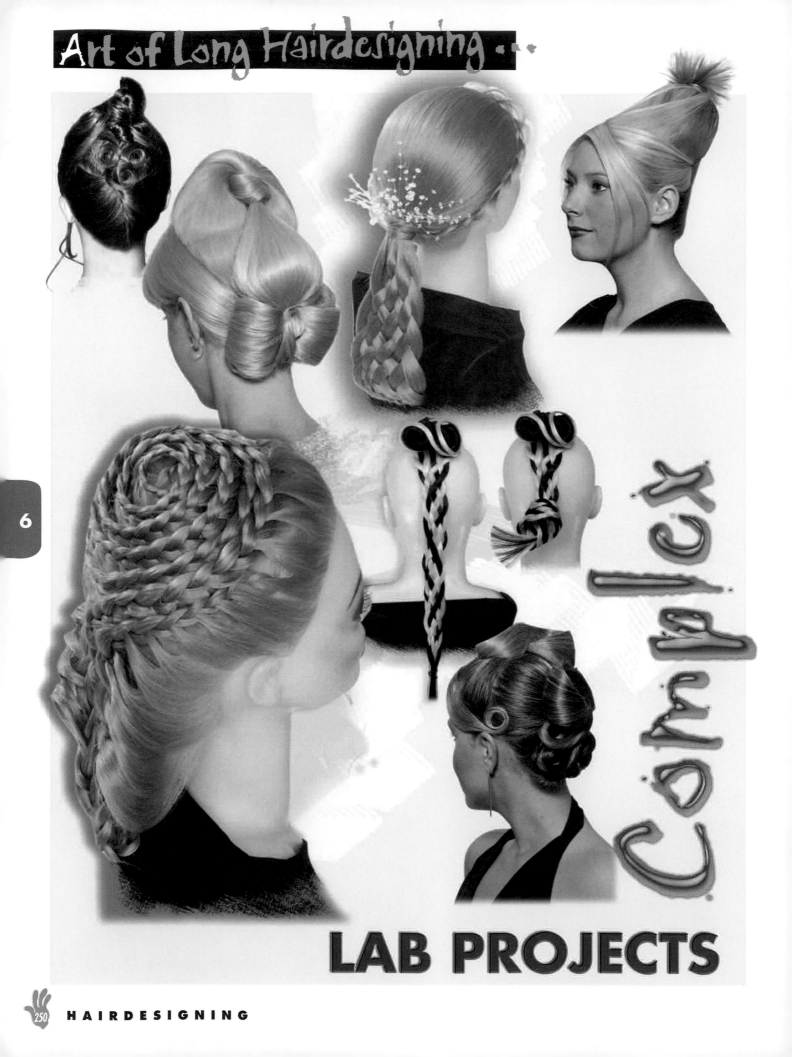

Complex

LAB PROJECTS

6

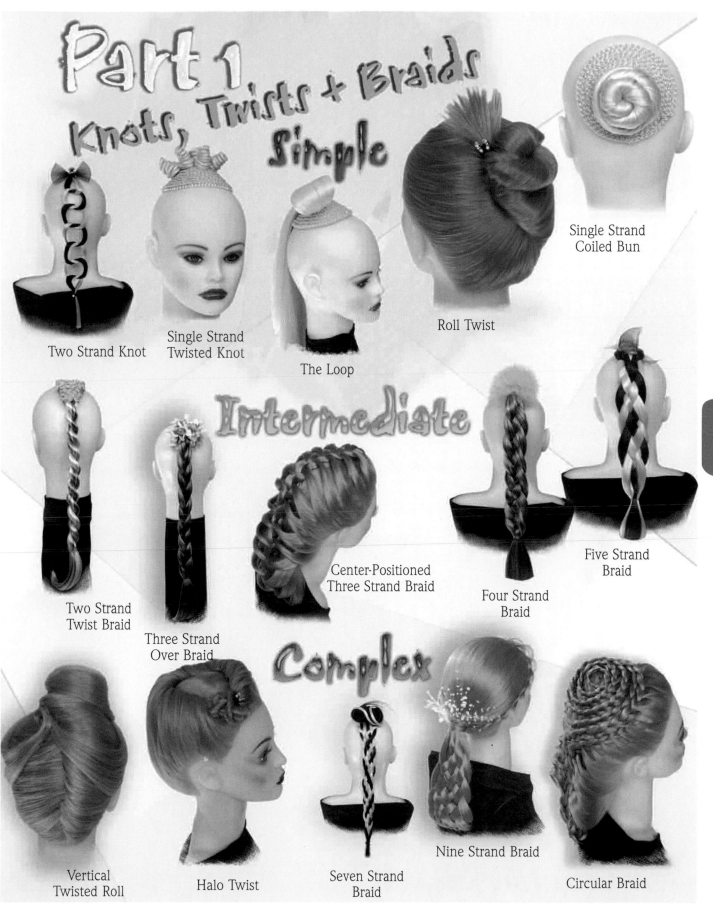

Part 1
Knots, Twists + Braids

Simple

Two Strand Knot

Single Strand
Twisted Knot

The Loop

Roll Twist

Single Strand
Coiled Bun

Intermediate

Two Strand
Twist Braid

Three Strand
Over Braid

Center-Positioned
Three Strand Braid

Four Strand
Braid

Five Strand
Braid

Complex

Vertical
Twisted Roll

Halo Twist

Seven Strand
Braid

Nine Strand Braid

Circular Braid

6

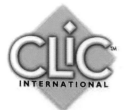
Two Strand Knot

OBJECTIVE To enhance the appearance of a basic knot by using two strand colors.

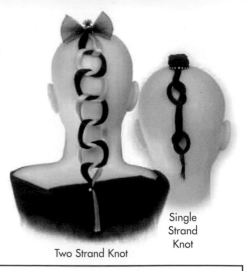

Two Strand Knot

Single Strand Knot

TOOLS & MATERIALS

- Neck strip and cape/smock
- Towels
- Pomade or other liquid styling tools
- Rattail comb
- Styling brushes
- Cleansing and conditioning products
- Client record card/file
- Airformer and/or flat iron
- Clips
- Small elastic band

PROCEDURE

"The client consultation is an important part of your professional service. Be sure to complete this step prior to each client service you provide. Your successful retail sales and customer satisfaction rates depend upon it!"

RETAIL RE-BOOK REFERRAL

1. Drape the client in preparation for the service.
2. Thoroughly brush the client's hair to remove knots, tangles and hairspray.
3. Cleanse and condition the hair according to the client's needs. Rinse thoroughly and towel dry.
4. Comb the hair to detangle. Apply an appropriate liquid styling tool and airform the hair.
5. The hair may be flat ironed if it is curly in texture.
6. Perform the style as shown.
7. Follow standard clean-up procedures.
8. Document the client record card/file.

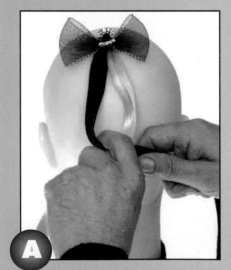

A Separate the hair into two strands, with one strand in each hand.

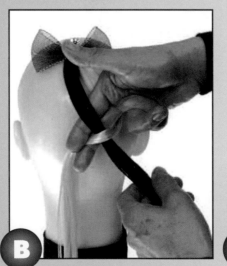

B Cross right strand over left. Place index and middle fingers between the two strands and grab the top strand between them from underneath.

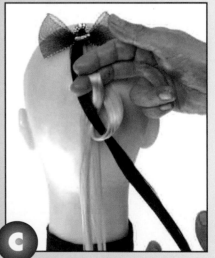

C Pull the hair through the center from underneath to form a knot.

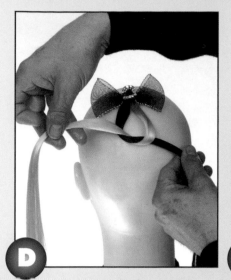

D

The first completed two strand knot.

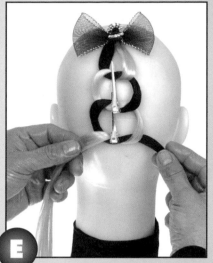

E

Place a clip in the center of each knot to hold it in place. Apply consistent, light tension to avoid changes in the knot size.

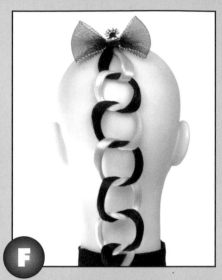

F

Continue this pattern for the next knots to complete the finished two strand knot design. Secure the ends with an elastic band.

Variation of Design: Single Strand Knot

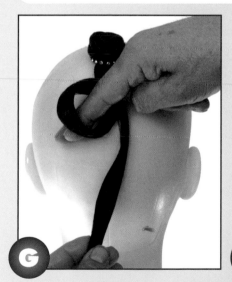

G

Forming the first loop.

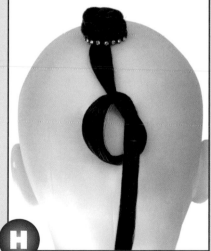

H

The first completed knot.

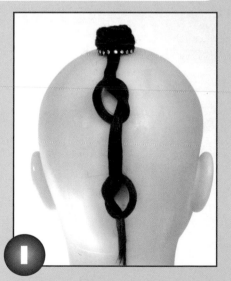

I

Finished design.

EVALUATION _____

_____

GRADE _____   STUDENT'S NAME _____   ID# _____

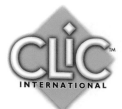

Single Strand Twisted Knot

OBJECTIVE

To design a simple twisted knot style using a single strand of hair.

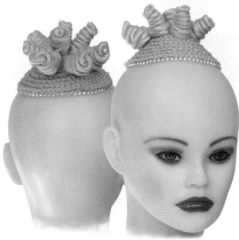

Single Strand Twisted Knot

TOOLS & MATERIALS

- Neck strip and cape/smock
- Towels
- Pomade or other liquid styling tools
- Styling combs and brushes
- Cleansing and conditioning products
- Client record card/file
- Airformer and/or flat iron
- Clips, bobbie pins, and hair pins

PROCEDURE

"The client consultation is an important part of your professional service. Be sure to complete this step prior to each client service you provide. Your successful retail sales and customer satisfaction rates depend upon it!"

RETAIL • RE-BOOK • REFERRAL

1. Drape the client in preparation for the service.
2. Thoroughly brush the client's hair to remove knots, tangles and hairspray.
3. Cleanse and condition the hair according to the client's needs. Rinse thoroughly and towel dry.
4. Comb the hair to detangle. Apply an appropriate liquid styling tool and airform the hair.
5. The hair may be flat ironed if it is curly in texture.
6. Perform the style as shown.
7. Follow standard clean-up procedures.
8. Document the client record card/file.

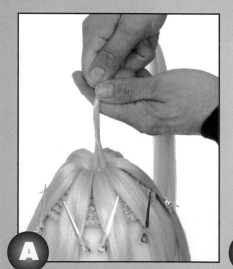

A Subdivide the hair to be styled into one half inch (1.3 cm) diameter strands.

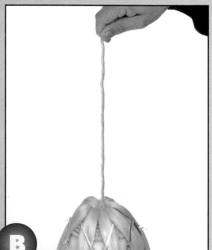

B With one hand, begin twisting the hair in a clockwise direction.

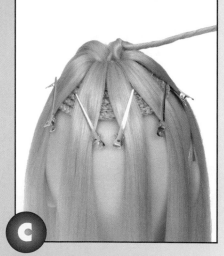

C Once the entire strand of hair is tightly twisted, begin winding in a clockwise direction at the base.

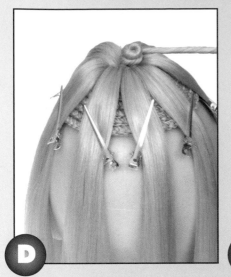

D Loosely wind the strand underneath the coil formation, enabling the knot to stand up.

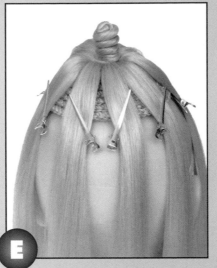

E When the hair is wrapped completely around the base of the knot, tuck the ends into the base.

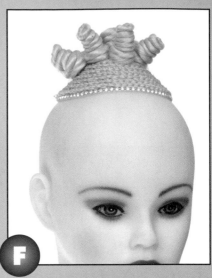

F Front view of the finished set of single strand twist knots.

Variations of Design:

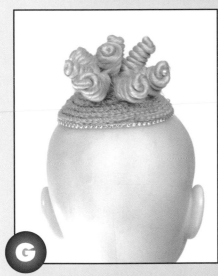

G Rear view of the finished knotted style.

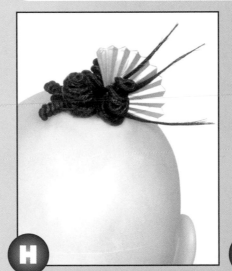

H **Ornamentation**
Adding ornamentation to enhance a twist knot.

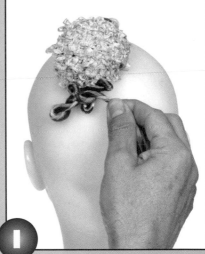

I **Multiple Strand Twisting**
Forming coil clusters creates dimensional texture.

EVALUATION

GRADE STUDENT'S NAME ID#

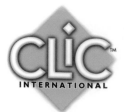

The Loop

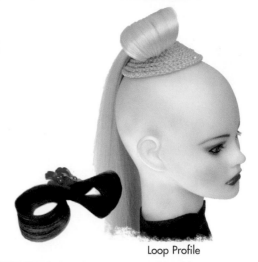

Loop Profile

OBJECTIVE

To enhance long hairdesigns with a soft and sophisticated loop.

TOOLS & MATERIALS

- Neck strip and cape/smock
- Towels
- Pomade or other liquid styling tools
- Styling combs and brushes
- Bobbie pins and hair pins
- Cleansing and conditioning products
- Client record card/file
- Airformer and/or flat iron
- Clips
- Ornamentation

PROCEDURE

"The client consultation is an important part of your professional service. Be sure to complete this step prior to each client service you provide. Your successful retail sales and customer satisfaction rates depend upon it!"

RETAIL • RE-BOOK • REFERRAL

1. Drape the client in preparation for the service.
2. Thoroughly brush the client's hair to remove knots, tangles and hairspray.
3. Cleanse and condition the hair according to the client's needs. Rinse thoroughly and towel dry.
4. Comb the hair to detangle. Apply an appropriate liquid styling tool and airform the hair.
5. The hair may be flat ironed if it is curly in texture.
6. Perform the style as shown.
7. Follow standard clean-up procedures.
8. Document the client record card/file.

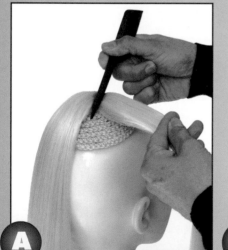

A Begin by taking a one inch (2.5 cm) section of hair.

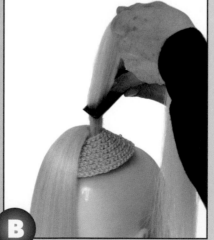

B Softly compact the hair by lacing at the base to stand hair up.

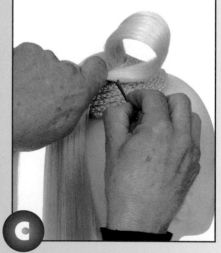

C Bend the hair under to form a loop, leaving ends out. Secure the loop base with a bobbie pin.

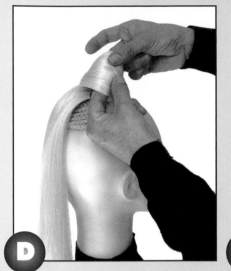

D Place the remaining ends inside the loop and secure with another bobbie pin.

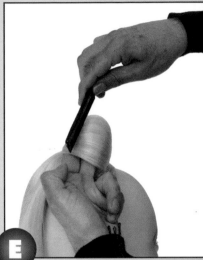

E Use a comb to evenly smooth the surface of the loop. Spray to hold the loop.

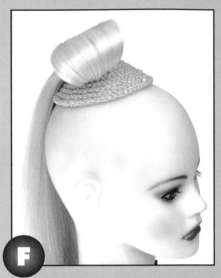

F The completed loop design component.

Variations of Design

6

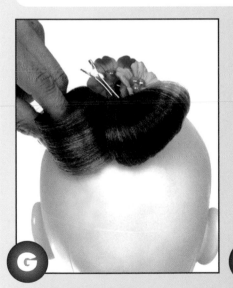

G **Double Roll Design**

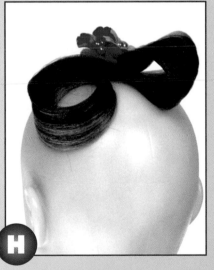

H **Double Roll Design**

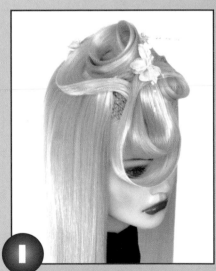

I **Complex Loop Design**
The loop may be placed on the head in any position. Varying the loop sizes creates a more interesting sophisticated style.

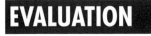

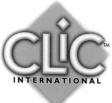

Roll Twist

OBJECTIVE

To create an elegantly finished roll twist.

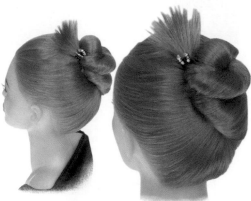

Roll Twist

TOOLS & MATERIALS

- Neck strip and cape/smock
- Towels
- Pomade or other liquid styling tools
- Styling combs and brushes
- Bobbie pins and hair pins
- Cleansing and conditioning products
- Client record card/file
- Airformer and/or flat iron
- Ornamentation
- Clips

PROCEDURE

"The client consultation is an important part of your professional service. Be sure to complete this step prior to each client service you provide. Your successful retail sales and customer satisfaction rates depend upon it!"

RETAIL • RE-BOOK • REFERRAL

1. Drape the client in preparation for the service.
2. Thoroughly brush the client's hair to remove knots, tangles and hairspray.
3. Cleanse and condition the hair according to the client's needs. Rinse thoroughly and towel dry.
4. Comb the hair to detangle. Apply an appropriate liquid styling tool and airform the hair.
5. The hair may be flat ironed if it is curly in texture.
6. Perform the style as shown.
7. Follow standard clean-up procedures.
8. Document the client record card/file.

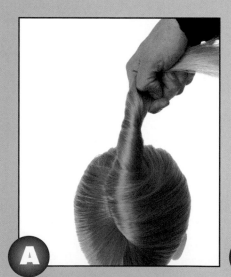

A Brush the hair together near the occipital bone. Twist upward to form a roll.

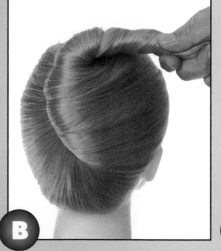

B Begin rotating twisted hair in a clockwise direction.

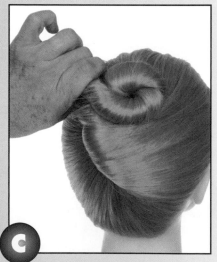

C The rotated roll will form a circular bun at the top of the twist.

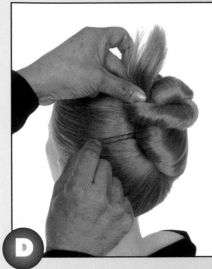

D

Holding the ends, place bobbie pins or hair pins along the side of the twist.

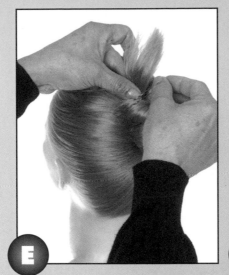

E

Loose ends may be tucked inside for a traditional twist or fanned out for a modern look. Spray well to hold the style.

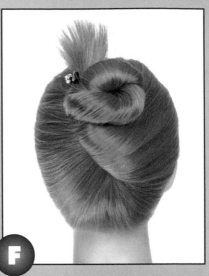

F

The finished roll twist may be detailed further with ornamentation.

Variation of Design: Comb Twist

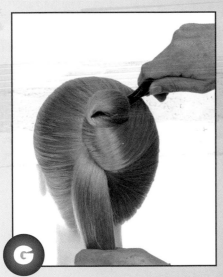

G

For hair past shoulder length: Place a tail comb in the middle of the gathered hair and begin to twist up toward the crown.

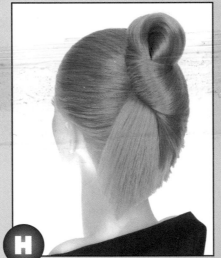

H

The finished style is secured with bobbie pins, leaving the ends of the hair out.

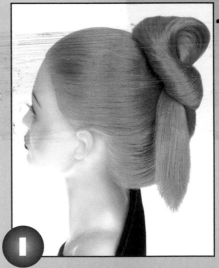

I

Profile detail of the finished style.

EVALUATION

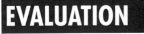

GRADE

STUDENT'S NAME

ID#

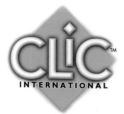

Single Strand Coiled Bun

OBJECTIVE

To create a circular bun by twisting a single strand.

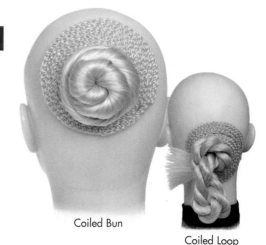

Coiled Bun

Coiled Loop

TOOLS & MATERIALS

- Neck strip and cape/smock
- Towels
- Pomade or other liquid styling tools
- Styling combs and brushes
- Clips
- Cleansing and conditioning products
- Client record card/file
- Airformer and/or flat iron
- Bobbie pins and hair pins
- Small elastic bands

PROCEDURE

"The client consultation is an important part of your professional service. Be sure to complete this step prior to each client service you provide. Your successful retail sales and customer satisfaction rates depend upon it!"

RETAIL RE-BOOK REFERRAL

1. Drape the client in preparation for the service.
2. Thoroughly brush the client's hair to remove knots, tangles and hairspray.
3. Cleanse and condition the hair according to the client's needs. Rinse thoroughly and towel dry. Apply a liquid styling tool. Comb the hair to detangle.
4. Airform the hair if desired (twisting the hair while damp may make it easier to style).
5. The hair may be flat ironed if it is curly in texture. Spray well to smooth and control all flyaway hair.
6. Perform the style as shown.
7. Follow standard clean-up procedures.
8. Document the client record card/file.

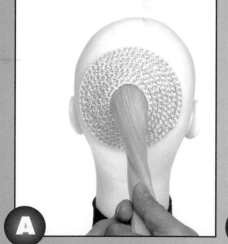

A Gather hair together at the occipital and start twisting in a clockwise direction. Work down the strand, using tension while twisting.

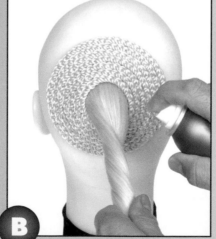

B Hold the hair taut. Spray flyaway hair to keep it smooth.

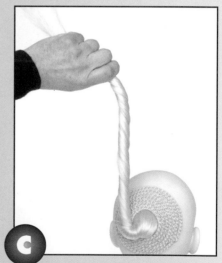

C Secure the ends of the completed twist with an elastic band. Bring the hair up and turn again in a clockwise direction to form a circular coil.

Single Strand Coiled Bun

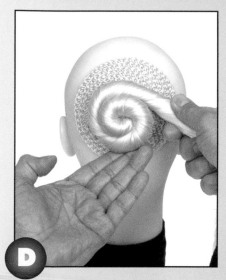

D

Continue adding to the three strand braid by alternating from right to left, picking hair up from the perimeter.

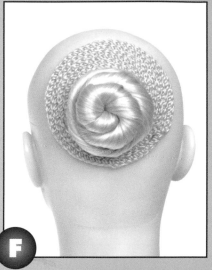

E

Secure the ends of the completed twist with an elastic band. Bring the hair up and turn again in a clockwise direction to form a circular coil.

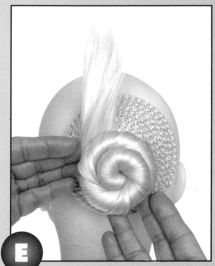

F

The completed single strand coiled bun style.

Variation of Design: Single Strand Coiled Loop

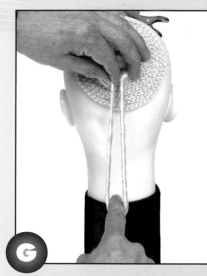

G

One half inch (1.3 cm) sections are twisted until hair coils on its own. Place the end of the strand with the beginning and form the hair into a loop.

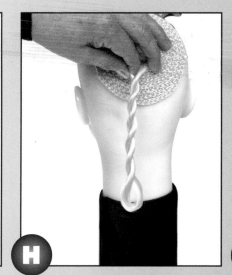

H

Twist and secure each loop with a bobbie pin.

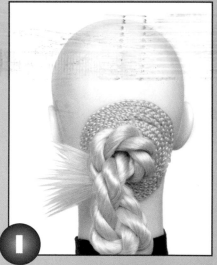

I

For variety of the finished look, stylists may choose to join single coils together or keep them separate.

EVALUATION

GRADE STUDENT'S NAME ID#

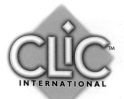

Two Strand Twist Braid

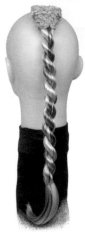

OBJECTIVE

To explore creative alternatives for twisting hair by completing the two strand twist braid.

Two Strand Twist Braid

TOOLS & MATERIALS

- Neck strip and cape/smock
- Towels
- Pomade or other liquid styling tools

- Styling combs and brushes
- Clips, bobbie pins, and hair pins
- Cleansing and conditioning products

- Client record card/file
- Airformer and/or flat iron
- Small elastic bands

- Ornamentation

PROCEDURE

"The client consultation is an important part of your professional service. Be sure to complete this step prior to each client service you provide. Your successful retail sales and customer satisfaction rates depend upon it!"

RETAIL · RE-BOOK
REFERRAL

1. Drape the client in preparation for the service.
2. Thoroughly brush the client's hair to remove knots, tangles and hairspray.
3. Cleanse and condition the hair according to the client's needs. Rinse thoroughly and towel dry. Apply a liquid styling tool. Comb the hair to detangle.
4. Airform the hair if desired (twisting the hair while damp may make it easier to braid).
5. The hair may be flat ironed if it is curly in texture. Spray well to smooth and control all flyaway hair.
6. Perform the style as shown.
7. Follow standard clean-up procedures.
8. Document the client record card/file.

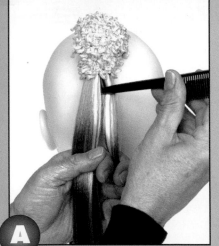

A Separate the ponytail into two equal sections using the tail of a comb.

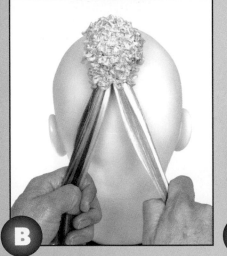

B Hold one strand in each hand and maintain equal tension.

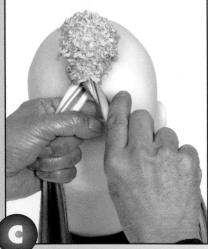

C Pick up approximately two inches (5 cm) of hair at the perimeter, using diagonal partings.

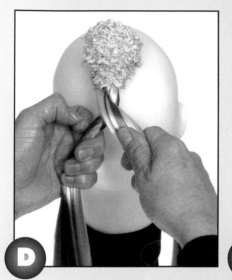

D

Starting again from the left side, twist the strand while crossing over the right.

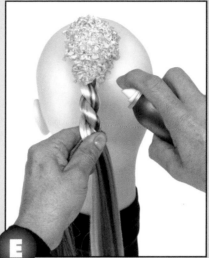

E

Spray the hair as needed to keep the twisted strand smooth.

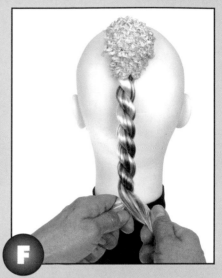

F

Continue to twist and cross the left over the right strand until the ends have been reached.

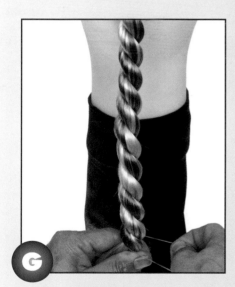

G

Use an elastic band to secure the twisted, rope-like ponytail.

H

The finished two strand twist braid.

EVALUATION

GRADE

STUDENT'S NAME

ID#

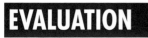

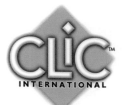

Three Strand Over Braid

OBJECTIVE

To create a casual 3-strand over braid by adding hair entirely from the outer perimeter.

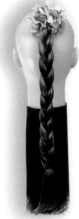

Three Strand Braid

TOOLS & MATERIALS

- Neck strip and cape/smock
- Towels
- Pomade or other liquid styling tools

- Styling combs and brushes
- Clips, bobbie pins, and hair pins
- Cleansing and conditioning products

- Client record card/file
- Airformer and/or flat iron
- Small elastic bands

- Ornamentation

PROCEDURE

"The client consultation is an important part of your professional service. Be sure to complete this step prior to each client service you provide. Your successful retail sales and customer satisfaction rates depend upon it!"

RETAIL · RE-BOOK · REFERRAL

1. Drape the client in preparation for the service.
2. Thoroughly brush the client's hair to remove knots, tangles and hairspray.
3. Cleanse and condition the hair according to the client's needs. Rinse thoroughly and towel dry. Apply a liquid styling tool. Comb the hair to detangle.
4. Airform the hair if desired (braiding the hair while damp may make it easier to braid).
5. The hair may be flat ironed if the hair is of a curly texture.
6. Perform the style as shown.
7. Follow standard clean-up procedures.
8. Document the client record card/file.

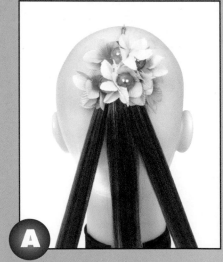

A Separate the hair into three equal sections.

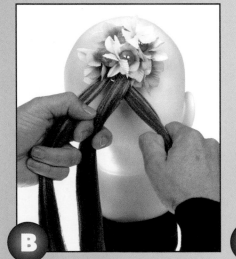

B Hold two strands of hair in the left hand and one strand in the right hand.

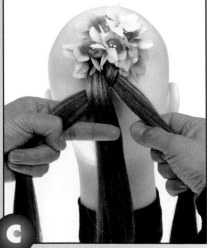

C The left outside strand is crossed over the center strand, placing it between the other two as the new center strand.

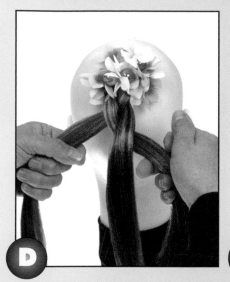

D Cross the right outside strand over the center strand; now this strand becomes the center.

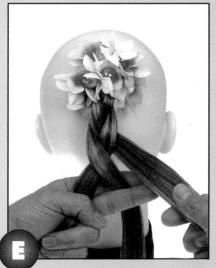

E Cross the left outside strand again over center, followed by the right outside strand over center.

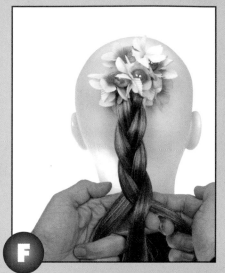

F Continue the pattern down to the hair ends and secure the remainder with an elastic band.

6

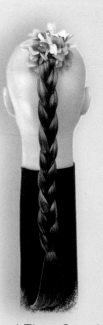

G The completed Three Strand Over Braid.

Variation of Design: Three Strand Under Braid

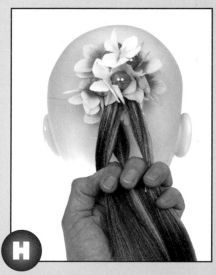

H The left outside strand is crossed under the center strand.

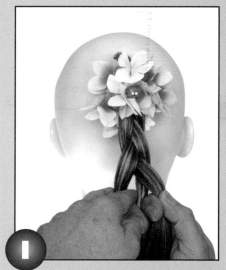

I Cross the right outside strand under the center strand and continue the pattern to the ends.

EVALUATION

GRADE

STUDENT'S NAME

ID#

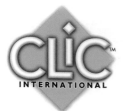

Center-Positioned Three Strand Braid

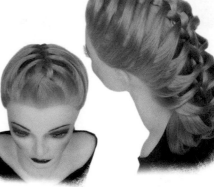

Center-Positioned Three Strand Braid

OBJECTIVE

To create a three strand braid down the center of the head by picking up and adding the hair from only the outer perimeter area to the center braid. This type of braid has two versions:
1. Flat center-positioned three strand braid **OR**
2. Raised center-positioned three strand braid

TOOLS & MATERIALS

- Neck strip and cape/smock
- Towels
- Pomade or other liquid styling tools
- Styling combs and brushes
- Clips, bobbie pins, and hair pins
- Cleansing and conditioning products
- Client record card/file
- Airformer and/or flat iron
- Small elastic bands
- Ornamentation

PROCEDURE

"The client consultation is an important part of your professional service. Be sure to complete this step prior to each client service you provide. Your successful retail sales and customer satisfaction rates depend upon it!"

RETAIL RE-BOOK REFERRAL

1. Drape the client in preparation for the service.
2. Thoroughly brush the client's hair to remove knots, tangles and hairspray.
3. Cleanse and condition the hair according to the client's needs. Rinse thoroughly and towel dry. Apply a liquid styling tool. Comb the hair to detangle.
4. Airform the hair if desired (braiding the hair while damp may make it easier to braid).
5. The hair may be flat ironed if the hair is of a curly texture.
6. Perform the style as shown.
7. Follow standard clean-up procedures.
8. Document the client record card/file.

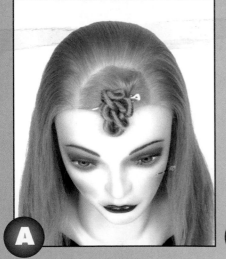

A Section a small half circle or triangular shape.

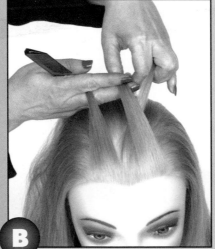

B Divide the hair into three strands and bring the hair from the left perimeter across the center strand. Maintaining tension, bring the hair at the right perimeter into the center by crossing over the new center strand.

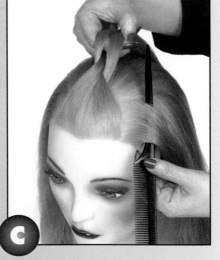

C Pick up approximately two inches (5 cm) of hair at the perimeter, using diagonal partings.

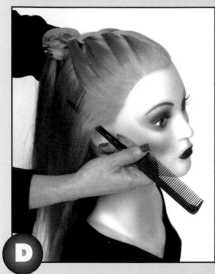

D

Continue adding to the three strand braid by alternating from right to left, picking hair up from the perimeter.

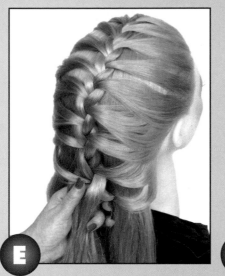

E

When braiding the hair from the occipital area to the nape, loosen the tension on the hair. Continue by adding hair sectioned alternately from the left and right outer perimeter.

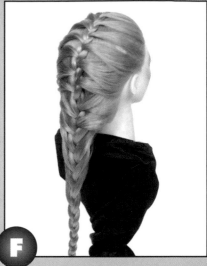

F

Finish the style with a basic three strand braid after all perimeter hair at the nape area has been inserted into the braid. Secure the braid with a small elastic band.

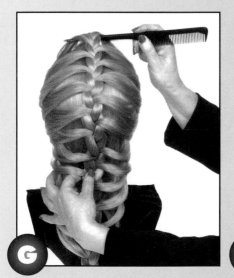

G

Visualize and adjust the balance points along the length of the braid.

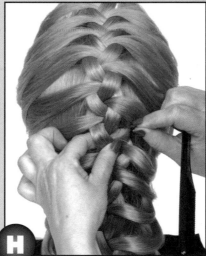

H

Unbraided hair ends that remain may be hidden under the center braid and pinned.

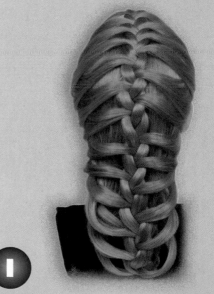

I

The finished braid may be adorned with flowers, small pearls or other ornamentation.

EVALUATION

GRADE

STUDENT'S NAME

ID#

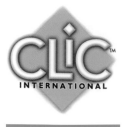

Four Strand Braid

OBJECTIVE

To take braiding skills to the next level by creating an intricate four strand braid.

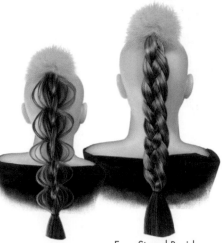

Creative Chain Braid   Four Strand Braid

TOOLS & MATERIALS

- Neck strip and cape/smock
- Towels
- Pomade or other liquid styling tools
- Styling combs and brushes
- Clips, bobbie pins, and hair pins
- Cleansing and conditioning products
- Client record card/file
- Airformer and/or flat iron
- Small elastic bands
- Ornamentation

PROCEDURE

"The client consultation is an important part of your professional service. Be sure to complete this step prior to each client service you provide. Your successful retail sales and customer satisfaction rates depend upon it!"

RETAIL • RE-BOOK REFERRAL

1. Drape the client in preparation for the service.
2. Thoroughly brush the client's hair to remove knots, tangles and hairspray.
3. Cleanse and condition the hair according to the client's needs.
   Rinse thoroughly and towel dry. Apply a liquid styling tool. Comb the hair to detangle.
4. Airform the hair if desired (braiding the hair while damp may make it easier to braid).
5. The hair may be flat ironed if it is curly in texture.
6. Perform the style as shown.
7. Follow standard clean-up procedures.
8. Document the client record card/file.

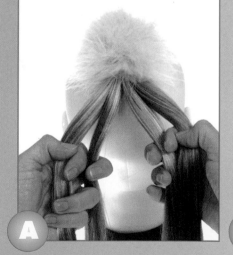

A Divide hair into four equal sections. Hold two separate strands in each hand.

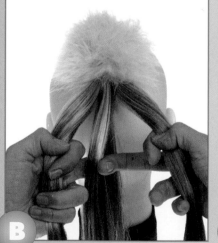

B The right hand inside strand is placed over the inside strand of the left hand.

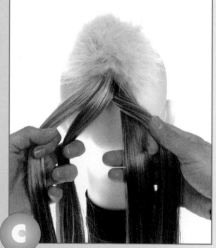

C The new inside right strand is crossed over the outside right strand.

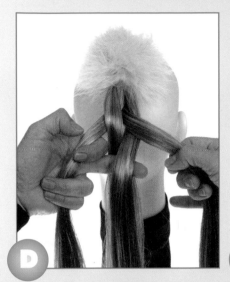

D Cross the new inner right strand over the inner left and under the outer left strand.

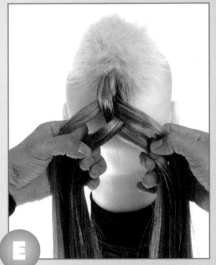

E The pattern should always have two strands in each hand. Place the outer left strand over the inner left strand and under the inner right strand.

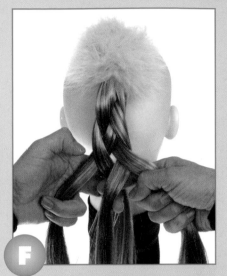

F Continue the pattern by placing the outside right strand under the inside right strand and over the inner left strand. The outside left strand goes over the inner left strand and under the inner right strand. Work from right to left down the length of the strand.

Variation of Design: Creative Chain Braid

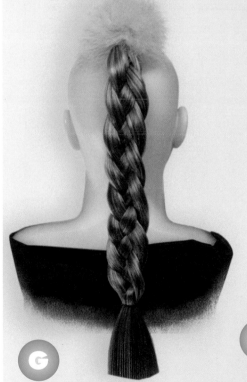

G The ends of the completed four strand braid are secured with an elastic band.

H Lightly pull a few strands of hair from the outer area of each link in the braid's chain.

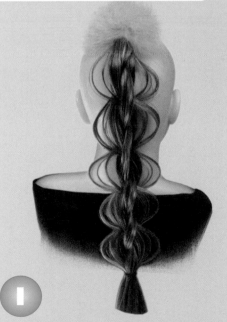

I The finished look adds flair to the basic, braided design.

EVALUATION

GRADE _____ STUDENT'S NAME _____ ID# _____

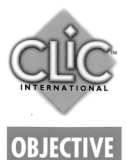

Five Strand Braid

OBJECTIVE

To further enhance creativity by designing a five strand braid.

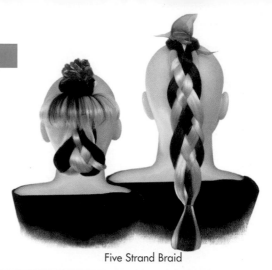

Five Strand Braid

TOOLS & MATERIALS

- Neck strip and cape/smock
- Towels
- Pomade or other liquid styling tools
- Styling combs and brushes
- Clips, bobbie pins, and hair pins
- Cleansing and conditioning products
- Client record card/file
- Airformer and/or flat iron
- Small elastic bands
- Ornamentation

PROCEDURE

"The client consultation is an important part of your professional service. Be sure to complete this step prior to each client service you provide. Your successful retail sales and customer satisfaction rates depend upon it!"

1. Drape the client in preparation for the service.
2. Thoroughly brush the client's hair to remove knots, tangles and hairspray.
3. Cleanse and condition the hair according to the client's needs. Rinse thoroughly and towel dry. Apply a liquid styling tool. Comb the hair to detangle.
4. Airform the hair if desired (braiding the hair while damp may make it easier to braid).
5. The hair may be flat ironed if it is curly in texture.
6. Perform the style as shown.
7. Follow standard clean-up procedures.
8. Document the client record card/file.

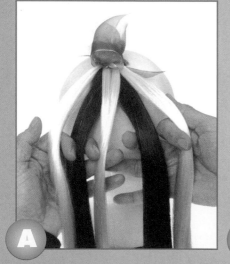

A Equally subdivide the hair into five strands.

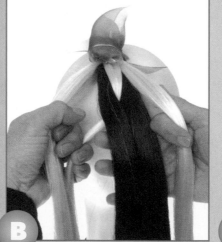

B Starting in the middle, cross the third strand from the left under the second.

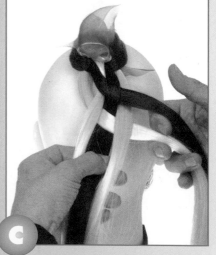

C Weave the left outside strand under and over the next two strands. The right hand is holding two strands.

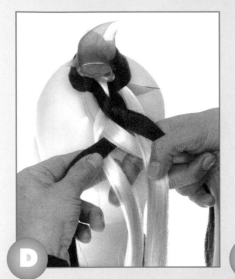

D

Cross the right outside strand under and over the next two strands from the right. The left hand now holds three strands.

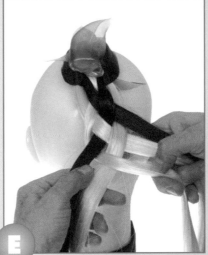

E

Repeat the left side pattern by crossing the outside left strand first under, then over the next two strands.

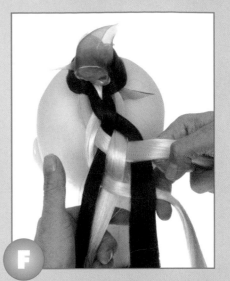

F

Continuing on the outside right, cross under the second strand and over the third strand.

Variation of Design

6

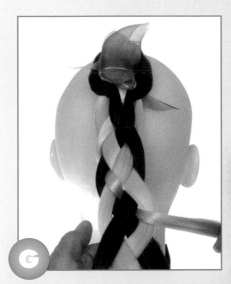

G

Alternate sides from left to right, starting with the side holding three strands. Always weave the outside strand toward the center, going under the first strand and then over the second strand.

H

Repeat the pattern down the length of the hair. The ends may be secured with an elastic band or pinned underneath the braid for a smoother finish.

I

Variation is achieved by changing ornamentation and folding the five strand braid under to crop the style.

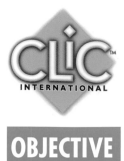

Vertical Twisted Roll

OBJECTIVE

To establish a rolled vertical twist with a supportive base form.

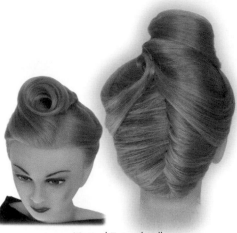

Vertical Twisted Roll

TOOLS & MATERIALS

- Neck strip and cape/smock
- Towels
- Pomade or other liquid styling tools
- Styling combs and brushes
- Bobbie pins and hair pins
- Cleansing and conditioning products
- Client record card/file
- Airformer and/or flat iron
- Clips
- Ornamentation

PROCEDURE

"The client consultation is an important part of your professional service. Be sure to complete this step prior to each client service you provide. Your successful retail sales and customer satisfaction rates depend upon it!"

1. Drape the client in preparation for the service.
2. Thoroughly brush the client's hair to remove knots, tangles and hairspray.
3. Cleanse and condition the hair according to the client's needs. Rinse thoroughly and towel dry.
4. Comb the hair to detangle. Apply an appropriate liquid styling tool and airform the hair.
5. The hair may be flat ironed if it is curly in texture.
6. Perform the style as shown.
7. Follow standard clean-up procedures.
8. Document the client record card/file.

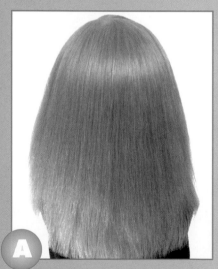

A Brush all hair smoothly back.

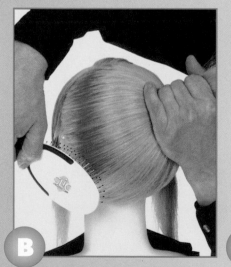

B Leave a small section of hair on either side by the front hairline to frame the face. Direct the remaining hair in the back over to one side.

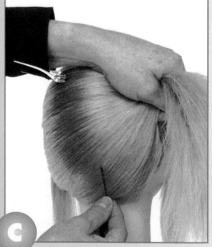

C Interlock bobbie pins vertically from the center nape to the crown area.

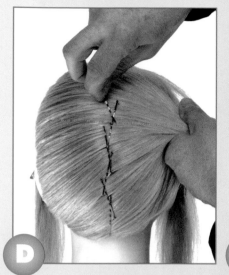

D Place the last bobbie pin downward to secure the base of the twist.

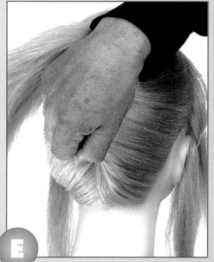

E Begin to twist the hair at the nape. Face the roll in toward the row of bobbie pins.

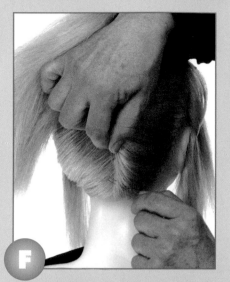

F Use hair pins to grab the twisted hair along the track of bobbie pins and secure the twist.

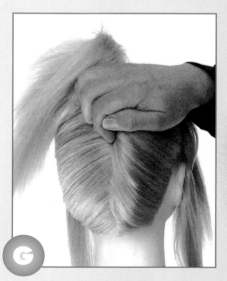

G Continue securing the twist with hair pins to the crown area. The hair ends and front hairline may be rolled into the style and pinned or finished separately.

H The completed twist is elegant with or without ornamentation.

EVALUATION

GRADE

STUDENT'S NAME

ID#

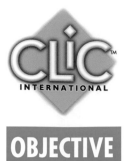

Halo Twist

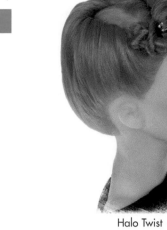

Halo Twist

OBJECTIVE

To refine artistic ability by creating the elegant halo twist.

TOOLS & MATERIALS

- Neck strip and cape/smock
- Towels
- Pomade or other liquid styling tools
- Styling combs and brushes
- Bobbie pins and hair pins
- Cleansing and conditioning products
- Client record card/file
- Airformer and/or flat iron
- Clips
- Ornamentation

PROCEDURE

"The client consultation is an important part of your professional service. Be sure to complete this step prior to each client service you provide. Your successful retail sales and customer satisfaction rates depend upon it!"

1. Drape the client in preparation for the service.
2. Thoroughly brush the client's hair to remove knots, tangles and hairspray.
3. Cleanse and condition the hair according to the client's needs. Rinse thoroughly and towel dry.
4. Comb the hair to detangle. Apply an appropriate liquid styling tool and airform the hair.
5. The hair may be flat ironed if it is curly in texture.
6. Perform the style as shown.
7. Follow standard clean-up procedures.
8. Document the client record card/file.

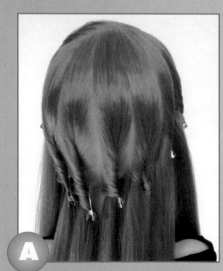

A Divide the hair into eight vertical subsections of equal size.

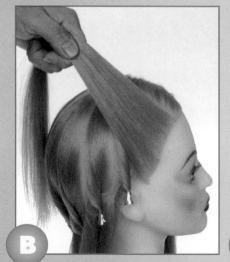

B Begin at the hairline on the right hand side.

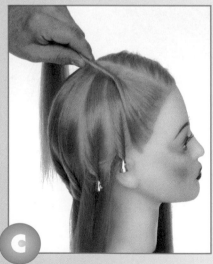

C Twist in a counter-clockwise direction, directing hair toward the crown.

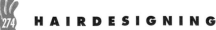

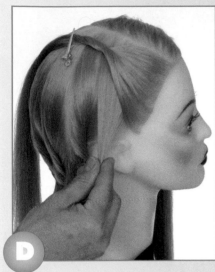

D

After securing the first subsection, pick up the second subsection of hair.

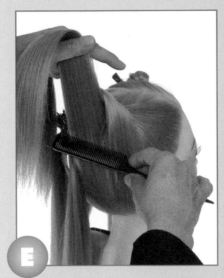

E

Twist the first and second subsections together.

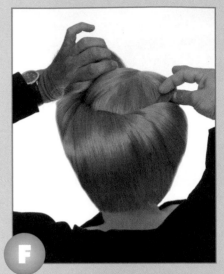

F

Continue working around the head. Twist and join each subsection until the left side is reached.

6

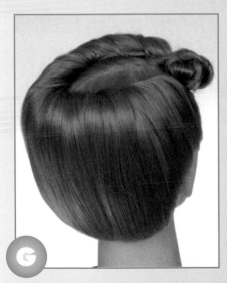

G

Direct the last subsection across the top of the forehead. Tuck ends underneath and secure the style with bobbie pins.

H

Lightly spray and smooth the finished design before adding ornamentation.

I

The completed Halo Twist with retro style ornamentation.

EVALUATION

GRADE

STUDENT'S NAME   ID#

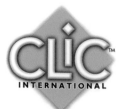

Seven Strand Braid

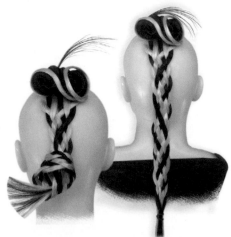

OBJECTIVE

To build manual dexterity by constructing an elaborate seven strand braid.

Seven Strand Braid Variations

TOOLS & MATERIALS

- Neck strip and cape/smock
- Towels
- Pomade or other liquid styling tools

- Styling combs and brushes
- Clips, bobbie pins, and hair pins
- Cleansing and conditioning products

- Client record card/file
- Airformer and/or flat iron
- Small coated elastic bands

- Ornamentation

PROCEDURE

"The client consultation is an important part of your professional service. Be sure to complete this step prior to each client service you provide. Your successful retail sales and customer satisfaction rates depend upon it!"

RETAIL · RE-BOOK · REFERRAL

1. Drape the client in preparation for the service.
2. Thoroughly brush the client's hair to remove knots, tangles and hairspray.
3. Cleanse and condition the hair according to the client's needs. Rinse thoroughly and towel dry. Apply a liquid styling tool. Comb the hair to detangle.
4. Airform the hair if desired (braiding the hair while damp may make it easier to braid).
5. The hair may be flat ironed if it is curly in texture.
6. Perform the style as shown.
7. Follow standard clean-up procedures.
8. Document the client record card/file.

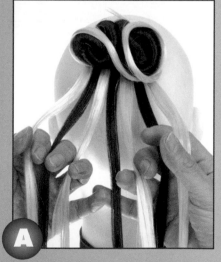

A Separate the hair into seven equal sections, with three strands in the middle and two strands on each side.

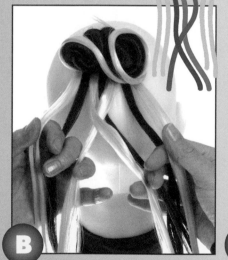

B Start with the three strands from the center section. Cross the middle section's right strand over center and then bring the middle left strand over the new center strand. There will be four strands on the right side and three on the left.

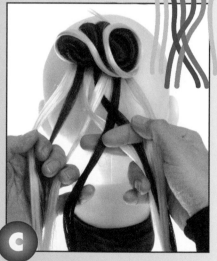

C Working toward the middle, take the inner right strand under and over the next two strands. Four strands are now on the left and three on the right.

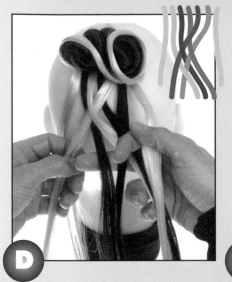

D

Still moving from outside to center, weave the inside left strand under and over the next two strands. Four strands are on the right and three on the left.

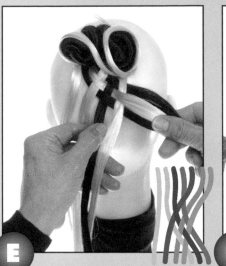

E

Cross the strand on the right outward perimeter over, under, and over the next three strands heading inward. There will now be four strands on the left side.

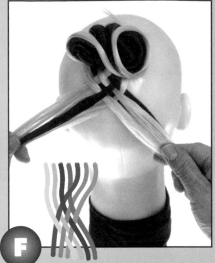

F

Plait the outside left strand over, under, and over the next three strands going toward the center. There will now be four strands on the right side.

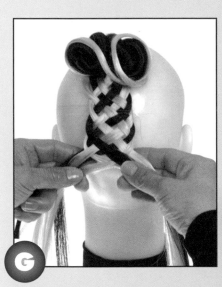

G

Repeat this over/under/over pattern, alternating from right side to left side until complete, always starting with the outside strand and working toward the center.

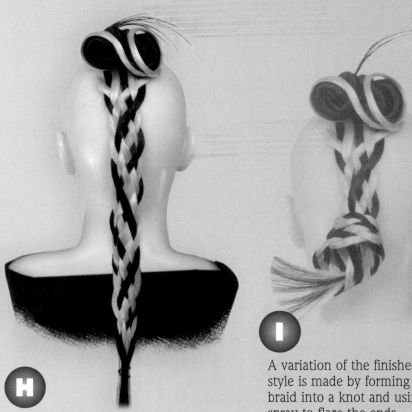

H

Ornamentation adds detail to the finished seven strand braid.

I

A variation of the finished style is made by forming the braid into a knot and using spray to flare the ends.

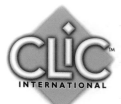

Nine Strand Braid

OBJECTIVE

To craft a basket weave or macramé style nine strand braid, suitable on hair shoulder-length or longer.

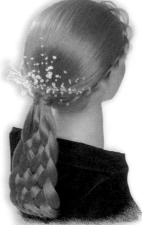

Nine Strand Braid Variation

TOOLS & MATERIALS

- Neck strip and cape/smock
- Towels
- Pomade or other liquid styling tools
- Styling combs and brushes
- Clips, bobbie pins, and hair pins
- Cleansing and conditioning products
- Client record card/file
- Airformer and/or flat iron
- One large and one small elastic band
- Ornamentation

PROCEDURE

"The client consultation is an important part of your professional service. Be sure to complete this step prior to each client service you provide. Your successful retail sales and customer satisfaction rates depend upon it!"

RETAIL · RE-BOOK · REFERRAL

1. Drape the client in preparation for the service.
2. Thoroughly brush the client's hair to remove knots, tangles and hairspray.
3. Cleanse and condition the hair according to the client's needs. Rinse thoroughly and towel dry. Apply a liquid styling tool. Comb the hair to detangle.
4. Airform the hair if desired (braiding the hair while damp may make it easier to braid).
5. The hair may be flat ironed if the hair is of a curly texture.
6. Perform the style as shown.
7. Follow standard clean-up procedures.
8. Document the client record card/file.

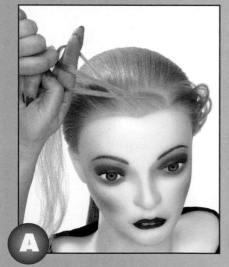

A Make two 3-strand braids in a two inch (5 cm) section on both sides of an off-center parting. The remaining hair is placed in a ponytail at the lower nape area. Wrap a small section of hair around the band and secure underneath with pins.

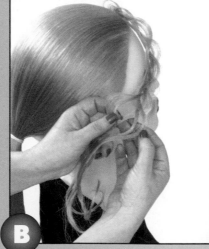

B While creating the 3-strand braid, spread the loops to form a loose, light and airy effect.

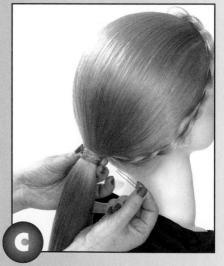

C Place the braid following the perimeter above the ear. Secure braids from both sides around the ponytail at the nape using either a bobbie pin or a hair pin.

Nine Strand Braid

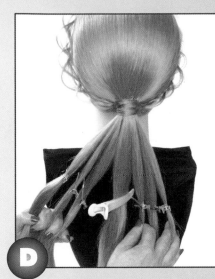

D

Begin making the 9-strand braid by separating the ponytail into three large sections and then dividing them into three smaller subsections. Place a clip on each one for better control and easier identification when incorporating that section into the braided style.

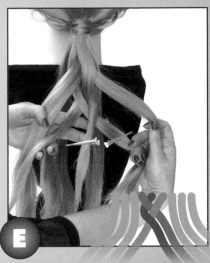

E

Start with the center section. Begin making a regular 3-strand braid by bringing the left strand over the center and then right over center, but then continue the right strand under the next strand to the left. Weave strands toward the center using tension that is firm but not excessive.

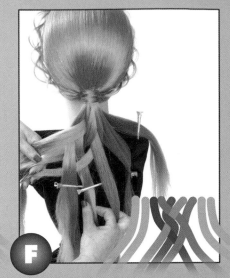

F

Working toward center, cross the left inner strand under then over the next two strands. Repeat the weave with the right middle strand going under and then over the next two strands. Use clips for control and apply a pomade to keep the strands as neat as possible.

6

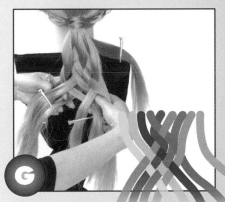

G

The next strand (the middle left) crosses over, under, and over the three strands going toward center. There will now be three strands on each side. Repeat this pattern with the right side. There will be four strands on the left, three on the right. Once the starting point for the under/over/under/over pattern reaches the outside strand, continue to alternate sides until the ponytail ends are reached.

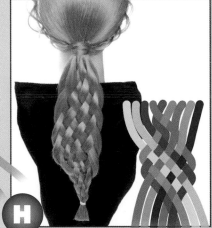

H

The stylist may choose to condense this pattern from nine to five strands and finish with a 3-strand braid. To condense the number of strands in the braid, combine the two outer strands from each side with the strand beside it before continuing the braid pattern.

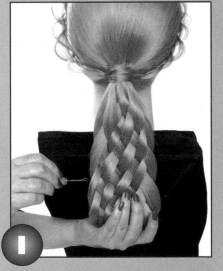

I

Fold the braid under and secure with bobbie pins. The overall look is clean and polished. Change the braid's shape or add ornamentation influenced by your own creativity.

EVALUATION

GRADE   STUDENT'S NAME   ID#

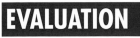

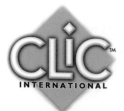

CLiC
INTERNATIONAL

Circular Braid
(3-strand one side pick-up)

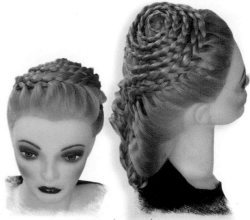

Circular Braid

OBJECTIVE

Create an intricate three strand circular braid with two side braids folded toward the center.

TOOLS & MATERIALS

- Neck strip and cape or smock
- Towels
- Pomade or other liquid styling tools
- Styling combs and brushes
- Bobbie pins and hair pins
- Cleansing and conditioning products
- Client record card/file
- Airformer and/or flat iron
- Small elastic bands
- Clips

PROCEDURE

"The client consultation is an important part of your professional service. Be sure to complete this step prior to each client service you provide. Your successful retail sales and customer satisfaction rates depend upon it!"

RETAIL · RE-BOOK · REFERRAL

1. Drape the client in preparation for the service.
2. Thoroughly brush the client's hair to remove knots, tangles and hairspray.
3. Cleanse and condition the hair according to the client's needs. Rinse thoroughly and towel dry. Apply a liquid styling tool. Comb the hair to detangle.
4. Airform the hair if desired (braiding the hair while damp may make it easier to braid).
5. The hair may be flat ironed if the hair is of a curly texture.
6. Perform the style as shown.
7. Follow standard clean-up procedures.
8. Document the client record card/file.

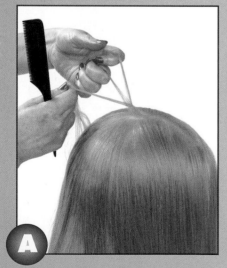

A Place the circular braid by starting a basic 3-strand braid at the center crown area of the head.

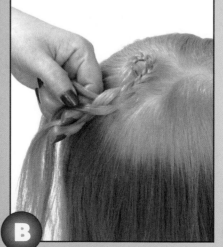

B Add hair into the center from only the right side of the braid, moving in a circular pattern.

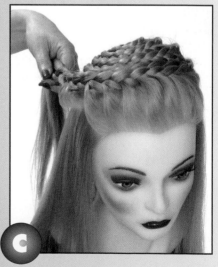

C Continue the braid, picking up hair only on the right side. Move down only where the circle meets. For this style, only the frontal fringe area was included.

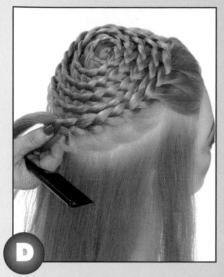

D

The pattern finishes in the occipital area, at the rear center of the head.

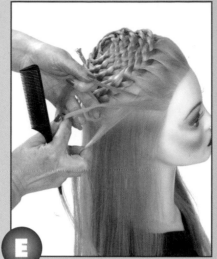

E

After temporarily securing the circular braid with clips, start another 3-strand braid. Using inch wide (2.5 cm) diagonal partings, continue to braid by adding hair only from the outer perimeter (left to center and right to center).

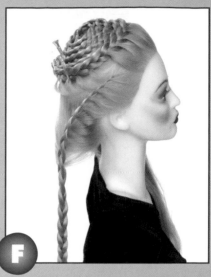

F

Continue the pattern until all hair is incorporated into the braided style. Secure finished side braids with an elastic band when hair runs out in the nape perimeter area.

6

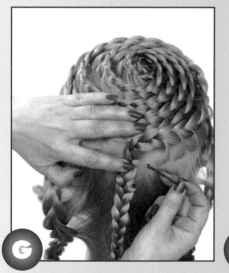

G

Secure the center braid (left over from the circular braid) with bobbie pins in the center of the head.

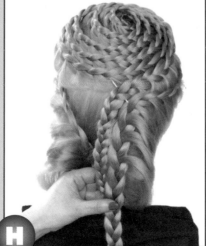

H

The outer braids may now be joined to the braid in the center with bobbie pins. Turn the remaining braid under and secure it to hide the ends.

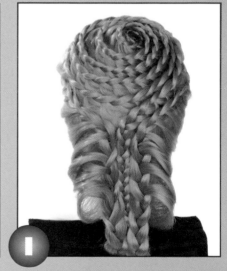

I

Check for balance. The end result depends on the length of the hair and the manner and location in which the braid is turned under. The finished intricate braid does not require ornamentation.

EVALUATION

GRADE

STUDENT'S NAME

ID#

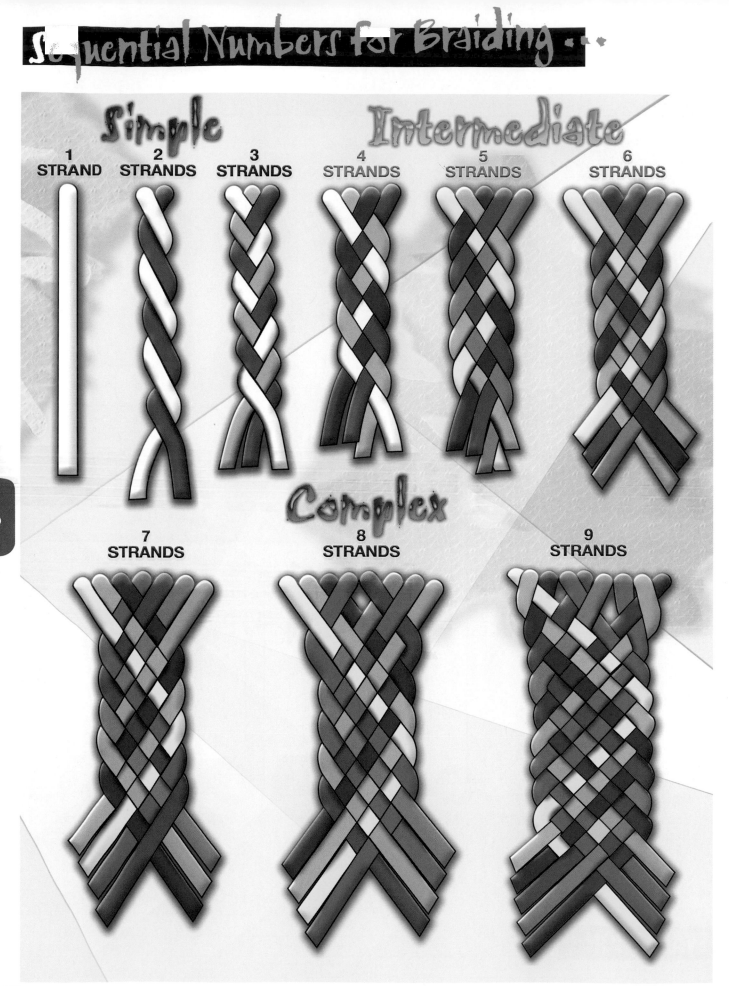

Simple

Intermediate

1 STRAND — **2 STRANDS** — **3 STRANDS** — **4 STRANDS** — **5 STRANDS** — **6 STRANDS**

Complex

7 STRANDS — **8 STRANDS** — **9 STRANDS**

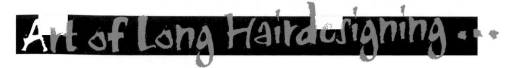

Art of Long Hairdesigning ...

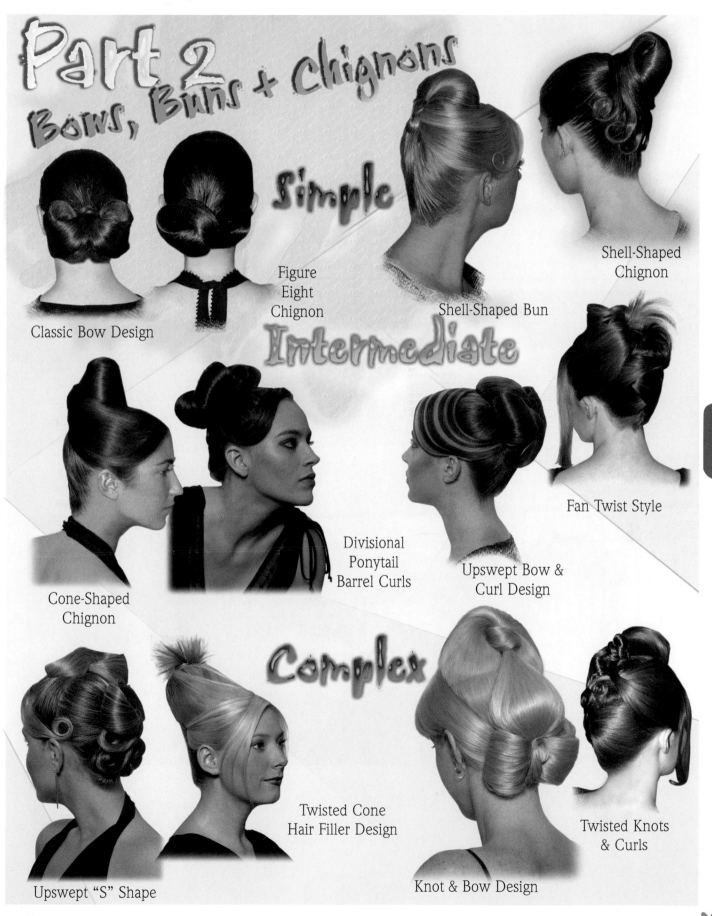

Part 2
Bows, Buns + Chignons

Simple

Classic Bow Design

Figure Eight Chignon

Shell-Shaped Bun

Shell-Shaped Chignon

Intermediate

Cone-Shaped Chignon

Divisional Ponytail Barrel Curls

Upswept Bow & Curl Design

Fan Twist Style

Complex

Upswept "S" Shape

Twisted Cone Hair Filler Design

Knot & Bow Design

Twisted Knots & Curls

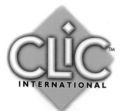

Classic Bow Design

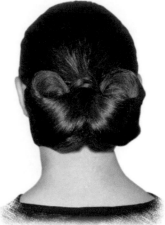

Classic Bow Design

OBJECTIVE

To create a classic bow style design at the nape of the neck that is simple, but has an elegant finish.

TOOLS & MATERIALS

- Neck strip and cape/smock
- Towels
- Finishing spray or other liquid styling tools

- Styling combs and brushes
- Bobbie pins and hair pins
- Cleansing and conditioning products

- Client record card/file
- Airformer and/or flat iron
- One large coated elastic band

- Clips

PROCEDURE

"The client consultation is an important part of your professional service. Be sure to complete this step prior to each client service you provide. Your successful retail sales and customer satisfaction rates depend upon it!"

RETAIL · RE-BOOK · REFERRAL

1. Drape the client in preparation for the service.
2. Thoroughly brush the client's hair to remove knots, tangles and hairspray.
3. Cleanse and condition the hair according to the client's needs. Rinse thoroughly and towel dry.
4. Comb the hair to detangle. Apply an appropriate liquid styling tool, and airform the hair.
5. The hair may be flat ironed if it is curly in texture.
6. Perform the style as shown.
7. Follow standard clean-up procedures.
8. Document the client record card/file.

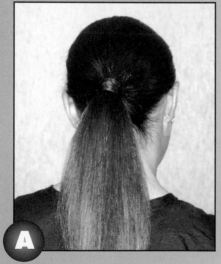

A Brush the hair into a smooth ponytail at the occipital bone and secure it with a large coated elastic band. Wrap a small section of hair around the band and secure underneath with pins.

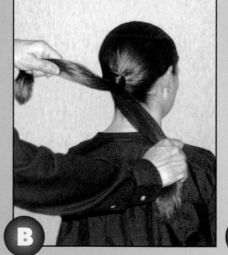

B Divide the ponytail vertically into two equal sections.

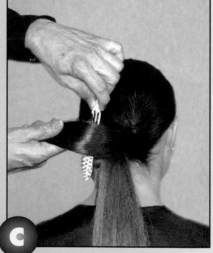

C Lightly lace the first section of hair from base to ends. This creates control for shaping the style.

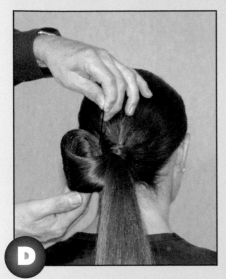

D

Create a vertical barrel curl with the hair. Secure by placing bobbie pins from both directions to interlock for strength at the inside of the barrel curl.

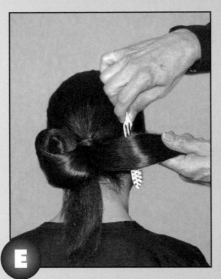

E

Repeat the two previous steps for the opposite barrel curl section.

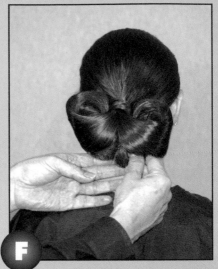

F

Tuck the remaining hair under the barrel curls, and secure with bobbie/hair pins.

6

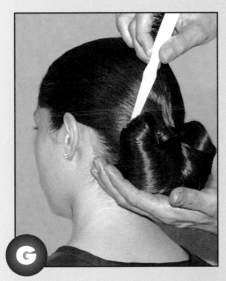

G

Smooth and polish all loose hair with the end of the brush before spraying into place.

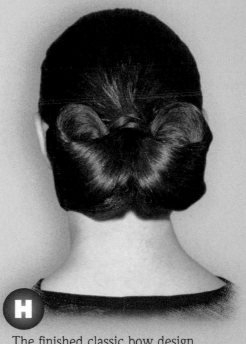

H

The finished classic bow design.

EVALUATION

GRADE

STUDENT'S NAME

ID#

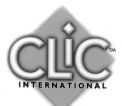

Figure Eight Chignon

OBJECTIVE

To create an elegant, figure eight chignon at the nape of the neck.

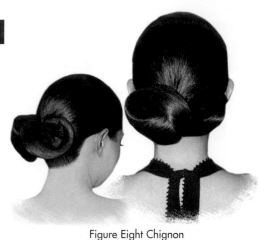

Figure Eight Chignon

TOOLS & MATERIALS

- Neck strip and cape/smock
- Towels
- Finishing spray or other liquid styling tools
- Styling combs and brushes
- Bobbie pins and hair pins
- Cleansing and conditioning products
- Client record card/file
- Airformer and/or flat iron
- One large coated elastic band
- Clips

PROCEDURE

"The client consultation is an important part of your professional service. Be sure to complete this step prior to each client service you provide. Your successful retail sales and customer satisfaction rates depend upon it!"

RETAIL · RE-BOOK · REFERRAL

1. Drape the client in preparation for the service.
2. Thoroughly brush the client's hair to remove knots, tangles and hairspray.
3. Cleanse and condition the hair according to the client's needs. Rinse thoroughly and towel dry.
4. Comb the hair to detangle. Apply an appropriate liquid styling tool, and airform the hair.
5. The hair may be flat ironed if it is curly in texture.
6. Perform the style as shown.
7. Follow standard clean-up procedures.
8. Document the client record card/file.

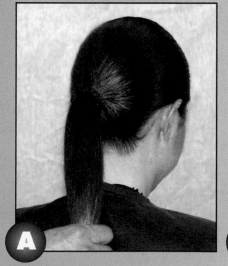

A Make a ponytail just below the occipital bone. Smooth the hair carefully and secure with a large coated elastic band.

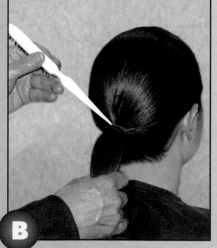

B Wrap a very small portion of hair around the elastic band, covering it for a more elegant look. Spray lightly.

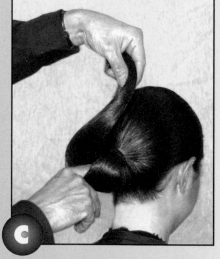

C Take the entire ponytail in the left hand. Place the right hand index finger at the base of the ponytail to form a loop. Wrap hair under and over fingers in a clockwise direction to start a figure eight.

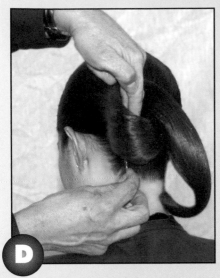

D

Secure the hair from the inside of the wrap with interlocking bobbie pins. Lightly spray to secure the style.

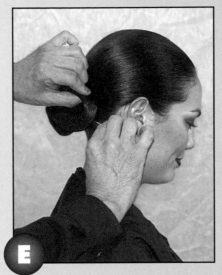

E

Complete the figure eight with the remaining hair. Secure with two interlocking bobbie pins.

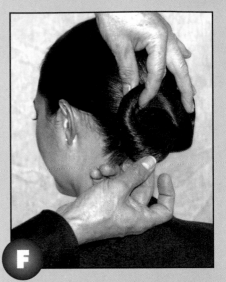

F

Smooth and polish all loose hair with the end of the brush before spraying into place.

G

Rear view of the finished elegant figure eight chignon.

H

The figure eight chignon in profile.

EVALUATION

GRADE STUDENT'S NAME ID#

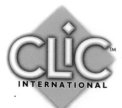

Shell-Shaped Bun

OBJECTIVE To create a traditional, shell-shaped bun in the crown area.

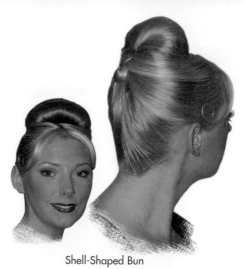

Shell-Shaped Bun

TOOLS & MATERIALS

- Neck strip and cape/smock
- Cleansing and conditioning products
- Towels
- Client record card/file
- Finishing spray or other liquid styling tools
- Airformer and/or flat iron
- Styling combs and brushes
- One large coated elastic band
- Bobbie pins and hair pins
- Clips

PROCEDURE

"The client consultation is an important part of your professional service. Be sure to complete this step prior to each client service you provide. Your successful retail sales and customer satisfaction rates depend upon it!"

RETAIL • RE-BOOK
REFERRAL

1. Drape the client in preparation for the service.
2. Thoroughly brush the client's hair to remove knots, tangles and hairspray.
3. Cleanse and condition the hair according to the client's needs. Rinse thoroughly and towel dry.
4. Comb the hair to detangle. Apply an appropriate liquid styling tool, and airform the hair.
5. The hair may be flat ironed if it is curly in texture.
6. Perform the style as shown.
7. Follow standard clean-up procedures.
8. Document the client record card/file.

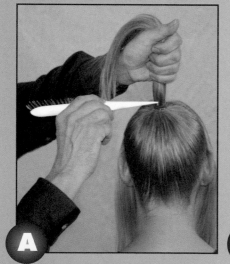

A Section hair from ear to ear. Create a ponytail at the base of the crown.

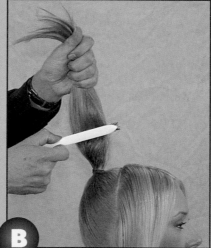

B Lightly lace the ponytail from base to ends.

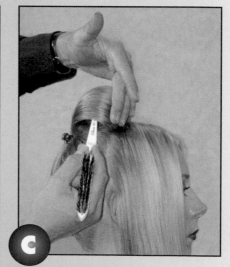

C Make a smooth bun at the back of the head by spreading the hair out to form a shell shape.

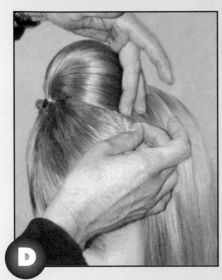

D

Secure the style with hair pins on both ends of the shell-shaped bun.

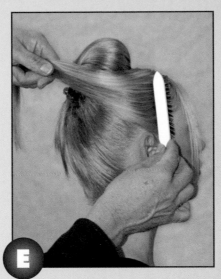

E

Brush one side section back, wrapping the ends around the elastic band, and tucking the ends underneath. Secure the hair with bobbie pins just below the bun.

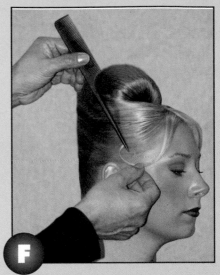

F

Brush the other side section back, loop around the previous placement, and fasten securely. Hair may be left out at the fringe area to create a special effect. Use finishing spray to hold the detail in place.

6

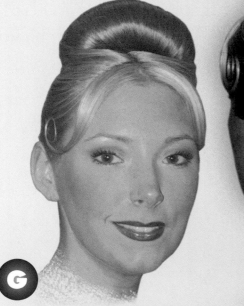

G

A finished traditional shell-shaped bun.

H

The full back view shows how the interlocked side strands conceal the base of the shell.

EVALUATION

GRADE

STUDENT'S NAME

ID#

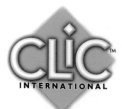
Shell-Shaped Chignon

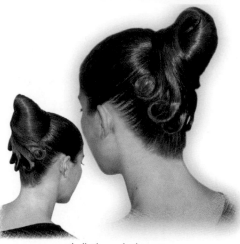

OBJECTIVE To create a dramatic, shell-shaped chignon in the crown and occipital areas.

Shell-Shaped Chignon

TOOLS & MATERIALS

- Neck strip and cape/smock
- Towels
- Finishing spray or other liquid styling tools
- Styling combs and brushes
- Bobbie pins and hair pins
- Cleansing and conditioning products
- Client record card/file
- Airformer and/or flat iron
- One large coated elastic band
- Clips

PROCEDURE

"The client consultation is an important part of your professional service. Be sure to complete this step prior to each client service you provide. Your successful retail sales and customer satisfaction rates depend upon it!"

RETAIL · RE-BOOK · REFERRAL

1. Drape the client in preparation for the service.
2. Thoroughly brush the client's hair to remove knots, tangles and hairspray.
3. Cleanse and condition the hair according to the client's needs. Rinse thoroughly and towel dry.
4. Comb the hair to detangle. Apply an appropriate liquid styling tool, and airform the hair.
5. The hair may be flat ironed if it is curly in texture.
6. Perform the style as shown.
7. Follow standard clean-up procedures.
8. Document the client record card/file.

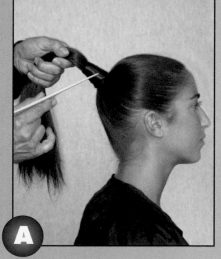

A

Brush hair into a smooth, neat ponytail just below the crown of the head. Wrap a very small section of hair around the base to cover the elastic hair band.

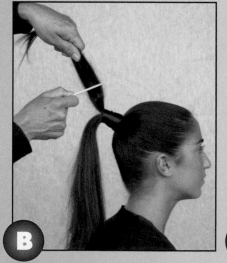

B

Separate the hair horizontally into two equal sections. French lace each section lightly from base to ends.

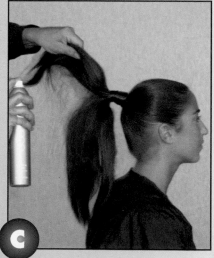

C

Lightly spray each section, and then gently smooth the hair while rejoining the sections.

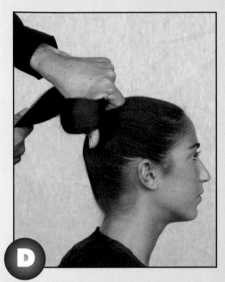

D

Place a thumb on the crown at a 90-degree angle. Wrap the hair around the thumb in a counterclockwise direction.

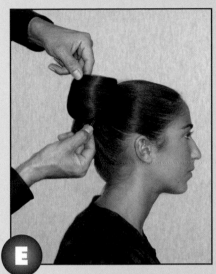

E

Secure the roll on the inside with two interlocking bobbie pins. Once the hair is taut and secure, pull lightly with thumbs and index fingers to create a cone effect.

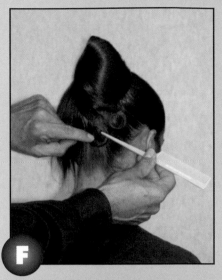

F

With the remaining ends of the hair, make five pin curls going along the bottom of the roll. Secure each with a hair pin. Smooth and polish all loose hair with a tail comb before spraying into place.

6

G

The finished dramatic shell-shaped chignon.

H

Another angle showing the shell-shaped detailing.

EVALUATION

GRADE　　　　STUDENT'S NAME　　　　　　　　ID#

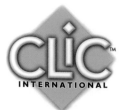

Cone-Shaped Chignon

OBJECTIVE

To create a timeless, cone-shaped chignon in the crown area.

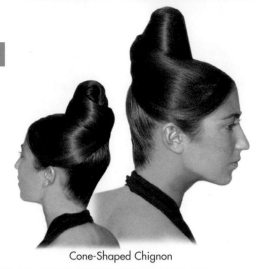

Cone-Shaped Chignon

TOOLS & MATERIALS

- Neck strip and cape/smock
- Towels
- Finishing spray or other liquid styling tools

- Styling combs and brushes
- Clips, bobbie pins, and hair pins
- Cleansing and conditioning products

- Client record card/file
- Airformer and/or flat iron
- One large coated elastic band

- One Scrunchi™ hair band or other filler

PROCEDURE

"The client consultation is an important part of your professional service. Be sure to complete this step prior to each client service you provide. Your successful retail sales and customer satisfaction rates depend upon it!"

RETAIL · RE-BOOK · REFERRAL

1. Drape the client in preparation for the service.
2. Thoroughly brush the client's hair to remove knots, tangles and hairspray.
3. Cleanse and condition the hair according to the client's needs. Rinse thoroughly and towel dry.
4. Comb the hair to detangle. Apply an appropriate liquid styling tool, and airform the hair.
5. The hair may be flat ironed if it is curly in texture.
6. Perform the style as shown.
7. Follow standard clean-up procedures.
8. Document the client record card/file.

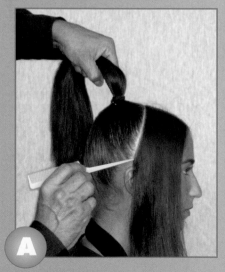

A Section the hair from ear to ear. Brush the back section into a ponytail at the top part of the crown.

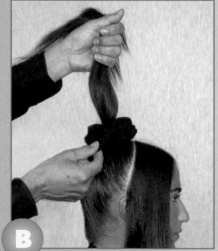

B Place a Scrunchi™ hair band around the ponytail to act as a hair filler.

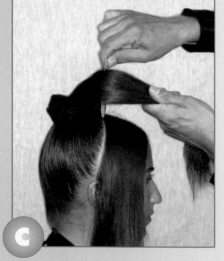

C French lace the ponytail lightly from base to ends. Wrap hair around the Scrunchi™ in a counter-clockwise direction to create a cone shape.

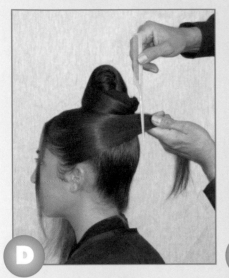

D

Take one front side section and wrap the hair around to the opposite side. Tuck the ends under the chignon. Secure with bobbie pins.

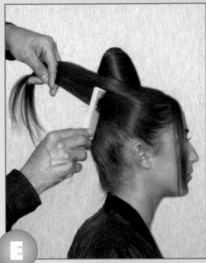

E

Repeat the previous step using hair from the opposite side.

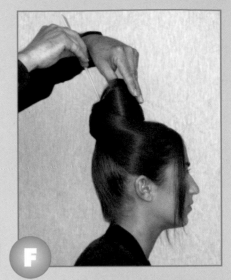

F

Smooth and polish all loose hair with a tail comb before spraying into place.

6

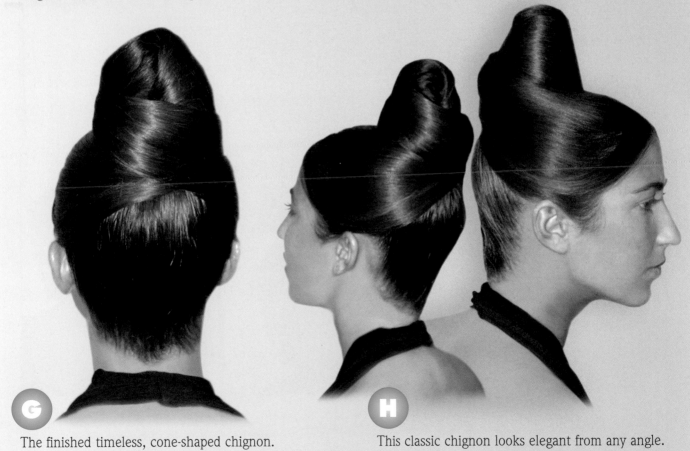

G

The finished timeless, cone-shaped chignon.

H

This classic chignon looks elegant from any angle.

EVALUATION

GRADE

STUDENT'S NAME

ID#

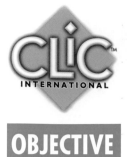

Divisional Ponytail Barrel Curls

OBJECTIVE

To create an upswept barrel curl design in the crown area.

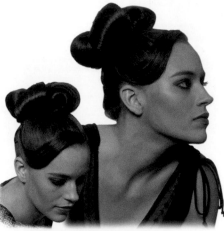

Divisional Ponytail Barrel Curls

TOOLS & MATERIALS

- Neck strip and cape/smock
- Towels
- Finishing spray or other liquid styling tools
- Styling combs and brushes
- Bobbie pins and hair pins
- Cleansing and conditioning products
- Client record card/file
- Airformer and/or flat iron
- One large coated elastic ban
- Clips

PROCEDURE

"The client consultation is an important part of your professional service. Be sure to complete this step prior to each client service you provide. Your successful retail sales and customer satisfaction rates depend upon it!"

RETAIL · RE-BOOK · REFERRAL

1. Drape the client in preparation for the service.
2. Thoroughly brush the client's hair to remove knots, tangles and hairspray.
3. Cleanse and condition the hair according to the client's needs. Rinse thoroughly and towel dry.
4. Comb the hair to detangle. Apply an appropriate liquid styling tool, and airform the hair.
5. The hair may be flat ironed if it is curly in texture.
6. Perform the style as shown.
7. Follow standard clean-up procedures.
8. Document the client record card/file.

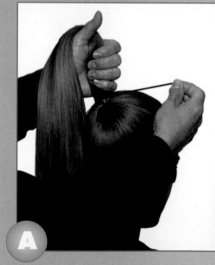

A Create a small fringe area at the front on one side, and form it into a counter-clockwise, flat, full stem pin curl. Use a clip to secure the curl before brushing all remaining hair into a ponytail at the crown area. Use a coated elastic band to secure the hair.

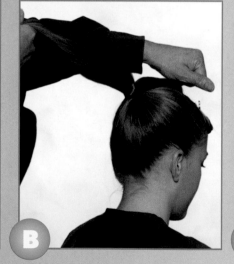

B Separate the ponytail into two sections, with one thick and the other smaller. Wrap the smaller section of hair around the ponytail's base to cover the elastic hair band.

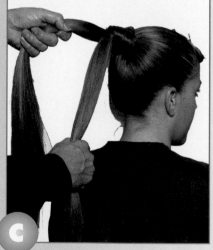

C Divide the thicker ponytail section vertically into two equal subsections.

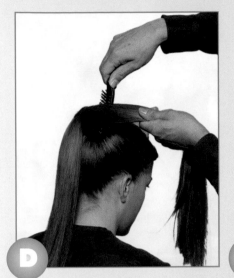

D Lightly lace each subsection from base to ends.

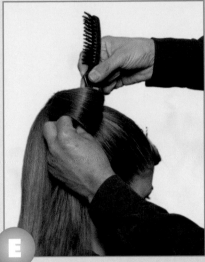

E Using the end of a brush as a center axis, roll the hair into two barrel curls, leaving the ends of the hair out.

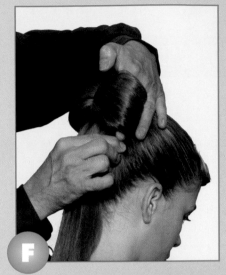

F Vertically interlock the bobbie pins in the center to secure the barrel curls.

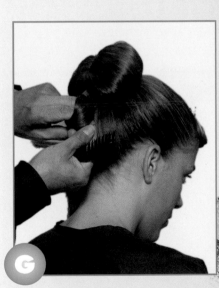

G Make one or more flat, rolled curls below the barrel curls with the remaining hair ends. If the hair is shorter, a "C" shape on the end will suit the style. Secure with hairpins.

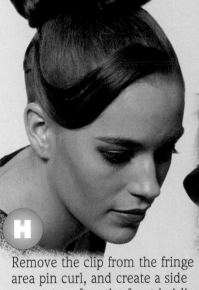

H Remove the clip from the fringe area pin curl, and create a side sweep to soften the front hairline. Secure the ends of the fringe behind the ear with a hairpin.

I The finished barrel curl design looks interesting from any angle.

EVALUATION

GRADE   STUDENT'S NAME   ID#

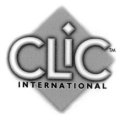

Upswept Bow + Curl Design

OBJECTIVE

To create a fashionable color-enhanced bow and curl design.

Upswept Bow & Curl Design

TOOLS & MATERIALS

- Neck strip and cape or smock
- Towels
- Finishing spray or other liquid styling tools
- Styling combs and brushes
- Bobbie pins and hair pins
- Cleansing and conditioning products
- Client record card/file
- Airformer and/or flat iron
- One large coated elastic band
- Clips

PROCEDURE

"The client consultation is an important part of your professional service. Be sure to complete this step prior to each client service you provide. Your successful retail sales and customer satisfaction rates depend upon it!"

RETAIL • RE-BOOK • REFERRAL

1. Drape the client in preparation for the service.
2. Thoroughly brush the client's hair to remove knots, tangles and hairspray.
3. Cleanse and condition the hair according to the client's needs. Rinse thoroughly and towel dry.
4. Comb the hair to detangle. Apply an appropriate liquid styling tool, and airform the hair.
5. The hair may be flat ironed if it is curly in texture.
6. Perform the style as shown.
7. Follow standard clean-up procedures.
8. Document the client record card/file.

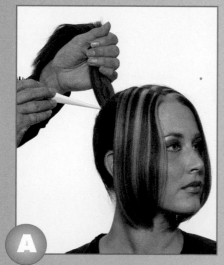

A Section the hair from ear to ear. Create a ponytail at the crown, secured with hair elastic.

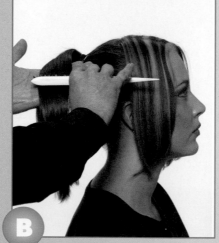

B Divide the ponytail into three equal sections.

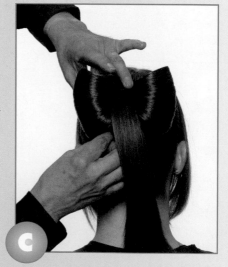

C Make a barrel curl on one side and secure it vertically in the style with interlocking bobbie pins. Make a second barrel curl in the same manner on the opposite side.

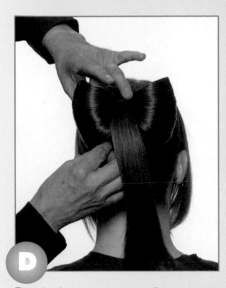

D Divide the center ponytail into two horizontal sections. Above the bow design, use the top section to make the beginning of the letter "S." Form the lower portion of the letter "S" below the bow using the bottom section of the center ponytail. Finish with a pin curl on each end, secured with bobbie pins and hairpins.

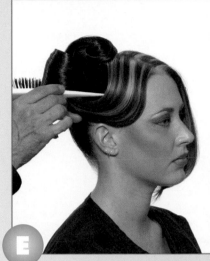

E Divide the front section in two. Sweep the hair back above the ear, creating an "S" shape. Secure with bobbie pins underneath the style in the back.

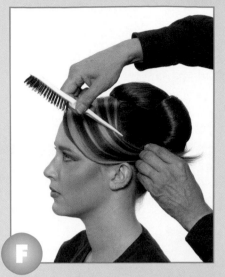

F Sweep the opposite front section back, creating a soft curve. Smooth the hair and spray while working. Secure the section underneath the bow design in the occipital area with bobbie pins.

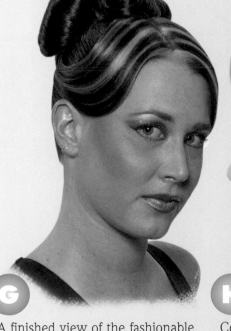

G A finished view of the fashionable bow and curl design.

H Color enhances the bow and curl design, requiring no further ornamentation.

EVALUATION

GRADE STUDENT'S NAME ID#

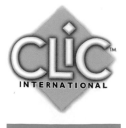
Fan Twist Style

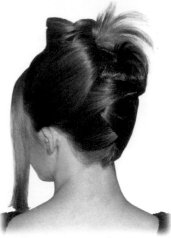

Fan Twist Style

OBJECTIVE

To create a contemporary fan twist design in the crown and occipital areas.

TOOLS & MATERIALS

- Neck strip and cape/smock
- Towels
- Finishing spray or other liquid styling tools
- Styling combs and brushes
- Cleansing and conditioning products
- Client record card/file
- Airformer and/or flat iron
- Clips, bobbie pins, and hair pins

PROCEDURE

"The client consultation is an important part of your professional service. Be sure to complete this step prior to each client service you provide. Your successful retail sales and customer satisfaction rates depend upon it!"

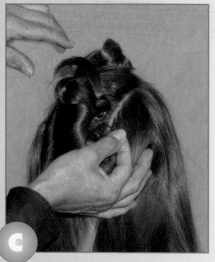

RETAIL RE-BOOK REFERRAL

1. Drape the client in preparation for the service.
2. Thoroughly brush the client's hair to remove knots, tangles and hairspray.
3. Cleanse and condition the hair according to the client's needs. Rinse thoroughly and towel dry.
4. Comb the hair to detangle. Apply an appropriate liquid styling tool, and airform the hair.
5. The hair may be flat ironed if it is curly in texture.
6. Perform the style as shown.
7. Follow standard clean-up procedures.
8. Document the client record card/file.

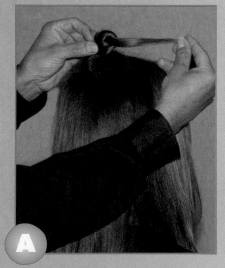

A Make a two inch (5 cm) diamond section at the crown of the head. Create a knot leaving the ends out.

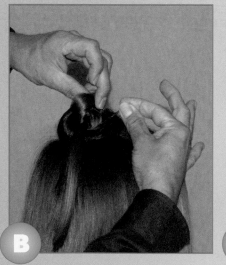

B Secure the knot with bobbie pins interlocked at the base.

C Continue making diamond sections about twice as large as the first. At approximately the occipital level, softly turn the hair into a twist. Create a knot near the ends, and secure with bobbie pins and hairpins.

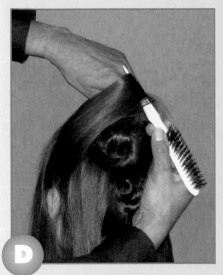

D Continue by making diagonal partings and softly twisting the hair toward the scalp. Secure the twist with bobbie pins and hair pins.

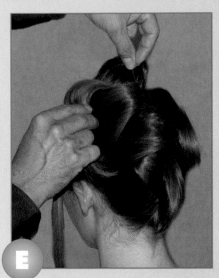

E Leaving out a few ends to make a fan effect, tuck the rest into the style. Make sure the fan size is in proportion to the head shape.

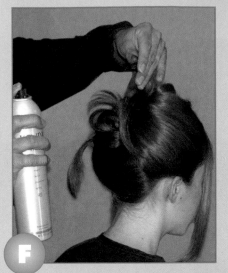

F Spray and set the fan shape into place.

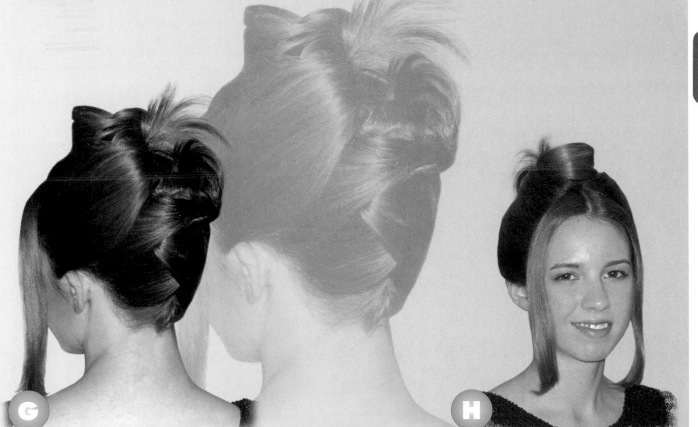

G A contemporary fan twist style.

H Front view of the style. A little hair was left to frame the face.

EVALUATION

GRADE

STUDENT'S NAME   ID#

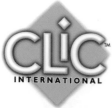

COMPLEX LAB PROJECT

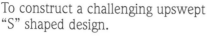

Upswept "S" Shape

OBJECTIVE To construct a challenging upswept "S" shaped design.

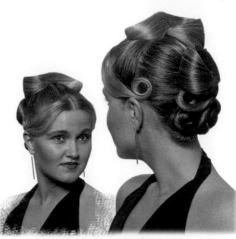

Upswept "S" Shape

TOOLS & MATERIALS

- Neck strip and cape/smock
- Towels
- Finishing spray or other liquid styling tools

- Styling combs and brushes
- Bobbie pins and hair pins
- Cleansing and conditioning products

- Client record card/file
- Airformer and/or flat iron
- Three large coated elastic bands

- Clips

PROCEDURE

"The client consultation is an important part of your professional service. Be sure to complete this step prior to each client service you provide. Your successful retail sales and customer satisfaction rates depend upon it!"

RETAIL RE-BOOK REFERRAL

1. Drape the client in preparation for the service.
2. Thoroughly brush the client's hair to remove knots, tangles and hairspray.
3. Cleanse and condition the hair according to the client's needs. Rinse thoroughly and towel dry.
4. Comb the hair to detangle. Apply an appropriate liquid styling tool, and airform the hair.
5. The hair may be flat ironed if it is curly in texture.
6. Perform the style as shown.
7. Follow standard clean-up procedures.
8. Document the client record card/file.

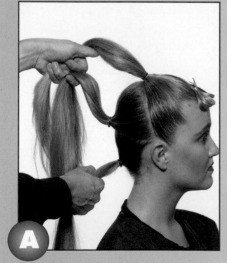

A Section the hair into three ponytail sections: one at the top of the crown, one at the occipital bone, and one at the lower part of the nape. Create a frontal fringe area with a one inch (2.5 cm) center part.

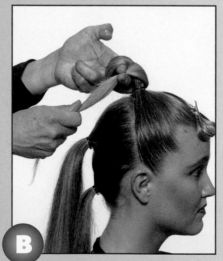

B Ribbon hair over and under index and middle fingers to create a loose knot, leaving ends out.

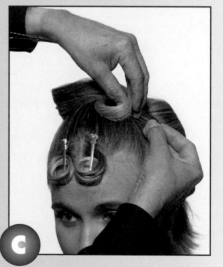

C Curve the ends in a clockwise direction to form the base of an "S" pattern, and secure with hair pins and bobbie pins. On either side of the part in the fringe area, place one flat, full stem pin curl. Rotate the pin curl directions to face each other at the part, with the right hand curl moving in a clockwise direction, and the left side pin curl moving counter-clockwise.

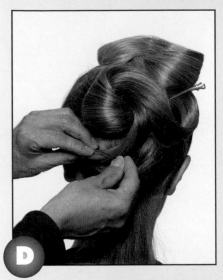

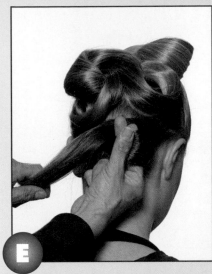

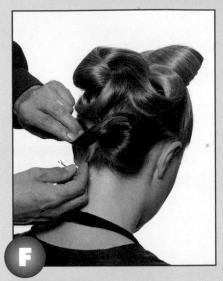

D Use the second ponytail section to form another loose knot, leaving the ends out. Secure with bobbie pins. The ends are coiled in a clockwise direction and secured with hairpins.

E With the last ponytail section at the nape, twist the hair into a figure "8" shape and tuck the ends securely underneath.

F As a final touch, smooth and secure loose ends as necessary using hairspray, bobbie pins or hairpins.

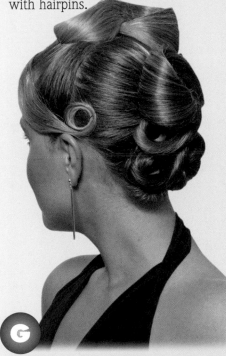

G Unfasten and redirect each pin curl from the fringe area along the side of the head. Secure the ends with hair pins to partially cover the part lines at the ears.

H The finished upswept "S" shaped style.

EVALUATION

GRADE

STUDENT'S NAME

ID#

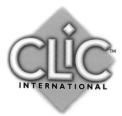

COMPLEX LAB PROJECT

Twisted Cone Hair Filler Design

OBJECTIVE To create a twisted, conical design using a hair filler to enhance volume.

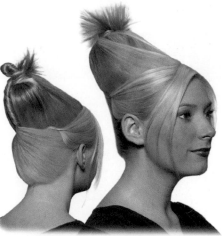

Twisted Cone Hair Filler Design

TOOLS & MATERIALS

- Neck strip and cape/smock
- Towels
- Finishing spray or other liquid styling tools
- Styling combs and brushes
- Clips, bobbie pins, and hair pins
- Cleansing and conditioning products
- Client record card/file
- Airformer and/or flat iron
- One large coated elastic band
- Hair fillers

PROCEDURE

"The client consultation is an important part of your professional service. Be sure to complete this step prior to each client service you provide. Your successful retail sales and customer satisfaction rates depend upon it!"

RETAIL · RE-BOOK · REFERRAL

1. Drape the client in preparation for the service.
2. Thoroughly brush the client's hair to remove knots, tangles and hairspray.
3. Cleanse and condition the hair according to the client's needs. Rinse thoroughly and towel dry.
4. Comb the hair to detangle. Apply an appropriate liquid styling tool, and airform the hair.
5. The hair may be flat ironed if it is curly in texture.
6. Perform the style as shown.
7. Follow standard clean-up procedures.
8. Document the client record card/file.

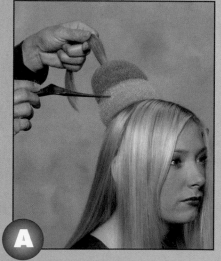

A Make a side parting, and then divide the hair across the top from ear to ear. Create a ponytail in the back crown with a three inch (7.5 cm) semi-circular section. Stack two hair fillers around the ponytail.

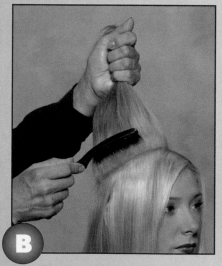

B Make a larger four inch (10 cm) circular section around the ponytail and brush the hair over the fillers. Merge this hair with the ponytail hair.

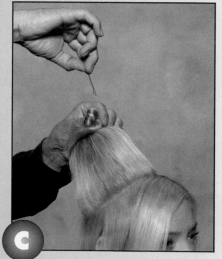

C Twist the ends of the hair covering the fillers. As it twists into a coil on top of the fillers, make a knot and secure with two hair pins.

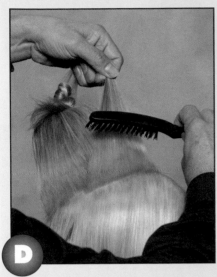

D

Working with the front section of the hair, make a two inch (5 cm) diagonal section on the top, approximately one inch (2.5 cm) from the front hairline. Smooth the hair up and over to the opposite side. This will create a crisscross look for the front of the style. Wrap the section up and around the filler.

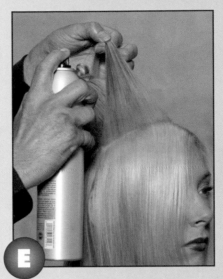

E

Use aerosol hairspray 12 inches (30 cm) from the head to help create the smooth finish of this design. (Pump action spray is too wet for this technique.)

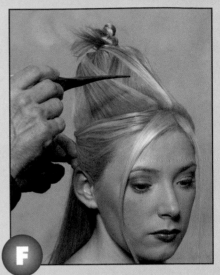

F

In order to create a crisscross effect, roll the back section in one direction and the front section in the opposite direction.

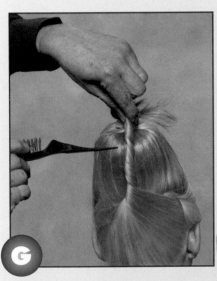

G

Gather all the nape area hair and twist tightly, knotting the strand at the end. Secure with pins, and choose to leave the ends either in or out.

H

The finished twisted cone design.

6

EVALUATION

GRADE

STUDENT'S NAME

ID#

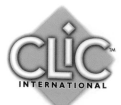

Twisted Knot + Curls

OBJECTIVE
To create an inverted triangle twist design with knots and curls.

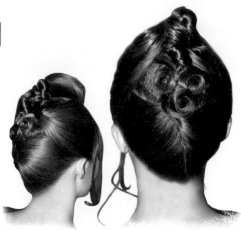

Twisted Knot & Curls

TOOLS & MATERIALS

- Neck strip and cape/smock
- Towels
- Finishing spray or other liquid styling tools
- Styling combs and brushes
- Cleansing and conditioning products
- Client record card/file
- Airformer and/or flat iron
- Clips, bobbie pins, and hair pins

PROCEDURE
"The client consultation is an important part of your professional service. Be sure to complete this step prior to each client service you provide. Your successful retail sales and customer satisfaction rates depend upon it!"

RETAIL RE-BOOK REFERRAL

1. Drape the client in preparation for the service.
2. Thoroughly brush the client's hair to remove knots, tangles and hairspray.
3. Cleanse and condition the hair according to the client's needs. Rinse thoroughly and towel dry.
4. Comb the hair to detangle. Apply an appropriate liquid styling tool, and airform the hair.
5. The hair may be flat ironed if it is curly in texture.
6. Perform the style as shown.
7. Follow standard clean-up procedures.
8. Document the client record card/file.

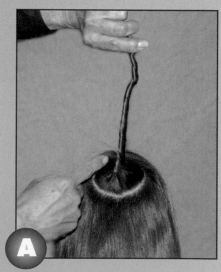

A Start with a classic center part. Make a 3 inch (7.5 cm) circular section in the crown area. Twist the hair very tightly all the way to the end.

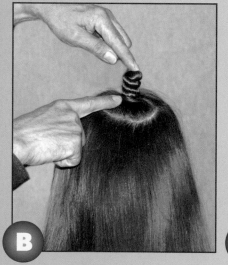

B Create a Zulu knot by continuing to twist the hair in a clockwise direction. Secure with bobbie pins at the base.

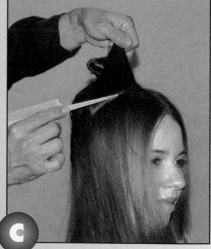

C Make another circular section about 2 inches (5 cm) wide surrounding the Zulu knot.

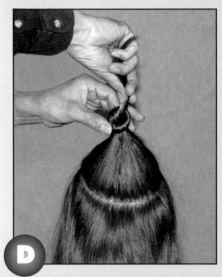

D

Brush the hair smoothly and knot in the middle, using the Zulu knot as a hair filler. Pin the knot securely in place, leaving the ends of the hair out.

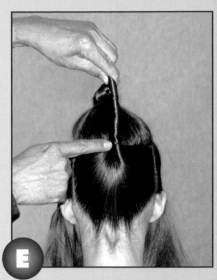

E

Part the hair at the ears, dividing the front section from the back. Brush to smooth the entire back section, and twist the hair while lifting the roll toward the crown. Continue twisting all the way to the ends. Form a loop with the ends, and secure with a bobbie pin.

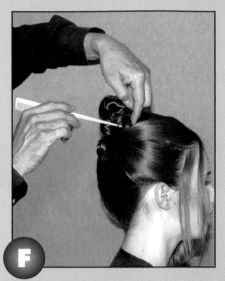

F

Select intermittent strands around the front hairline to leave out and frame the face. Lightly lace the front section on both sides of the part, smooth the sides upward and back toward the center of the occipital.

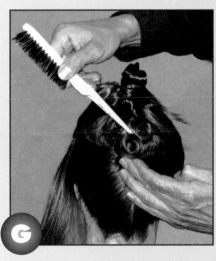

G

Separate both side sections into two strands. Loop one strand on each side into a pin curl rotating away from center going upward. The other strand from each side is formed into a pin curl loop rotating away from center and facing downward toward the neckline, creating an inverted triangle. Secure each pin curl with a hair pin.

H

The finished twisted knot and curls design.

EVALUATION

GRADE   STUDENT'S NAME   ID#

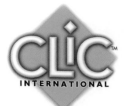

COMPLEX LAB PROJECT

Knot + Bow Design

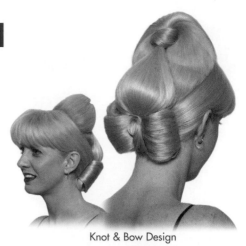

Knot & Bow Design

OBJECTIVE

To create a whimsical knot and bow design in the crown and nape areas.

TOOLS & MATERIALS

- Neck strip and cape/smock
- Towels
- Finishing spray or other liquid styling tools
- Styling combs and brushes
- Bobbie pins and hair pins
- Cleansing and conditioning products
- Client record card/file
- Airformer and/or flat iron
- One large coated elastic band
- Hair clips or clamps

PROCEDURE

"The client consultation is an important part of your professional service. Be sure to complete this step prior to each client service you provide. Your successful retail sales and customer satisfaction rates depend upon it!"

RETAIL · RE-BOOK · REFERRAL

1. Drape the client in preparation for the service.
2. Thoroughly brush the client's hair to remove knots, tangles and hairspray.
3. Cleanse and condition the hair according to the client's needs. Rinse thoroughly and towel dry.
4. Comb the hair to detangle. Apply an appropriate liquid styling tool, and airform the hair.
5. The hair may be flat ironed if it is curly in texture.
6. Perform the style as shown.
7. Follow standard clean-up procedures.
8. Document the client record card/file.

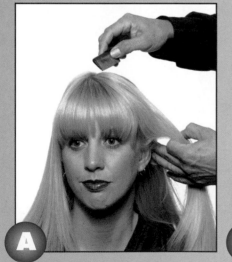

A Leaving a fringe in front, part the first section from ear to ear.

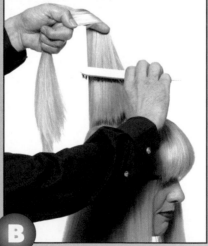

B Make a 4 inch (10 cm) circular section on the crown. Lightly lace the hair, directing it straight up into 90-degrees.

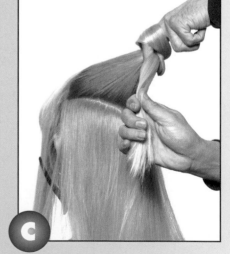

C Create a knot mid-shaft, about 4 inches (10 cm) from the scalp.

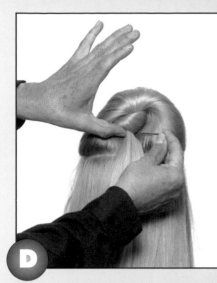

D Loosely fold the knot into the base and secure with bobbie pins, creating height for the style. Leave the ends of the hair out.

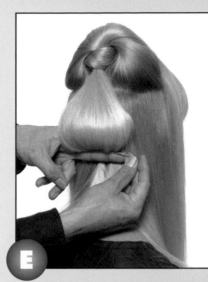

E While holding the hair at the mid-shaft, use your index finger to find the indentation of the occipital bone. Let the hair hang loose and push up about 1 inch (2.5 cm). Secure with bobbie pins, pinning the ends out of the way to later create the center loop of the bow.

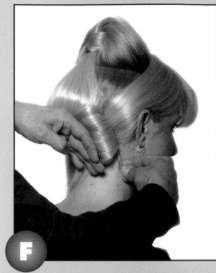

F Pull the sides back and downward. Without lifting, bring remaining hair in a ponytail at the nape of the neck and secure with an elastic band. Divide the ponytail in half. French lace one section lightly toward the face. Grasp the hair about 2 inches (5 cm) from the ends, roll the hair and secure the roll directly behind the ear with interlocking bobbie pins. Repeat on other side.

6

The finished knot and bow design in profile.

H Take the remaining small section and attach a bobbie pin approximately 1 inch (2.5 cm) from the ends. Form the hair ends into a loop, and secure with hair pins in the center of the two rolls to complete the design.

EVALUATION

GRADE

STUDENT'S NAME

ID#

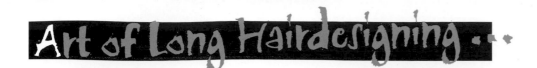
Ornamental combs

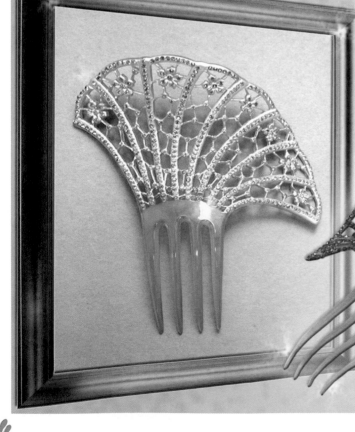

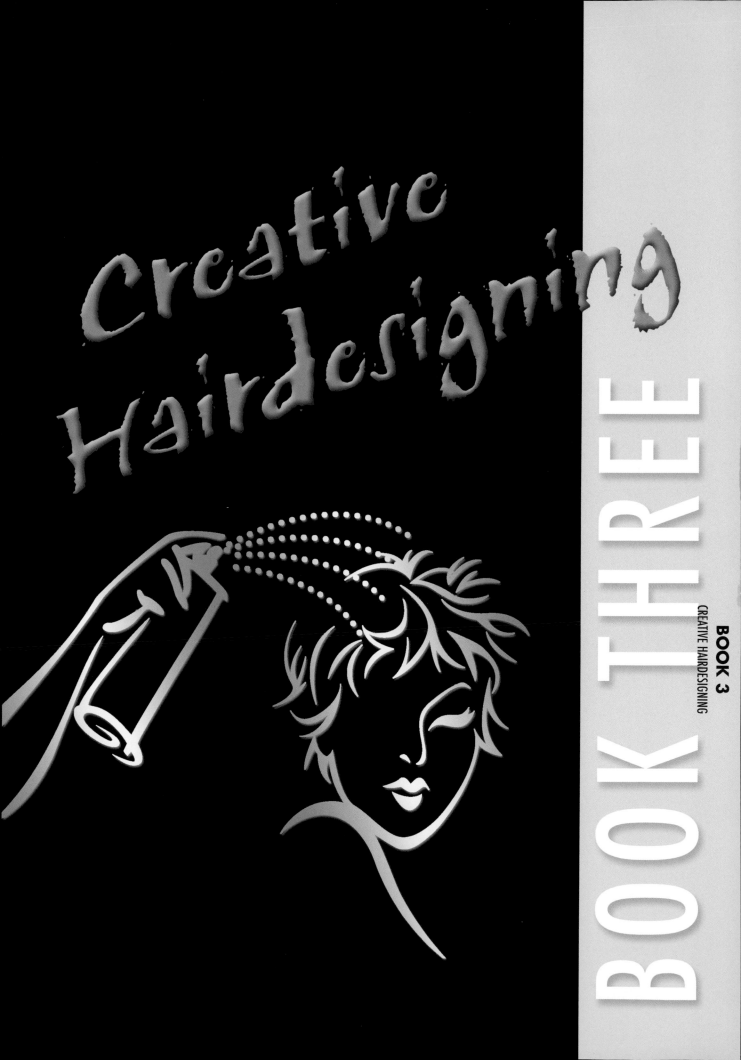

scrunching

curling

setting

smoothing

innovate

styling

lacing

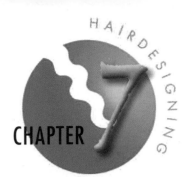

Art of Finishing

FINISHING

 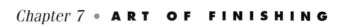

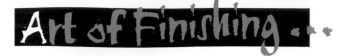

Art of Finishing
LAB PROJECTS

Simple

Intermediate

Complex

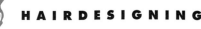

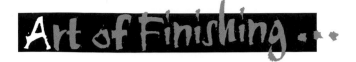

Art of Finishing...

Hairdesign *is the key to success in our industry. All clients receiving hair services will have to be finished in some way in order to leave the salon looking their best. If you can create a great haircut foundation but not a strong finished hairdesign, your clients may not return. Being able to artistically plan and execute the complete hairdesign instills their confidence in you, resulting in repeat business and referrals.*

"The design patterns in this chapter were created to fit on CLiC mannequins. Adjust the setting instructions that follow according to the head size you design upon, since the size and form of our clients' heads and different manufacturers' mannequins may vary."

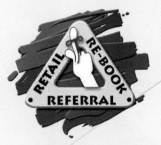

This chapter takes each haircut learned in the CLiC Haircutting module and breaks it down into lab projects for each hairdesign skill level, changing the styling tools used for each level of complexity.

The three lab projects for finishing skill levels are:

Simple	Intermediate	Complex
Airform Design	**Airform Design Finished with Diffuser or Curling/Flat Iron**	**Design Set with Rollers, Pin Curls, or Thermal Tools, or Finished with Hair Additions**
Use the airformer with styling brushes to provide movement or direction to the hair while drying.	Add curls or waves in the hair to support the airformed design with softness and moderate to accelerated texture changes.	Set hair in rollers or pin curls to increase style strength and provide additional texture. To supplement creativity, apply hair additions, flat iron or thermal tongs.

Review the list of styling tools in the chart above. For each lab project in this chapter, determine your choice of styling tool based on the client's expectations for the style's durability along with her lifestyle or skill at maintaining the hairdesign.

Hairspray and liquid styling tools add texture and control. Taking time to prepare the hair properly enables the client to maintain the design.

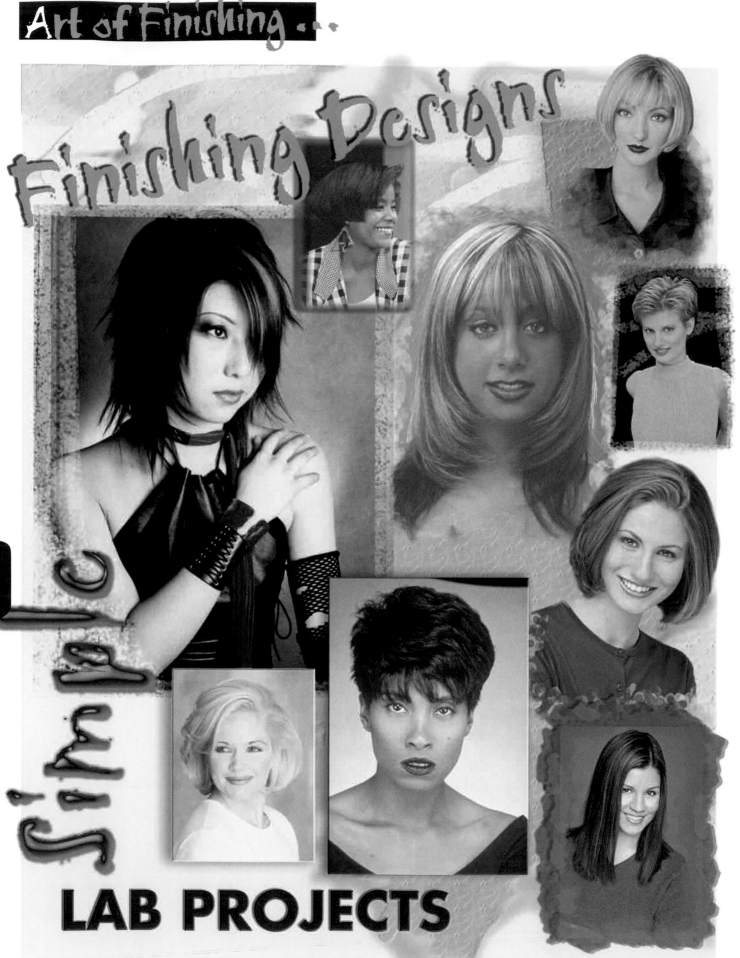

Art of Finishing...

Finishing Designs

LAB PROJECTS

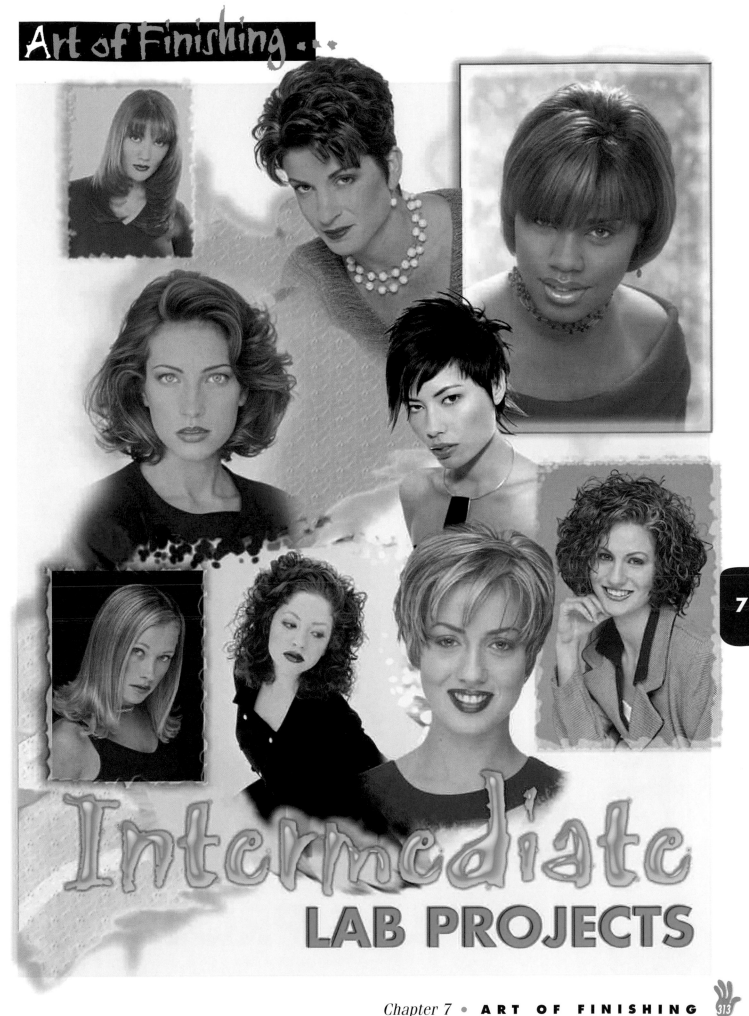

Art of Finishing...

Intermediate LAB PROJECTS

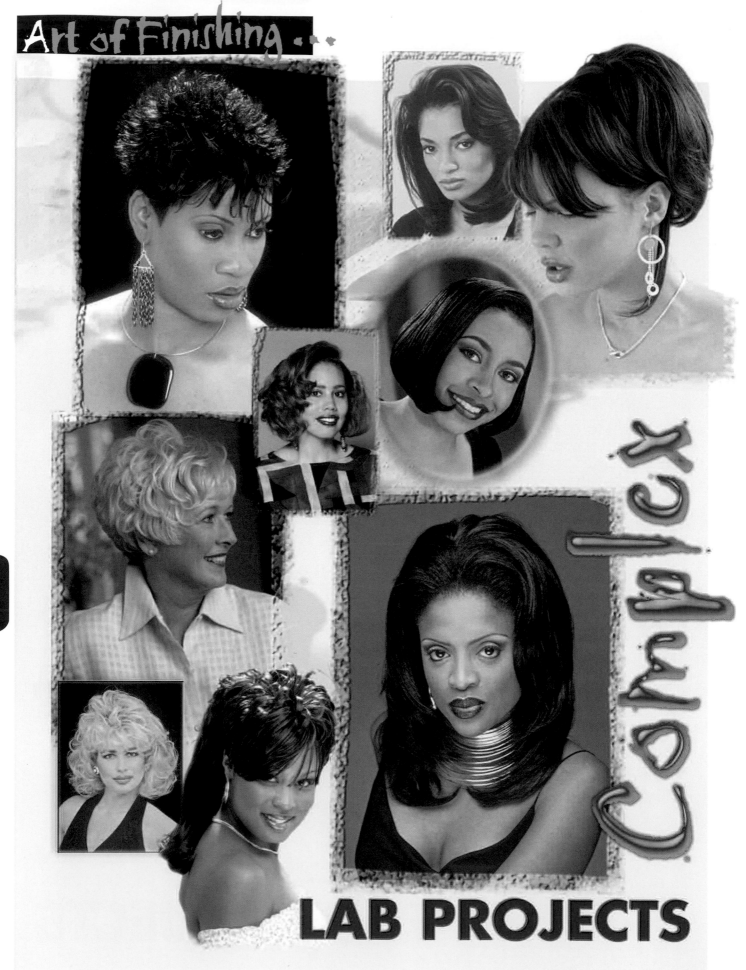

Art of Finishing...

Complex

LAB PROJECTS

7

Zones of the Head...

The head is categorized into zones, each with a distinct feature and relationship to the hairdesigning process. For the final form, understand each zone to implement creative and innovative hairdesigns.

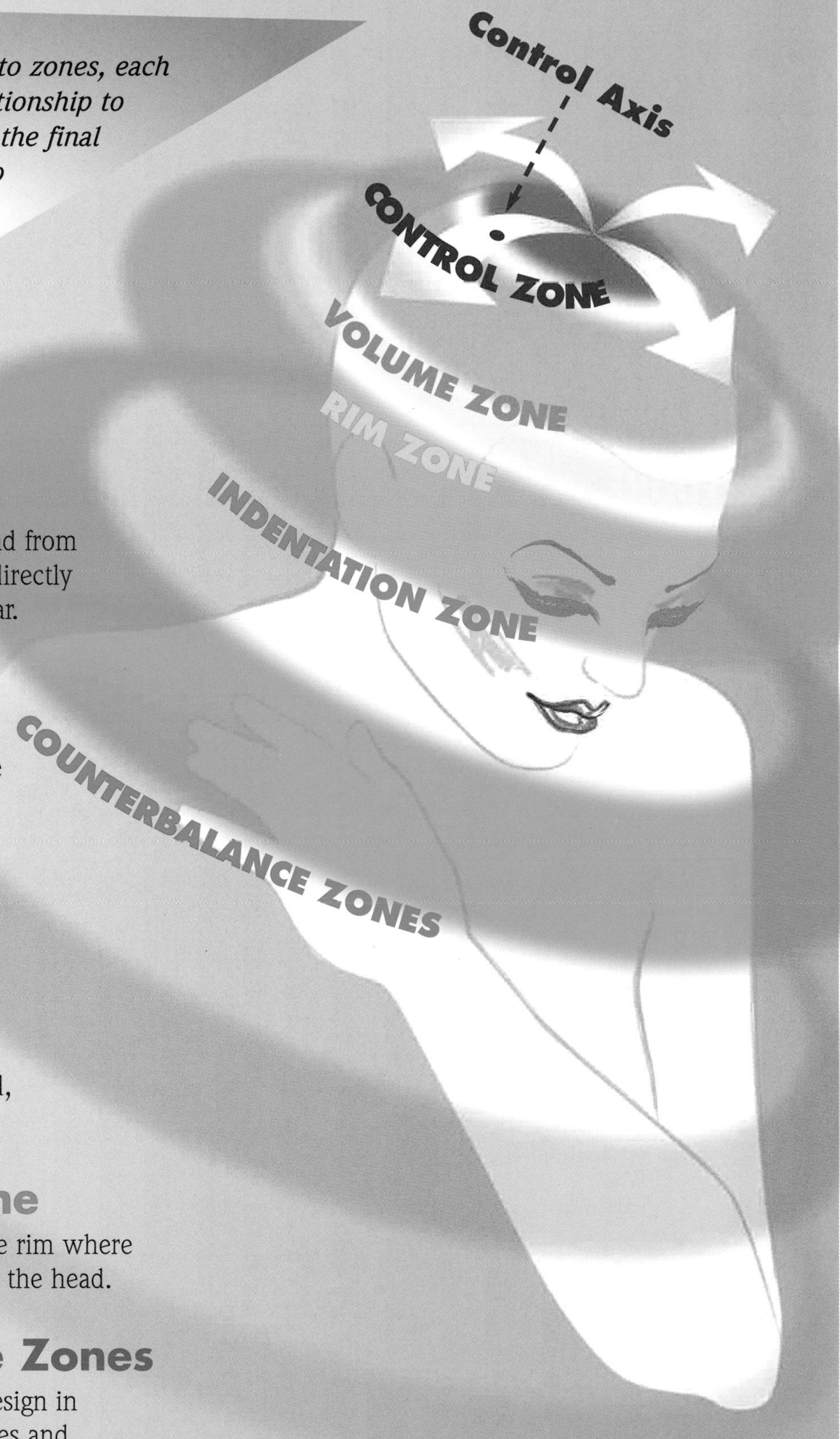

Control Axis

The point at the top of the head from which the hair is distributed, directly aligned with the back of the ear.

Control Zone

The area where a hairdesign begins or ends; the area where elevation angles are blended.

Volume Zone

The upper mass area located above the rim zone.

Rim Zone

The widest portion of the head, where it curves.

Indentation Zone

The lower mass area below the rim where hair can be designed closest to the head.

Counterbalance Zones

The areas for adapting a hairdesign in harmony with the facial features and body proportions.

Control Axis

CONTROL ZONE

VOLUME ZONE

RIM ZONE

INDENTATION ZONE

COUNTERBALANCE ZONES

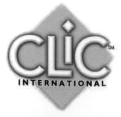

COMPLEX LAB PROJECT

Page Bob

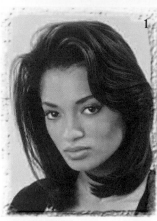

HAIRCUT A1
PROJECT DESIGN

OBJECTIVE

Style this classic, shoulder-length design by using the airformer, curling iron, or rollers. Determine which of the three styling variations will be required based on your client's expectations for the style's durability along with her lifestyle or skill at maintaining the hairdesign. Tools placed in a convex (volume) position and followed by a concave (indentation) placement bring lift into the base of the design with a subtle turn at the ends.

TOOLS & MATERIALS

- Neck strip and cape/smock
- Towels
- Styling brushes and combs
- Rollers and roller clips
- Client record card/file
- Sectioning clips or clamps
- Airformer
- Curling iron/flat iron
- Cleansing and conditioning products
- Finishing spray or other liquid styling tools

PROCEDURE

"The client consultation is an important part of your professional service. Be sure to complete this step prior to each client service you provide. Your successful retail sales and customer satisfaction rates depend upon it!"

1. Drape the client in preparation for the service.
2. Thoroughly brush the client's hair to remove knots, tangles and hairspray.
3. Cleanse and condition the hair according to the client's needs. Rinse thoroughly and towel dry.
4. Comb the hair to detangle. Apply an appropriate liquid styling tool.
5. Perform the style as shown.
6. Each subsection should remain clipped until the hair is cool after drying and then brushed thoroughly in the direction of the style's design plan. Finish with the appropriate lacing techniques and liquid styling tools.
7. Suggest appropriate retail tools for the client's at-home hairdesign maintenance.
8. Follow standard clean-up procedures.
9. Document the client record card/file.

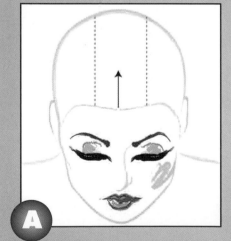

A Mold and scale a centered rectangle from the front hairline to the nape of the neck using the length of your tool (roller, round brush or curling iron) as a guide for the section's width.

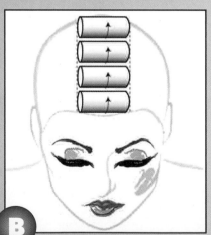

B The first four convex (volume) placements are on base and equal to the diameter of your styling tool.

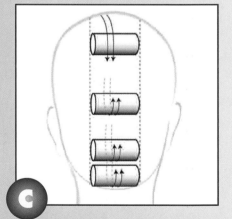

C The fifth convex (volume) placement is 1/2 under-directed in a 1 1/2 diameter base size. The sixth placement is full under-directed for concave (indentation) in a base 1 1/2 times the diameter of your styling tool. The seventh is concave 1/2 under-directed, 1 1/2 diameters. The eighth is also concave 1/2 under-directed, but uses the remaining hair in the nape as its base width.

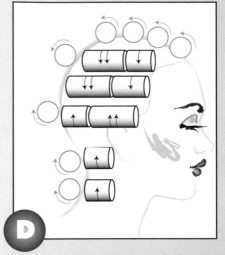

D

Both sides form a bricklayer pattern, beginning with two rows of convex (volume) movement 1/2 over-directed, 1 1/2 diameters in width. The third row is full concave (indentation) under-directed and 1 1/2 diameters. The fourth row is concave 1/2 under-directed, 1 1/2 diameters. The fifth placement is also concave 1/2 under-directed using all remaining hair.

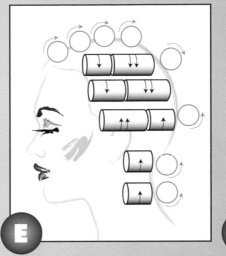

E

Repeat the bricklayer pattern on the opposite side of the head.

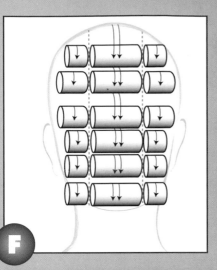

F

Convex (volume) can replace the concave (indentation) placements to move hair in any direction according to the desired finish.

Variations of Design

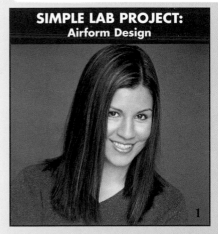

SIMPLE LAB PROJECT:
Airform Design

The airformer, a round brush and the addition of a liquid tool such as styling mousse will lift the hair at the base. This style has a smooth, decelerated tempo.

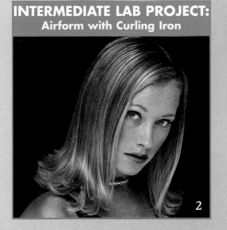

INTERMEDIATE LAB PROJECT:
Airform with Curling Iron

The finished airformed style can be enhanced with the use of a curling iron to create an end flip with a moderate design tempo.

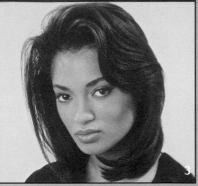

COMPLEX LAB PROJECT:
Roller Design

A longer-lasting design with more volume and tempo can be achieved by setting the hair with rollers and a styling lotion or gel.

EVALUATION

GRADE   STUDENT'S NAME   ID#

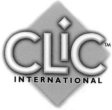

CLiC
INTERNATIONAL

Career Bob

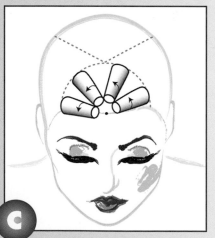

HAIRCUT A3

PROJECT DESIGN

OBJECTIVE

Enhance a change in direction at the fringe area of the face using curvature rotation in a design. Determine which of the three convex (volume) styling variations will be required based on your client's expectations for the style's durability along with her lifestyle or skill at maintaining the hairdesign.

TOOLS & MATERIALS

- Neck strip and cape/smock
- Towels
- Styling brushes and combs

- Rollers and roller clips
- Client record card/file
- Sectioning clips or clamps

- Airformer
- Curling iron/flat iron
- Cleansing and conditioning products

- Finishing spray or other liquid styling tools

PROCEDURE

"The client consultation is an important part of your professional service. Be sure to complete this step prior to each client service you provide. Your successful retail sales and customer satisfaction rates depend upon it!"

RETAIL · RE-BOOK · REFERRAL

1. Drape the client in preparation for the service.
2. Thoroughly brush the client's hair to remove knots, tangles and hairspray.
3. Cleanse and condition the hair according to the client's needs. Rinse thoroughly and towel dry.
4. Comb the hair to detangle. Apply an appropriate liquid styling tool.
5. Perform the style as shown.
6. Each subsection should remain clipped until the hair is cool after drying and then brushed thoroughly in the direction of the style's design plan. Finish with the appropriate lacing techniques and liquid styling tools.
7. Suggest appropriate retail tools for the client's at-home hairdesign maintenance.
8. Follow standard clean-up procedures.
9. Document the client record card/file.

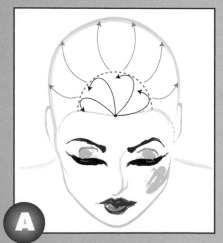

A Mold and scale a centered 1/2 circle measured from the arch in one eyebrow to the other, and moving either clockwise or counter-clockwise. Use roller diameter plus length as a guide for the section.

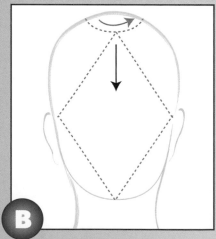

B Mold and scale a centered diamond starting directly behind the circle, moving down to the nape hairline. The varying lengths of cylinder rollers determine the width of the diamond.

C The circle is set with convex (volume) base placements. The first roller is 1/2 under-directed, 1 1/2 diameters; second roller is on base, 1 diameter; third roller is 1/2 under-directed, 1 1/2 diameters; the fourth roller is 1/2 under-directed, using the remaining hair.

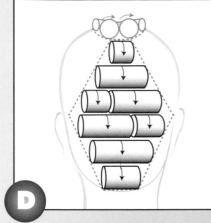

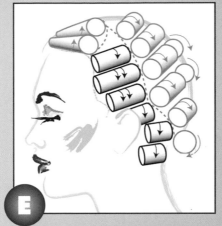

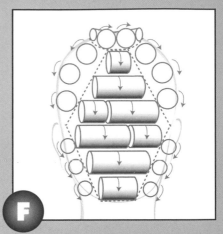

D The diamond is set with convex (volume) rollers. The length of the rollers used in this shape is determined by the size of the client's head. The first roller is on base, 1 diameter; second and third rows of rollers are 1/2 under-directed, 1 1/2 diameters; fourth and fifth rows of rollers are 1/2 under-directed, 1 diameter; and sixth roller is full under-directed, with remaining hair.

E Left side continues using convex (volume) placements to complete the design. First roller (which fits behind the circle) is 1/2 over-directed, 1 1/2 diameters; second roller is on base, 1 diameter; third roller is 1/2 under-directed, 1 1/2 diameters. The first and second rollers behind the ear are 1/2 under-directed 1 diameter, and the third roller is full under-directed with remaining hair. Follow the same pattern on the right side.

F The completed design viewed from the back.

Variations of Design

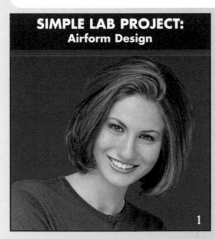

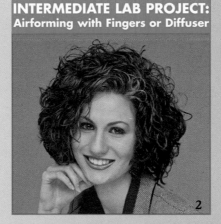

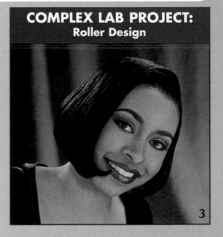

SIMPLE LAB PROJECT: Airform Design

1 The airformer and a round styling brush help create the curvature rotation within this decelerated volume design. A liquid tool such as styling mousse helps to lift the hair at the scalp.

INTERMEDIATE LAB PROJECT: Airforming with Fingers or Diffuser

2 Enhance the basic airformed style by finger scrunching the hair or using a diffuser to create more textural fullness and a moderately accelerated tempo. Add a curl activator to keep curls or waves from getting frizzy.

COMPLEX LAB PROJECT: Roller Design

3 Large diameter rollers create a slow, decelerated tempo. A styling lotion or gel increases design hold and improves the style's definition.

EVALUATION

GRADE STUDENT'S NAME ID#

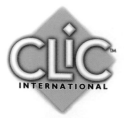
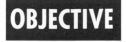

COMPLEX LAB PROJECT

Windblown Bob

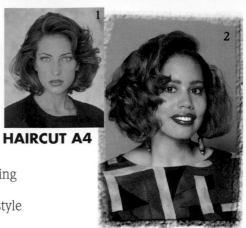

HAIRCUT A4

PROJECT DESIGN

OBJECTIVE

Create a design consisting of a curvature motion along the front hairline, influencing the hair's directional flow toward the face. Determine which of the three styling variations will be required based on your client's expectations for the style's durability along with her lifestyle or skill at maintaining the hairdesign.

TOOLS & MATERIALS

- Neck strip and cape/smock
- Towels
- Pomade or other liquid styling tools
- Styling combs and brushes
- Clips, bobbie pins, and hair pins
- Cleansing and conditioning products
- Client record card/file
- Airformer and/or flat iron
- Small elastic bands
- Ornamentation

PROCEDURE

"The client consultation is an important part of your professional service. Be sure to complete this step prior to each client service you provide. Your successful retail sales and customer satisfaction rates depend upon it!"

RETAIL · RE-BOOK · REFERRAL

1. Drape the client in preparation for the service.
2. Thoroughly brush the client's hair to remove knots, tangles and hairspray.
3. Cleanse and condition the hair according to the client's needs. Rinse thoroughly and towel dry.
4. Comb the hair to detangle. Apply an appropriate liquid styling tool.
5. Perform the style as shown.
6. Each subsection should remain clipped until the hair is cool after drying and then brushed thoroughly in the direction of the style's design plan. Finish with the appropriate lacing techniques and liquid styling tools.
7. Suggest appropriate retail tools for the client's at-home hairdesign maintenance.
8. Follow standard clean-up procedures.
9. Document the client record card/file.

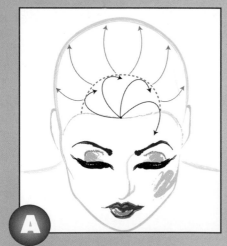

A Section a small half circle or triangular shape.

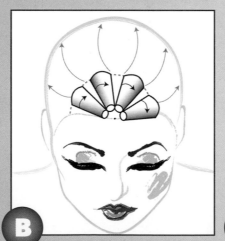

B The circle is set with convex (volume) base placements. The first roller is 1/2 under-directed, 1 1/2 diameters; second roller is on base, 1 diameter; third roller is 1/2 under-directed, 1 1/2 diameters; the fourth roller is 1/2 under-directed, using the remaining hair.

C On the right side, mold and scale a counter-clockwise 1/4 circle (the control axis is the corner of the eye) using a short conical roller as a guide for the depth and width of the shape.

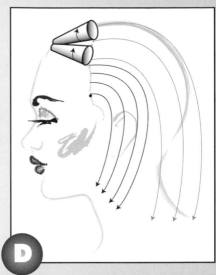

D

On the left side, mold and scale a 1/4 circle moving in a clockwise direction (the control axis is the corner of the eye) using a short conical roller as a guide for the shape's depth and width.

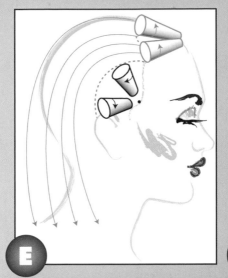

E

Using convex (volume) base placements, the first roller is 1/2 under-directed, 1 1/2 diameters and the second roller is 1/2 under-directed, 1 diameter or with remaining hair. The 1/4 circles are set with two short conical rollers in the rotational directions shown for each side.

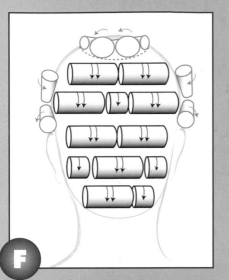

F

A bricklayer pattern using convex (volume) base placements is applied in the back. The first row of rollers is on base, 1 diameter, second and third rows of rollers are 1/2 under-directed, 1 diameter and fourth and fifth rows of rollers are 1/2 under-directed 1 1/2 diameters with remaining hair.

Variations of Design

SIMPLE LAB PROJECT:
Airform Design

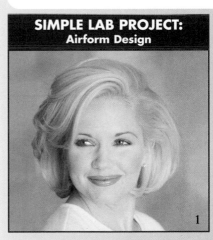

The airformer and a round styling brush help create a curvature rotational movement along the front hairline. A smoothing lotion can be used to add a sleek, soft finished look.

INTERMEDIATE LAB PROJECT:
Airforming with Curling Iron

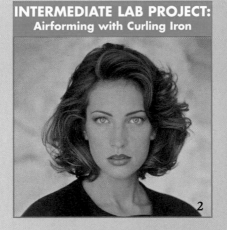

Introducing a curling iron to the finished airformed style can enhance the design's curl or wave. Using a thermal spray provides heat protection and also helps add body to the design.

COMPLEX LAB PROJECT:
Roller Design

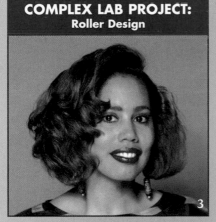

For a fuller, longer-lasting design with a stronger curl pattern, set the hair with rollers and a styling lotion or gel to support the design.

EVALUATION

GRADE STUDENT'S NAME ID#

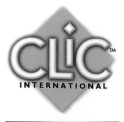

COMPLEX LAB PROJECT

Savàge

OBJECTIVE

Design this stylish shag utilizing oblongs along the front sides and across the back to create varied movement and texture. Determine which of the three styling variations will be required based on your client's expectations for the style's durability along with her lifestyle or skill at maintaining the hairdesign.

PROJECT DESIGN

TOOLS & MATERIALS

- Neck strip and cape/smock
- Towels
- Styling brushes and combs
- Rollers and roller clips
- Client record card/file
- Sectioning clips or clamps
- Airformer
- Curling iron/flat iron
- Cleansing and conditioning products
- Finishing spray or other liquid styling tools

PROCEDURE

"The client consultation is an important part of your professional service. Be sure to complete this step prior to each client service you provide. Your successful retail sales and customer satisfaction rates depend upon it!"

RETAIL • RE-BOOK • REFERRAL

1. Drape the client in preparation for the service.
2. Thoroughly brush the client's hair to remove knots, tangles and hairspray.
3. Cleanse and condition the hair according to the client's needs. Rinse thoroughly and towel dry.
4. Comb the hair to detangle. Apply an appropriate liquid styling tool.
5. Perform the style as shown.
6. Each subsection should remain clipped until the hair is cool after drying and then brushed thoroughly in the direction of the style's design plan. Finish with the appropriate lacing techniques and liquid styling tools.
7. Suggest appropriate retail tools for the client's at-home hairdesign maintenance.
8. Follow standard clean-up procedures.
9. Document the client record card/file.

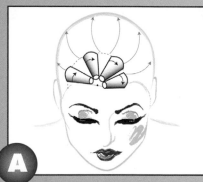

A Mold and scale a clockwise 1/2 circle centered from the inside corner of the right eyebrow, using a long conical roller's diameter plus length as a guide for the section. Create convex (volume) base placements as follows: The first roller is 1/2 under-directed, 1 1/2 diameters; second roller is on base, 1 diameter; third roller is 1/2 under-directed, 1 1/2 diameters; and fourth roller is placed 1/2 under-directed with the remaining hair.

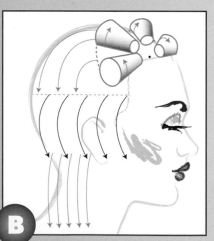

B Again guided by a long conical roller's diameter plus its length, mold and scale a counter-clockwise concave (indentation) oblong on the right side moving toward the face. The opposite side is molded and scaled toward the face using a clockwise concave oblong.

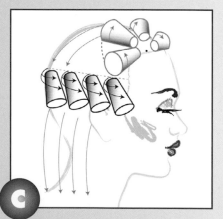

C The first three conical rollers on the right side of the head are set on base with 1 diameter and the fourth roller is 1/2 under-directed with 1 diameter or remaining hair. All rollers are placed with diagonal partings and are directed toward the face. Repeat this pattern using the same roller guides on the left side, directing all rollers toward the face.

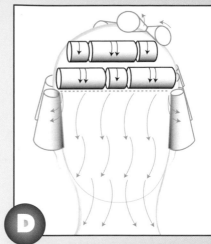

D

Directly behind the circle, set a bricklayer pattern using cylinder rollers with convex (volume) base placements. The first and second rows of rollers are on base with 1 diameter spacing.

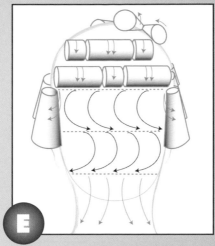

E

Below the rows of cylinder rollers, mold and scale one counter-clockwise and one clockwise concave (indentation) oblong, leaving hair below the second oblong shape. The diameter plus length of a short conical roller is used for scaling.

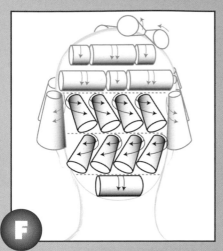

F

Set both oblongs with the first three conical rollers on base, 1 diameter within diagonal partings. The fourth roller is 1/2 under-directed with 1 diameter or remaining hair. Reverse the roller direction of the second oblong to follow the wave formation scaling. The hair below the second oblong is set in cylinder rollers placed horizontally using the remaining hair and 1/2 under-directed convex (volume) roller base placements.

Variations of Design

SIMPLE LAB PROJECT:
Airform Design

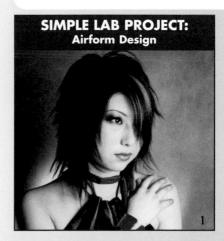

1

The airformer and a pin type brush are used to create closeness and smoothness within the design. A smoothing lotion and styling wax help define texture in the finished style.

INTERMEDIATE LAB PROJECT:
Airform with Curling Iron

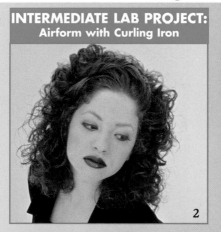

2

The use of a curling iron through-out the finished airformed style accelerates the design's tempo. A thermal spray applied before styling detangles and provides protection from the curling iron's heat.

COMPLEX LAB PROJECT:
Roller Design

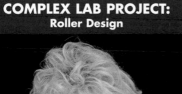
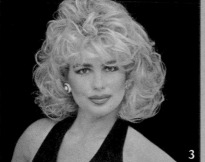

3

A styling lotion or gel increases the design's holding power when setting the hair for maximum volume with rollers.

EVALUATION

GRADE

STUDENT'S NAME

ID#

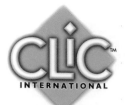

SIMPLE LAB PROJECT

Wedgette

OBJECTIVE

Create lift and soft texture in the volume area of this hairdesign, with closeness at the sides and nape. Determine which of the three styling variations will be required based on your client's expectations for the style's durability along with her lifestyle or skill at maintaining the hairdesign.

TOOLS & MATERIALS

- Neck strip and cape/smock
- Towels
- Styling brushes and combs
- Rollers and single/double prong clips
- Client record card/file
- Sectioning clips or clamps
- Curling iron/flat iron
- Airformer
- Cleansing and conditioning products
- Finishing spray or other liquid styling tools

PROCEDURE

"The client consultation is an important part of your professional service. Be sure to complete this step prior to each client service you provide. Your successful retail sales and customer satisfaction rates depend upon it!"

RETAIL · RE-BOOK · REFERRAL

1. Drape the client in preparation for the service.
2. Thoroughly brush the client's hair to remove knots, tangles and hairspray.
3. Cleanse and condition the hair according to the client's needs. Rinse thoroughly and towel dry.
4. Comb the hair to detangle. Apply an appropriate liquid styling tool.
5. Perform the style as shown.
6. Each subsection should remain clipped until the hair is cool after drying and then brushed thoroughly in the direction of the style's design plan. Finish with the appropriate lacing techniques and liquid styling tools.
7. Suggest appropriate retail tools for the client's at-home hairdesign maintenance.
8. Follow standard clean-up procedures.
9. Document the client record card/file.

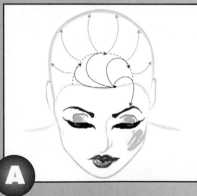

A

Use a long, medium and short conical roller to determine the width of the oval. Mold and scale a clockwise 1/2 oval, centered from the inside corner of the left eyebrow. Airform the hair using small subsections determined by the diameter of the styling brush used. Create either on base or 1/2 under-directed placements, and clip to secure the hair until cool.

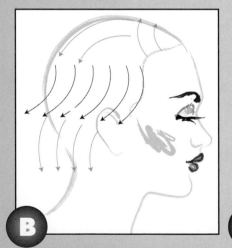

B

Mold and scale a counter-clockwise oblong on the right side. Airform hair toward the back center of the head. **Variation:** Hair may move toward the face or be rolled down.

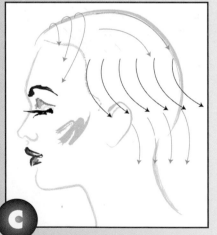

C

On the left side, mold and scale a clockwise oblong. Airform hair toward the back center of the head.

Variation – Pin Curl Set

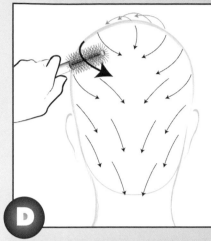

D

In the occipital area, mold hair into the back center of the head to the nape hairline. Airform the hair using small subsections with full under-directed base placements.

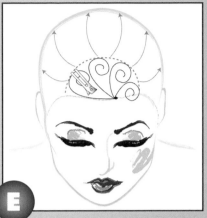

E

Set the 1/2 oval from step "A" using convex (volume) pin curls. Use the diameter of a conical roller to determine the amount of hair taken per pin curl, and secure each one with a single prong clip. The first pin curl is 1/2 under-directed with 1 1/2 diameters; second pin curl is on base with 1 diameter; third pin curl is 1/2 under-directed with 1 1/2 diameters; fourth pin curl is 1/2 under-directed using the remaining hair.

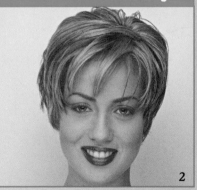

F

To set the side oblongs for this wet style, use full stem flat pin curls, and secure the pin curls off base using a single prong clip. The variation in "B" from previous page and step "D" replaces curved bases with square bases if the hairdesign movement is rolled downward instead of toward or away from the face.

Variations of Design

SIMPLE LAB PROJECT:
Airform Design

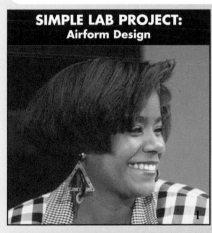

Airform using either a vent brush or your fingers to help add base lift in the crown. Move hair back or downward along the sides. Use styling wax or pomade to create a wispy end texture.

INTERMEDIATE LAB PROJECT:
Airform with Flat Iron Design

The addition of a flat iron is used on the finished airform which will provide the desired straightness and smoothness to this design. Styling wax can be used on the wispy ends.

COMPLEX LAB PROJECT:
Pin Curl Design

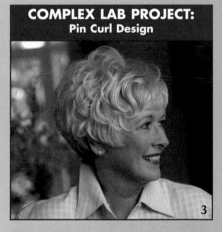

Pin curls enhance the design movement by providing additional support and wave or curl. A smoothing lotion will help control and form the ends into pin curls.

EVALUATION

GRADE

STUDENT'S NAME

ID#

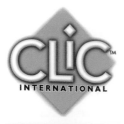

SIMPLE LAB PROJECT

Brush Cut

OBJECTIVE

Create base lift with either a smooth finish or a slight end flip for a carefree, sassy finish. Determine which of the three styling variations will be required based on your client's expectations for the style's durability along with her lifestyle or skill at maintaining the hairdesign.

HAIRCUT B3

PROJECT DESIGN VARIATION

TOOLS & MATERIALS

- Neck strip and cape/smock
- Towels
- Styling brushes and combs
- Rollers and roller clips
- Hair additions
- Client record card/file
- Sectioning clips or clamps
- Airformer and curling iron/flat iron
- Cleansing and conditioning products
- Finishing spray or other liquid styling tools

PROCEDURE

"The client consultation is an important part of your professional service. Be sure to complete this step prior to each client service you provide. Your successful retail sales and customer satisfaction rates depend upon it!"

RETAIL • RE-BOOK • REFERRAL

1. Drape the client in preparation for the service.
2. Thoroughly brush the client's hair to remove knots, tangles and hairspray.
3. Cleanse and condition the hair according to the client's needs. Rinse thoroughly and towel dry.
4. Comb the hair to detangle. Apply an appropriate liquid styling tool.
5. Perform the style as shown.
6. Finish with the appropriate lacing techniques and liquid styling tools.
7. Suggest appropriate retail tools for the client's at-home hairdesign maintenance.
8. Follow standard clean-up procedures.
9. Document the client record card/file.

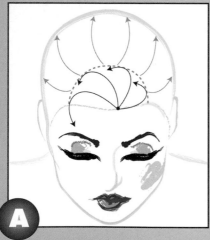

A Mold and scale a counter-clockwise 1/2 oval centered using the inside corner of the left eye-brow as the control axis. Determine the oval's section size using conical rollers by measuring with one short roller, followed by two medium rollers and one long roller.

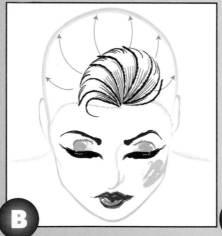

B Using the airformer and a brush, place counter-clockwise convex (volume) "C" curls in the oval. The first is 1/2 under-directed, second and third subsections are on base with 1 diameter base sizes, and with the remaining hair, use a full under-directed placement for the fourth subsection.

C On right side, use a bricklayer pattern to divide the hair into subsections. Airform each subsection, moving in a downward direction with 1/2 under-directed base placements. Continue this pattern on the left side.

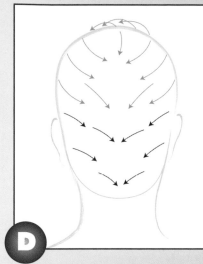

D

The design plan in the back starts below the occipital, sketch (mold) the hair into a dovetailing line moving toward the center of the head.

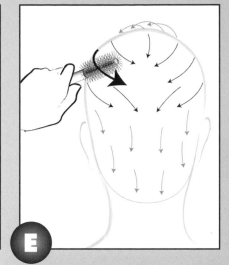

E

Continue in the back area using 1/2 under-directed base placements and changing to on base placements going from occipital to crown. Finish the design using the appropriate liquid styling tools.

Variation

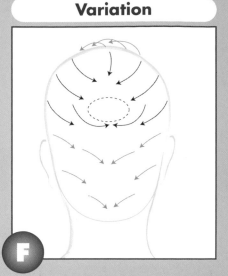

F

Apply a flat iron to the hair to provide additional smoothness and shine. Use a ponytail hair addition along with the design plan's convex (volume) base placements. Center the ponytail addition between crown and occipital. Pull the back area hair together to serve as a base for securing the hair addition.

Variations of Design

SIMPLE LAB PROJECT:
Airform Design

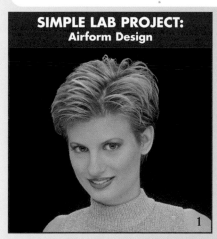

1

The airformer and a styling vent brush will create the movements within the design. Finish with a styling wax or pomade on the hair ends for added texture.

INTERMEDIATE LAB PROJECT:
Airform with Curling Iron

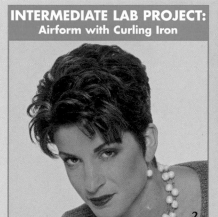

2

An ends to base curling iron technique creates more definition of movement on the ends of the airformed hair. Finish by texturizing the ends of the hair with a styling wax or pomade.

COMPLEX LAB PROJECT:
Airform with Flat Iron and a Ponytail Addition

3

The use of the flat iron will allow a base lift with a slight bend to the hair. The addition of a ponytail to this short hairdesign provides a unique, versatile long hair variation.

EVALUATION

GRADE

STUDENT'S NAME

ID#

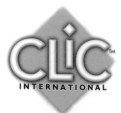

COMPLEX LAB PROJECT

Forward Fringe Bob

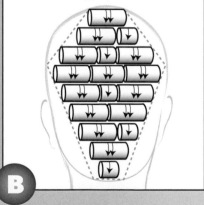

HAIRCUT C2

PROJECT DESIGN

OBJECTIVE

Design short, caressing layers coming toward the face in a three-dimensional style with rotational curvature. Determine which of the three styling variations will be required based on your client's expectations for the style's durability along with her lifestyle or skill at maintaining the hairdesign.

TOOLS & MATERIALS

- Neck strip and cape/smock
- Towels
- Styling brushes and combs
- Rollers and roller clips
- Client record card/file
- Sectioning clips or clamps
- Airformer/hood dryer
- Curling iron/flat iron
- Cleansing and conditioning products
- Finishing spray or other liquid styling tools

PROCEDURE

"The client consultation is an important part of your professional service. Be sure to complete this step prior to each client service you provide. Your successful retail sales and customer satisfaction rates depend upon it!"

RETAIL · RE-BOOK · REFERRAL

1. Drape the client in preparation for the service.
2. Thoroughly brush the client's hair to remove knots, tangles and hairspray.
3. Cleanse and condition the hair according to the client's needs. Rinse thoroughly and towel dry.
4. Comb the hair to detangle. Apply an appropriate liquid styling tool.
5. Perform the style as shown.
6. Each subsection should remain clipped until the hair is cool after drying and then brushed thoroughly in the direction of the style's design plan. Finish with the appropriate lacing techniques and liquid styling tools.
7. Suggest appropriate retail tools for the client's at-home hairdesign maintenance.
8. Follow standard clean-up procedures.
9. Document the client record card/file.

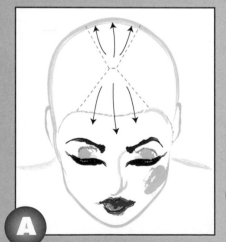

A

Section a triangle fringe from the frontal hairline. The triangle fringe will be dried under a hood dryer. Mold and scale a centered kite from behind the fringe back to the nape. The width of the kite section shape is determined by the lengths of long and short cylinder rollers.

B

Use convex (volume) base place-ments to set the kite. The first roller and the next three rows are 1 diameter on base place-ments. The fifth, sixth and seventh rows of rollers are 1/2 under-directed with 1 1/2 diameters. The eighth and ninth rows of rollers are 1/2 under-directed using a 1 diameter width subsection or the remaining hair.

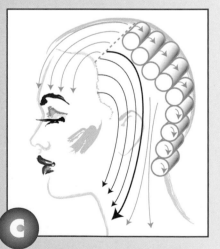

C

On the left side, a clockwise 1/2 oval is molded and scaled. Use one short, two medium and one long conical roller to measure the depth of the 1/2 oval shape.

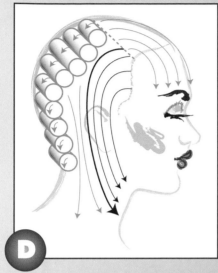

D

Mold and scale a counter-clockwise 1/2 oval on the right side using the same conical roller pattern.

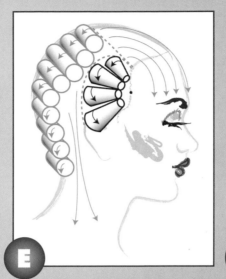

E

To set the 1/2 oval, the first conical roller (short length) is 1/2 under-directed with 1 1/2 diameters; second roller (medium) is on base, 1 diameter; third roller (medium) is on base, 1 diameter; the fourth roller (long) is 1/2 under-directed using the remaining hair.

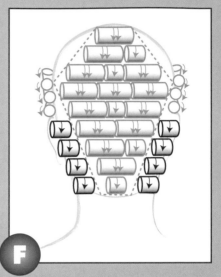

F

To set the side back area: The first cylinder roller is 1/2 under-directed with a 1 diameter, second roller is 1/2 under-directed with a 1 1/2 diameters, third and fourth rollers are 1/2 under-directed with 1 diameter.

Variations of Design

SIMPLE LAB PROJECT:
Airform Design

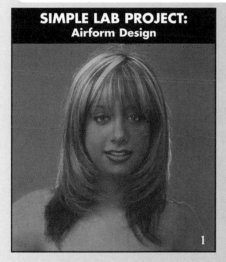

The airformer and a pin type styling brush provide the control and softness needed for this design. The use of a smoothing lotion or styling wax will give the style added texture.

INTERMEDIATE LAB PROJECT:
Airform with Curling Iron

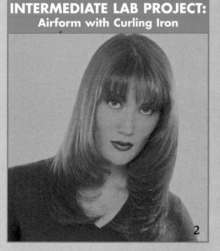

Softness around the face with a gently accelerating tempo is created with the use of a curling iron and a thermal protectant on the airformed style.

COMPLEX LAB PROJECT:
Roller Design

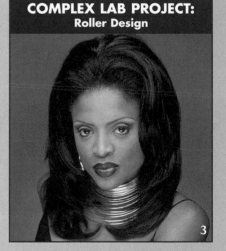

A style variation without the triangle fringe uses rollers and a styling lotion to provide the base lift and support necessary for added design durability.

EVALUATION

GRADE   STUDENT'S NAME   ID#

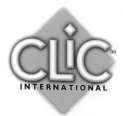

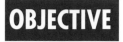

Boxed Bob

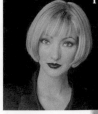

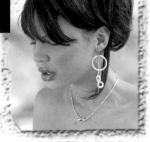

HAIRCUT C3

PROJECT DESIGN VARIATION

OBJECTIVE

Emphasize the smooth texture and sharp detail line in this design with the use of a flat iron. A hair addition in the crown area enhances convexity (volume) in the design. Determine which of the three styling variations will be required based on your client's expectations for the style's durability along with her lifestyle or skill at maintaining the hairdesign.

TOOLS & MATERIALS

- Neck strip and cape/smock
- Towels
- Styling brushes and combs

- Rollers and roller clips
- Hair additions
- Sectioning clips or clamps

- Airformer and curling iron/flat iron
- Finishing spray or other liquid styling tools
- Cleansing and conditioning products

- Client record card/file

PROCEDURE

"The client consultation is an important part of your professional service. Be sure to complete this step prior to each client service you provide. Your successful retail sales and customer satisfaction rates depend upon it!"

RETAIL · RE-BOOK · REFERRAL

1. Drape the client in preparation for the service.
2. Thoroughly brush the client's hair to remove knots, tangles and hairspray.
3. Cleanse and condition the hair according to the client's needs. Rinse thoroughly and towel dry.
4. Comb the hair to detangle. Apply an appropriate liquid styling tool.
5. Perform the style as shown.
6. Finish with the appropriate lacing techniques and liquid styling tools.
7. Suggest appropriate retail tools for the client's at-home hairdesign maintenance.
8. Follow standard clean-up procedures.
9. Document the client record card/file.

7

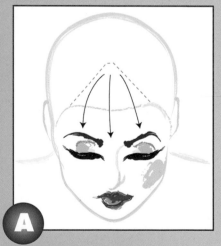

A

Mold and scale a triangle at the front hairline. The width of the triangle is determined by the desired amount of fringe area. Airform using small diameter partings with 1/2 under-directed base placements.

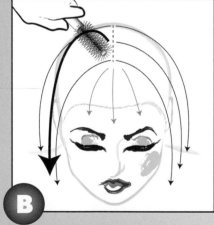

B

Create a vertical center part from the tip of the triangle, ending at the control axis, and another vertical parting down to the ear. Add base lift to these two subsections by taking small diameter partings while styling. Use 1/2 under-directed base placements with 1 1/2 diameters as determined by the diameter of the tool used (brush, roller or flat iron).

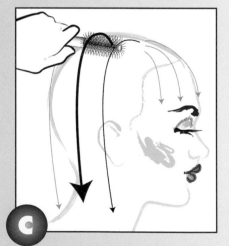

C

The side sections are airformed to come down over the ears.

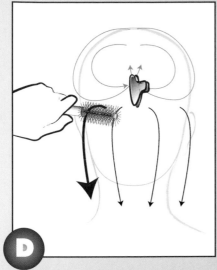

D

In the back, continue to airform using convex (volume) and/or concave (indentation) base placements. Create 1/2 under-directed placements on a 1 1/2 diameter width base section, which is determined by the diameter of the tool being used.

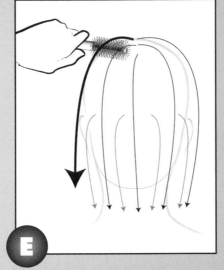

E

To complete the back, use 1 to 1 1/2 diameter widths determined by the tool being used. Create on base placements above the occipital and 1/2 under-directed placements below.

Variation

F

Part a triangle from the control axis in the crown area, with triangle's point facing the nape. Attach a hair addition to this point in the crown area by pulling the back area hair together to serve as a base for securing the hair addition. Blend the client's remaining hair into the hair addition.

Variations of Design

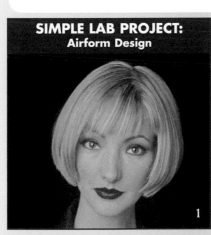

SIMPLE LAB PROJECT:
Airform Design

1

The airformer and a pin type styling brush help create a slight bevel on the ends of this smooth design. Using a lotion and taking small, horizontal partings when styling helps control and support the design's textured appearance.

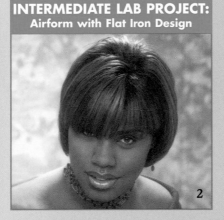

INTERMEDIATE LAB PROJECT:
Airform with Flat Iron Design

2

Smoothing lotion or glaze will control curls, waves or damaged ends in the airformed style. The flat iron details the design's finish.

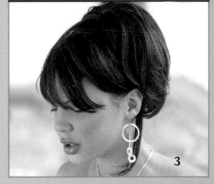

COMPLEX LAB PROJECT:
Airform with Hair Addition

3

Airform the hair to create a decelerated tempo. Supplementing this style with the placement of a hair addition in the crown area will provide base lift.

EVALUATION

GRADE

STUDENT'S NAME

ID#

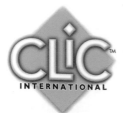

CLIC INTERNATIONAL

Audacé

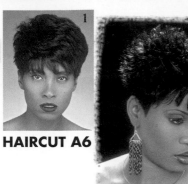

HAIRCUT A6

OBJECTIVE

Enhance this short, tapered design with long lengths along the front hairline and by detailing the texture while finishing. Determine which of the three styling variations will be required based on your client's expectations for the style's durability along with her lifestyle or skill at maintaining the hairdesign.

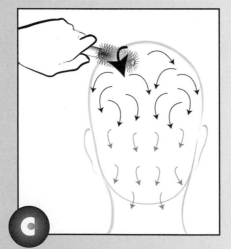

PROJECT DESIGN VARIATION

TOOLS & MATERIALS

- Neck strip and cape/smock
- Towels
- Styling brushes and combs
- Rollers and roller clips
- Sectioning clips or clamps
- Airformer
- Curling iron/flat iron/thermal iron (tongs)
- Cleansing and conditioning products
- Finishing spray or other liquid styling tools
- Client record card/file

PROCEDURE

"The client consultation is an important part of your professional service. Be sure to complete this step prior to each client service you provide. Your successful retail sales and customer satisfaction rates depend upon it!"

RETAIL · RE-BOOK · REFERRAL

1. Drape the client in preparation for the service.
2. Thoroughly brush the client's hair to remove knots, tangles and hairspray.
3. Cleanse and condition the hair according to the client's needs. Rinse thoroughly and towel dry.
4. Comb the hair to detangle. Apply an appropriate liquid styling tool.
5. Perform the style as shown.
6. Finish with the appropriate liquid styling tools.
7. Suggest appropriate retail tools for the client's at-home hairdesign maintenance.
8. Follow standard clean-up procedures.
9. Document the client record card/file.

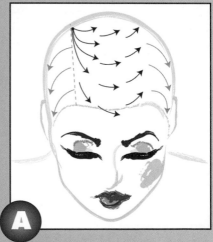

A

Mold and scale a counter-clockwise 1/2 oval, centered from the middle of the right eyebrow. The control axis for the 1/2 oval is placed at end of the part. Use long, medium and short conical rollers to determine the width of the oval. Section the remaining hair by area: frontal, crown, and occipital.

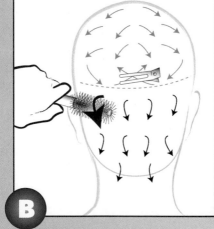

B

Start in the occipital, taking a parting size determined by the diameter of the brush used. Airform the hair using convex (volume) 1/2 or full under-directed base placements with 1 1/2 diameter widths.

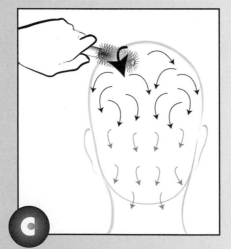

C

In reaching the volume area, begin using on base placements with 1 diameter widths.

7

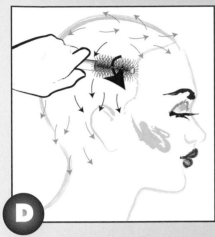

D

Repeat the control applications in "B" and "C" on the side sections.

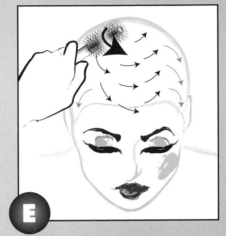

E

When back and side sections are complete, form a 1/2 oval at the top using convex (volume) base placements. The first subsection is 1/2 under-directed with 1 1/2 diameters; the second and third subsections are placed on base with a width of 1 diameter. Hair in the fourth subsection is blended with the crown area using 1/2 under-directed placements and remaining hair.

Variation – Tongs

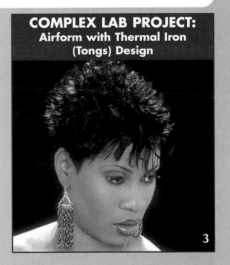

F

Follow scaling in "A" and applications in "B" through "E" when using tongs (thermal iron). Use smaller partings to allow for a more controlled and detailed finish. Replace the 1/2 oval shape with a rectangle if the style's direction requires movement away from the face.

Variations of Design

SIMPLE LAB PROJECT:
Airform Design

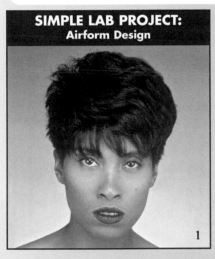

1

Airform using either a vent brush or your fingers to help add base lift in the crown. Move hair along the sides either down or back. Use styling wax or pomade to create a wispy end texture.

INTERMEDIATE LAB PROJECT:
Airform with Flat Iron Design

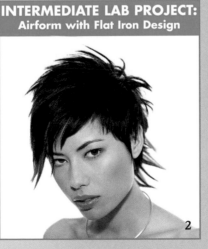

2

The use of a flat iron on the airformed design provides straightness and smoothness. Styling wax further defines the wispy ends.

COMPLEX LAB PROJECT:
Airform with Thermal Iron (Tongs) Design

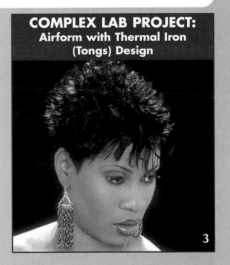

3

Tongs or an ends to base curling iron technique will create a curved end texture in this design. A thermal spray protects hair from heat appliances, while styling oil creates sheen and softness.

7

EVALUATION

GRADE

STUDENT'S NAME

ID#

No, art is not an imitation of nature; art is better than nature. It is nature illuminated.
- F. Delsarte

The great artist is the simplifier.
-Henri Amiel

TAKE NATURE FOR A MODEL...
- FRANCOIS-JOSEPH TALMA

The hand that follows intellect can achieve.
-Michelangelo

A thing of beauty is a joy forever.
-Keats

All the world's a stage...
-Shakespeare

PLAYBILL

TAKE ACTION ON YOUR DREAMS, OR THEY WILL REMAIN JUST DREAMS.
-ARNOLD ZEGARELLI

... and to look as beautiful as you can is a part of your art.
-Plato

It is by logic that we prove, but by intuition that we discover. To know how to criticize is good, but to know how to create is better.
Henri Poincare

HE THAT IS NOT WISE WILL NOT BE TAUGHT.
-ECCLESIASTICUS

THE STAGE IS THE MEETING PLACE OF ALL THE ARTS.
-OSCAR WILDE

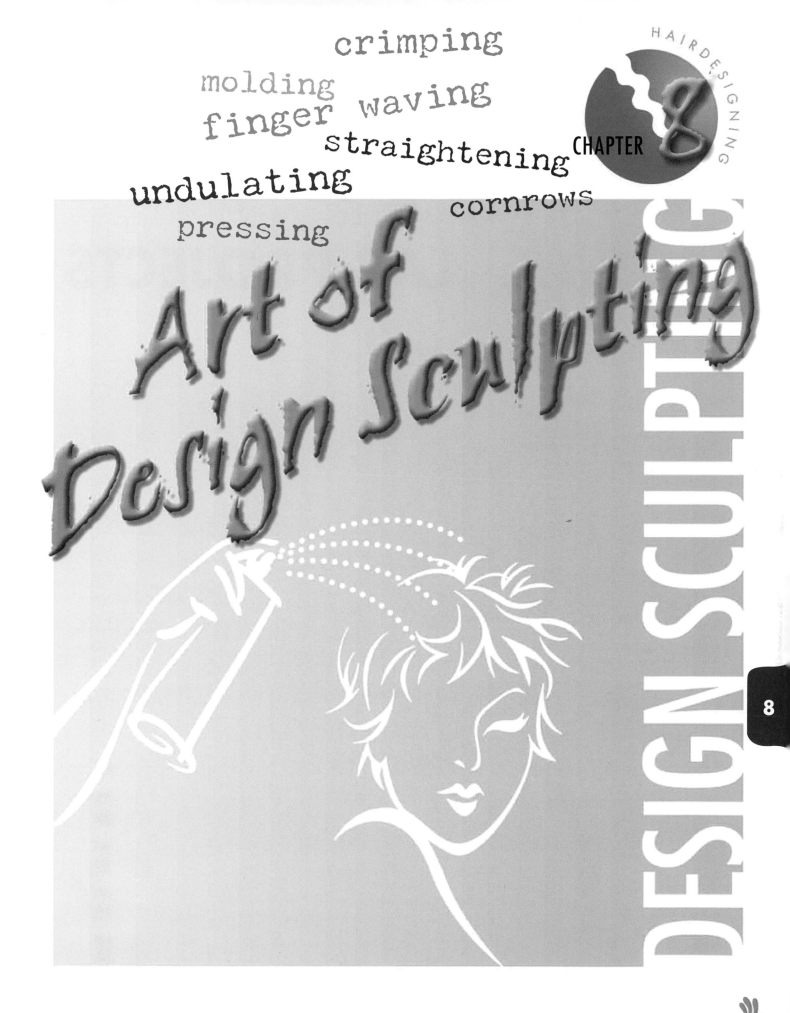

crimping

molding

finger waving

straightening

undulating

pressing

cornrows

HAIRDESIGNING

CHAPTER **8**

Art of
Design Sculpting

DESIGN SCULPTING

8

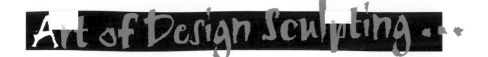

Design Sculpting LAB PROJECTS

8

Sculpting *shapes or forms creates a three-dimensional work of art. Design sculpting may construct a two-dimensional finished hairdesign. It may also be the structural framework to build upon toward the development of a more complex result, which creates a three-dimensional art form (length, width and depth).*

With the use of various thermal tools, design sculpting builds upon combing concepts and techniques to create designs that emphasize precision and detail.

The three lab projects for design sculpting skill levels are:

Simple

Work with fingers and a comb on the head to sketch or mold the hair into waves or create a hairdesign that conforms to the curve of the head.

Intermediate

Upgrade basic manual dexterity skills by twisting and pinning the hair or by expanding knowledge of comb and thermal iron techniques.

Complex

Advance finger and comb manipulation techniques and improve thermal iron skills by placing wave formations on the head form in various directional design patterns.

"Practice, Practice, Practice!"

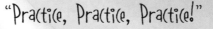

Design Sculpting

Simple

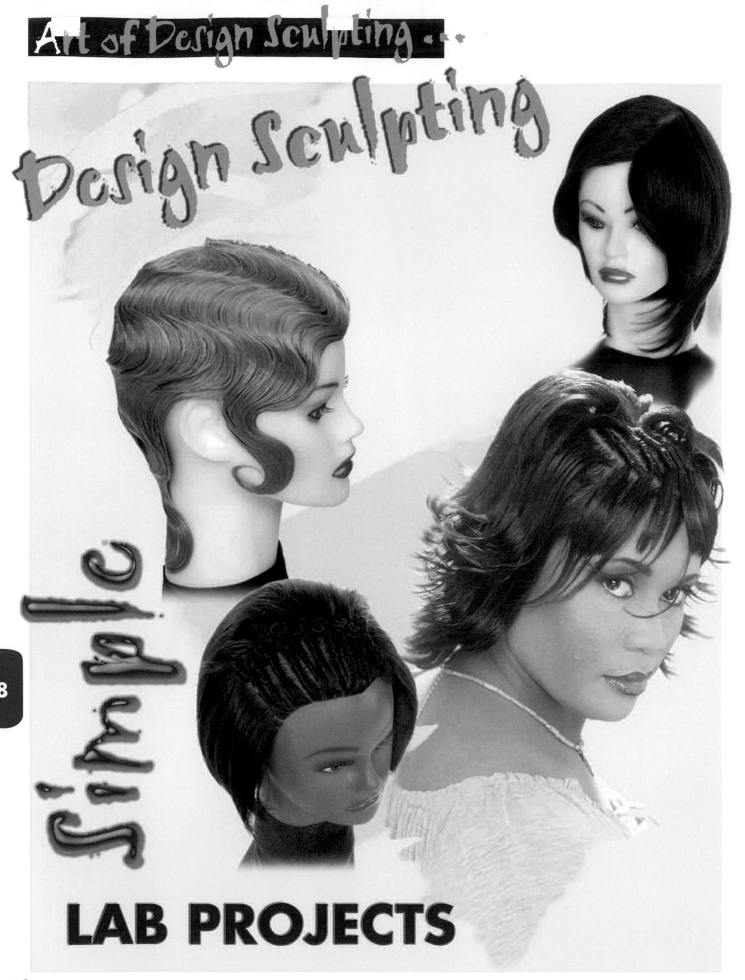

LAB PROJECTS

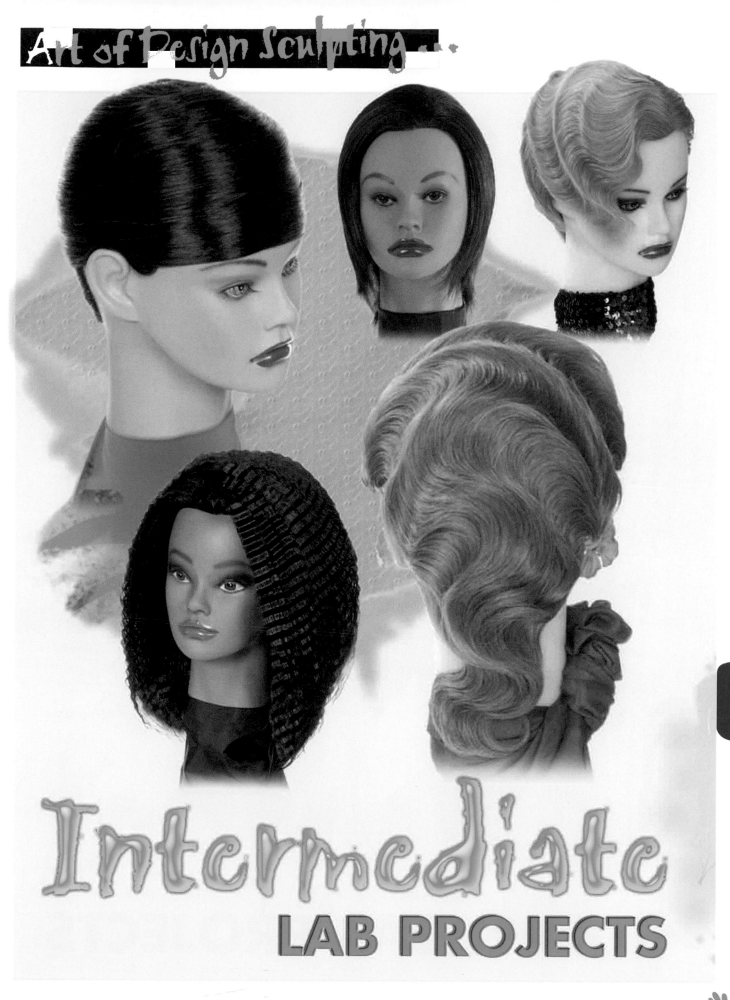

Intermediate
LAB PROJECTS

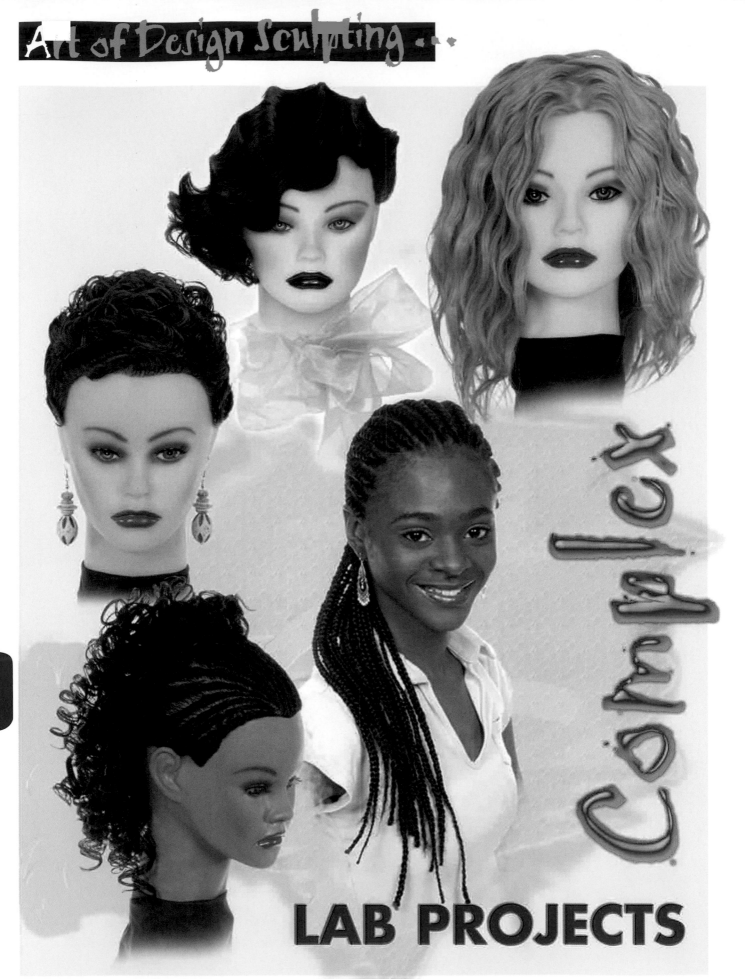

Complex

LAB PROJECTS

Art of Design Sculpting...

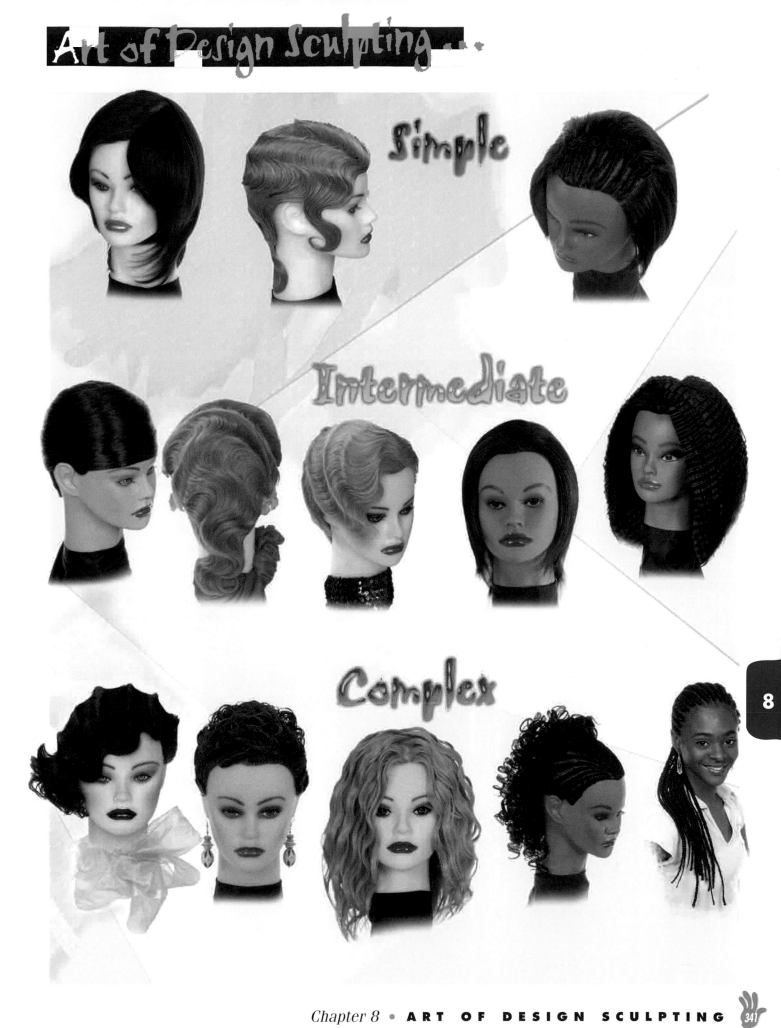

Simple

Intermediate

Complex

8

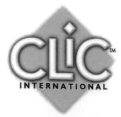

SIMPLE LAB PROJECT

Design Wrap

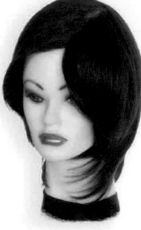

OBJECTIVE

Perform a low maintenance wrap set styling technique which utilizes the natural structure of the head as a tool to create a unique, two-dimensional setting pattern to manage and control the hair. This style will frame the face and have little to no elevation.

Design Wrap

TOOLS & MATERIALS

- Neck strip and cape/smock
- Towels and a hairnet
- Liquid styling tools

- Sectioning clips or clamps
- Airformer and/or hood dryer
- Cleansing and conditioning products

- Styling combs and brushes
- Rollers and picks or clips
- Flat/thermal/curling iron

- Client record card/file

PROCEDURE

"The client consultation is an important part of your professional service. Be sure to complete this step prior to each client service you provide. Your successful retail sales and customer satisfaction rates depend upon it!"

RETAIL RE-BOOK REFERRAL

1. Drape the client in preparation for the service. Hair should be naturally straight or chemically relaxed in order to achieve the best result.
2. Thoroughly brush the client's hair to remove knots, tangles, and hairspray.
3. Cleanse and condition the hair according to the client's needs. Rinse thoroughly and towel dry.
4. Comb the hair to detangle. Apply gel or another appropriate liquid styling tool.
5. Perform the style as shown.
6. Follow standard clean-up procedures.
7. Document the client record card/file.

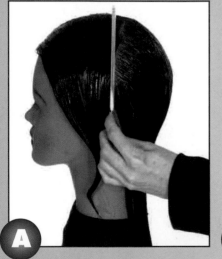

A

The design plan should establish the direction of the wrap, and determine whether or not the style contains a part. Determine the axis point in the crown area.

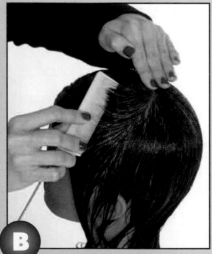

B

Placing a finger at the axis, use a comb to sketch (mold) the hair in either a clockwise or counter-clockwise radial distribution from the axis.

C

Follow the contour of the head, moving the comb and hair in the desired rotational direction.

8

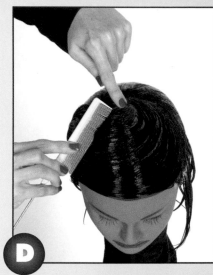

D Continue sketching the hair to fit the head form, working downward from the volume zone to the indentation zone.

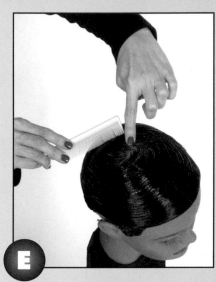

E Make sure the hair stays smooth while moving the hair with a comb around the circumference of the head.

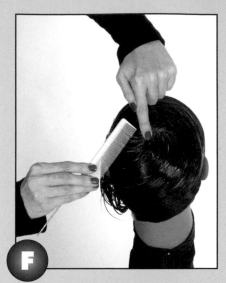

F The hair continues to form to the contour of the head, and is smoothed with the fine teeth of a comb or a natural bristle brush.

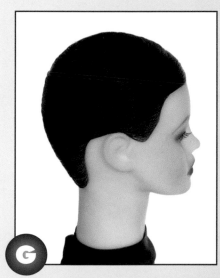

G Reapply gel if necessary to help hold the hair in place. When the hair is in the desired position, secure and support the pattern with neck strips and a hairnet or scarf.

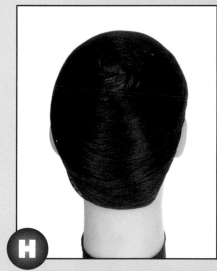

H Place the client under a hood dryer. Once dry, allow the hair to cool before brushing thoroughly in the direction of the style's design plan.

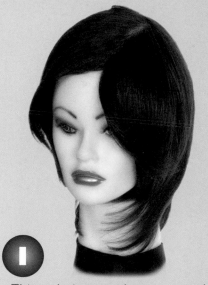

I This technique produces a smooth circular style which can be worn "as is" or thermal curled. Finish with detailing techniques and liquid styling spray.

EVALUATION

GRADE _____

STUDENT'S NAME _____   ID# _____

Variation of DESIGN

WRAP

LAB PROJECTS

Determine which of the three styling variations will be required based on your client's expectations for the style's durability along with her lifestyle or skill at maintaining the hairdesign.

Simple
Wet Design Wrap

Designed on wet, clean hair, this trouble-free style allows clients to manage and maintain the condition of their hair. A smoothing lotion or gel is applied to control curls or waves and assist in the straightening process.

Intermediate
Dry Design Wrap

If more straightening is desired, airform the hair using a smoothing lotion, then follow with a flat iron. An oil sheen adds smoothness and luster to the finished design. Use the wrap for clients who desire more volume or do not want to be placed under a hood dryer.

Complex
Roller Design Wrap

For the client who requires more base lift, place rollers at the crown, and start radial sketching around the roller perimeter. Gel supports and holds the finished style.

8

Five step method: forming the finger wave ridge

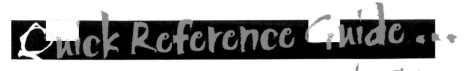

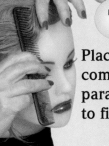
1 Place comb parallel to finger.

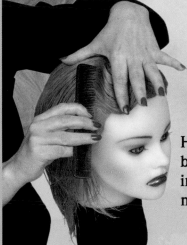

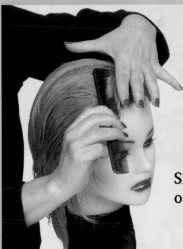
2 Slide hair about one inch (2.5 cm).

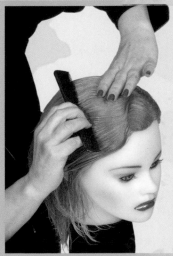
4 Hold the ridge between the index and middle fingers.

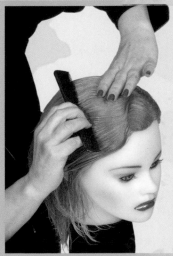
3 Lay the comb against the scalp to raise the ridge without pushing it up.

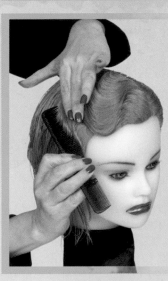
5 Comb the hair to the opposite side to prepare for the next direction.

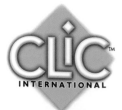

Basic Side Part Horizontal Finger Wave

OBJECTIVE

Create a side part horizontal finger wave with flat pin curls at the perimeter. This style from the 1920's continues to fascinate and remind us historical fashion repeats itself. Finger waves are best performed on 6" uniform hairdesigns or short bobs.

RA

Basic Side Part Horizontal Finger Wave

TOOLS & MATERIALS

- Neck strip and cape/smock
- Towels and a hairnet
- Single prong clips
- Client record card/file
- Cleansing and conditioning products
- Styling combs and brushes
- Liquid styling tools
- Hood dryer

PROCEDURE

"The client consultation is an important part of your professional service. Be sure to complete this step prior to each client service you provide. Your successful retail sales and customer satisfaction rates depend upon it!"

RETAIL • RE-BOOK • REFERRAL

1. Drape the client in preparation for the service.
2. Thoroughly brush the client's hair to remove knots, tangles and hairspray.
3. Cleanse and condition the hair according to the client's needs. Rinse thoroughly and towel dry.
4. Comb the hair to detangle. Apply gel or another appropriate liquid styling tool.
5. Perform the finger wave as shown.
6. Follow standard clean-up procedures.
7. Document the client record card/file.

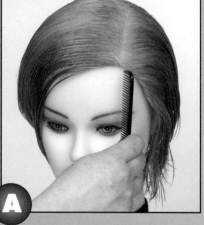

A Make a side part. Begin at the high point of the eyebrow, and finish the part where the end of a comb leaves the curve of the head at the crown. Direct the hair back toward the crown area, and mold an elongated "C" shaping on the heavy side of the part line. **Caution:** If the side part is too low, the design will be unbalanced.

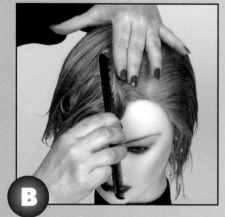

B Using a two finger measurement guide from the part, make the ridge of the finger wave by placing the comb's teeth parallel to your fingers and the part. Draw the comb forward along the index finger with the wide teeth facing slightly upward. Slide the hair about an inch (2.5 cm) toward the open end of the "C" shape. **Caution:** Do not push the hair up to form the ridge.

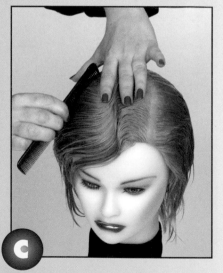

C Place the teeth of the comb flat against the scalp. Slide the middle finger to the index finger position. Apply pressure and redirect the hair downward, connecting into the next "C" shaped indentation to form a hollow.

8

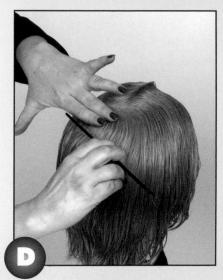

D Mold the hair in the opposite direction without disturbing the ridge by holding the ridge tightly with the index and middle fingers. Use the fine teeth of the comb to smooth the hair while retracing the movement. Continue forming the "C" shape around to the left side.

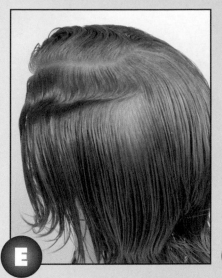

E The next finger wave will begin on the left side of the head, which will be lighter in weight due to the side placement of the part. Start the ridge two finger widths from the part. This ridge line will travel completely around the head form, creating the second ridge on the heavy side.

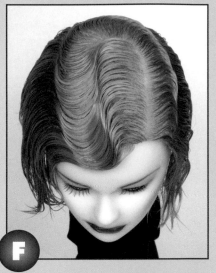

F Repeat the steps above for forming the ridge consistently throughout the finger wave. Work in small panels as measured from the second knuckle to the tip of the index finger. Hold each ridge with pressure between the index and middle fingers. Without lifting the fingers, remove the comb while rotating the teeth toward the scalp to smooth the hair.

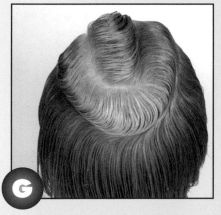

G Continue to use the two finger measurement guide, especially in this crucial connection area at the crown. Remember to slide the hair only about one inch (2.5 cm) to connect the ridges. Repeat the pattern from side to side on the head until the entire wave formation has been created.

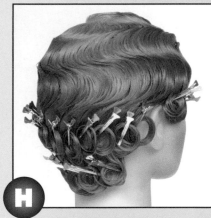

H Follow the finger wave below the occipital area with alternating oblong rows of counter-clockwise and clockwise pin curls (For instruction on making pin curls, see Chapter 4). Secure the design with a hairnet, and place the client under a hood dryer.

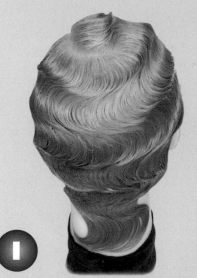

I The finished view is a timeless classic finger wave. It may be brushed, relaxed and dry molded for a softer look. Apply finishing spray to hold the style.

EVALUATION

GRADE

STUDENT'S NAME

ID#

8

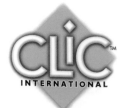

SIMPLE LAB PROJECT

Twisties Technique

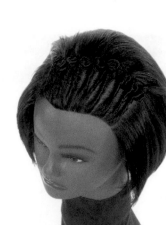

Twisties Technique

OBJECTIVE

To twist narrow subsections of hair close to the scalp and create a trendy design.

TOOLS & MATERIALS

- Neck strip and cape/smock
- Towels
- Liquid styling tools
- Small elastic bands
- Airformer
- Cleansing and conditioning products
- Styling combs and brushes
- Clips and bobbie pins
- Client record card/file
- Flat iron

PROCEDURE

"The client consultation is an important part of your professional service. Be sure to complete this step prior to each client service you provide. Your successful retail sales and customer satisfaction rates depend upon it!"

RETAIL RE-BOOK REFERRAL

1. Drape the client in preparation for the service.
2. Thoroughly brush the client's hair to remove knots, tangles and hairspray.
3. Cleanse and condition the hair according to the client's needs. Rinse thoroughly and towel dry.
   Variation: Perform this procedure on dry hair smoothed by an airformer and/or flat iron.
4. Comb the hair to detangle. Apply gel or another appropriate liquid styling tool.
5. Perform the style as shown.
6. Follow standard clean-up procedures.
7. Document the client record card/file.

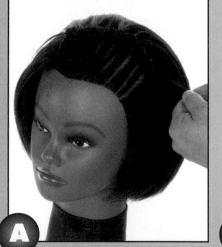

A

Part a thin subsection of hair approximately 1/4 inch wide (0.6 cm).

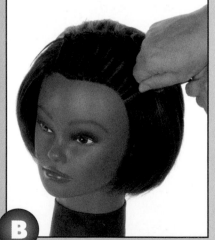

B

Start with a small portion of hair at the base of the subsection by the scalp.

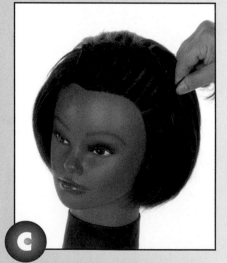

C

Using your thumb and index finger, twist the hair in either a clockwise or a counter-clockwise direction. Maintain low elevation by keeping very close to the head.

8

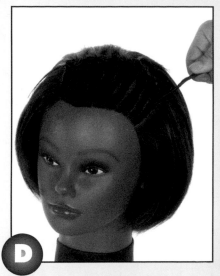

D Work down each subsection, from base to ends. Continue taking small amounts of hair and twisting the hair tightly to the scalp.

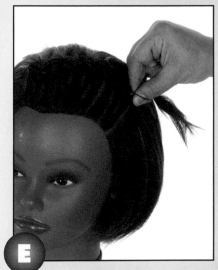

E At the end of each 1/4 inch (0.6 cm) subsection, secure the hair with an elastic band.

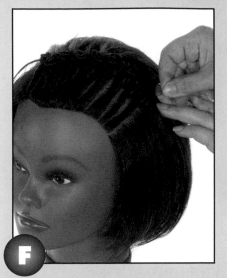

F Depending on the desired look, each subsection of hair may also be coiled at the base and secured with bobbie pins.

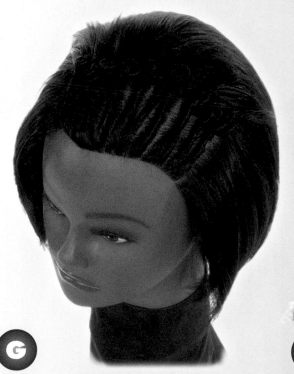

G The finished twisties design trend.

H Gel or finishing spray may be used for a wet look.

EVALUATION

_____

_____

GRADE _____ STUDENT'S NAME _____ ID# ____

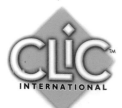

Vertical Finger Wave

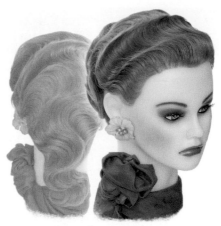

OBJECTIVE

Create a challenging vertical finger wave with a continuous flowing movement. The procedure is similar to a basic horizontal wave, except the comb is inserted vertically parallel to the head form rather than horizontally. This directional technique forms a vertical panel on the side or back plane of the head with waves traveling up and down the head form instead of forward and backward.

Vertical Finger Wave

TOOLS & MATERIALS

- Neck strip and cape/smock
- Towels and a hairnet
- Single prong clips
- Client record card/file
- Cleansing and conditioning products
- Styling combs and brushes
- Liquid styling tools
- Hood dryer

PROCEDURE

"The client consultation is an important part of your professional service. Be sure to complete this step prior to each client service you provide. Your successful retail sales and customer satisfaction rates depend upon it!"

RETAIL • RE-BOOK • REFERRAL

1. Drape the client in preparation for the service. Finger waves are best performed on 6" (15 cm) uniform hairdesigns or short bobs.
2. Thoroughly brush the client's hair to remove knots, tangles and hairspray.
3. Cleanse and condition the hair according to the client's needs. Rinse thoroughly and towel dry.
4. Comb the hair to detangle. Apply gel or another appropriate liquid styling tool.
5. Perform the finger wave as shown.
6. Follow standard clean-up procedures.
7. Document the client record card/file.

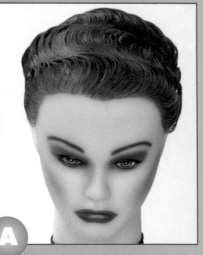

A

The "C" shaping may be started on either side. Develop the first ridge in the front by drawing the comb down vertically from the open end of the shaping. Work in 1 to 1.5 inch (2.5 – 3.8 cm) panels while creating each ridge. Follow the five step method for forming the ridge of a finger wave outlined earlier in this chapter.

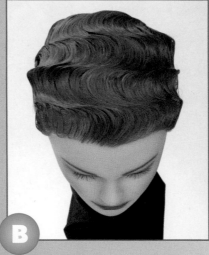

B

Form the finger wave until the crown has been reached with each ridge parallel and at an equal distance as measured by the width of two fingers. The formation of the vertical finger wave pattern actually appears to be horizontal when viewed only from the front hairline.

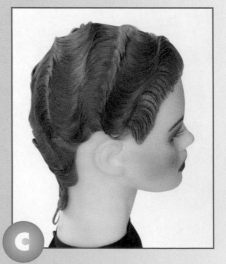

C

The profile view shows the vertical flow of the finger wave.

8

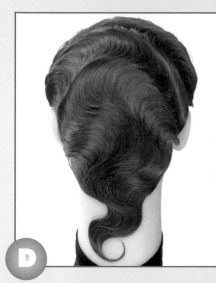

D At the crown area, continue forming the rest of the hair to the nape area into a smaller wave pattern to fit the head form. Place pin curls at the ends if needed. Secure the finger waves with a hairnet, and use a hood dryer to set the style.

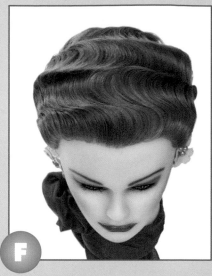

E Brush the hair gently to relax the wave pattern, starting at the nape and continuing to the front perimeter.

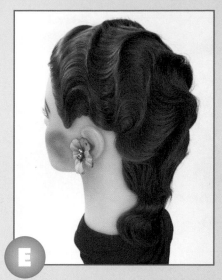

F Dry mold the waves, arranging them smoothly into their original directions.

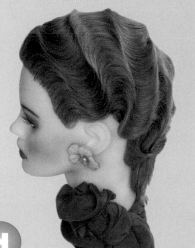

G The back should have a continuous flowing movement.

H Use finishing spray for hold as needed at the sides over the ear area.

EVALUATION

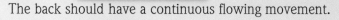

GRADE   STUDENT'S NAME   ID#

8

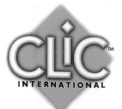

Diagonal Finger Wave

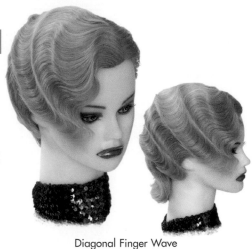

OBJECTIVE

Create a diagonal finger wave, placing the ridges parallel to each other at a 45-degree angle. Eliminating the part from this finger wave formation contributes to the diagonal feel of these waves.

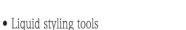

Diagonal Finger Wave

TOOLS & MATERIALS

- Neck strip and cape/smock
- Towels and a hairnet
- Single prong clips

- Client record card/file
- Cleansing and conditioning products
- Styling combs and brushes

- Liquid styling tools
- Hood dryer

PROCEDURE

"The client consultation is an important part of your professional service. Be sure to complete this step prior to each client service you provide. Your successful retail sales and customer satisfaction rates depend upon it!"

RETAIL · RE-BOOK
REFERRAL

1. Drape the client in preparation for the service.
2. Thoroughly brush the client's hair to remove knots, tangles and hairspray.
3. Cleanse and condition the hair according to the client's needs. Rinse thoroughly and towel dry.
4. Comb the hair to detangle. Apply gel or another appropriate liquid styling tool.
5. Perform the finger wave as shown.
6. Follow standard clean-up procedures.
7. Document the client record card/file.

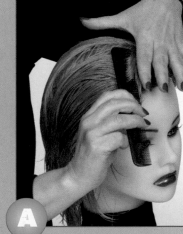

A

Start on the right side of the head to mold an elongated "C" shape from one recession line to the other. Begin forming the ridge on a 45-degree angle at the open end of the shaping.

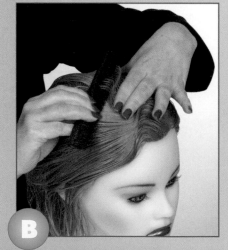

B

Follow the five step method for forming the ridge of a finger wave outlined earlier in this chapter. The second ridge starts again at the open end of the shaping on a 45-degree angle, but on the left side of the head, opposite the first ridge.

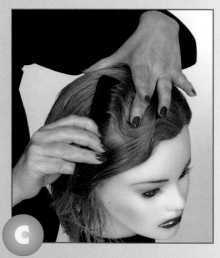

C

Connect the diagonal finger wave pattern under the first ridge using the distance of two fingers' width as a guide to maintain even spacing.

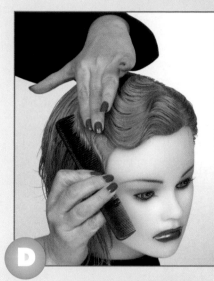

D Using the fine teeth of the comb, smooth the hair in the opposite direction to prepare for the next wave formation. Begin forming the third ridge at the open end of the shaping, reversing the directional flow used for the second ridge.

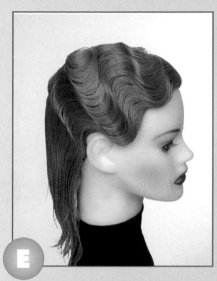

E Continue this pattern around the back of the head, always working from one side of the head toward the other side. Maintain a consistent 45-degree angle and a width measurement of two fingers for each wave pattern.

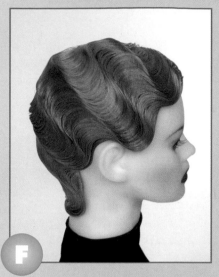

F Complete the pattern of alternating ridges and hollows in the lower nape.

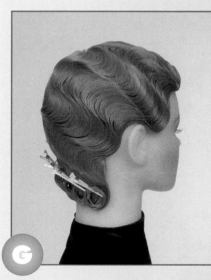

G The ends of the hair may be finished with pin curls. Place a hairnet over the finger waves, and use a hood dryer to set the style.

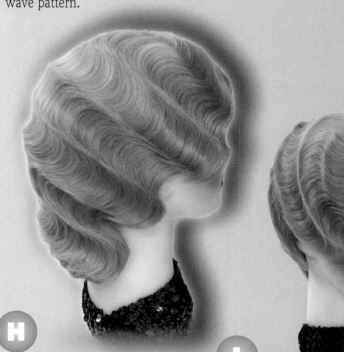

H Once dry, the diagonal finger wave may be brushed, relaxed, and dry molded for a softer finished look.

I Apply finishing spray to add definition and hold the waved style.

EVALUATION

GRADE   STUDENT'S NAME   ID#

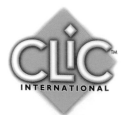

INTERMEDIATE LAB PROJECT

Thermal Pressing

OBJECTIVE To temporarily straighten overly curly or wavy hair using a conventional heater and pressing comb.

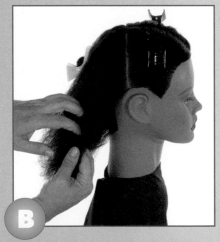

Thermal Pressing

TOOLS & MATERIALS

- Neck strip and cape/smock
- Clips or clamps
- Pressing comb and heater
- Airformer/hood dryer
- Marcel iron
- Cleansing and conditioning products
- Towels
- Styling combs and brushes
- Pressing cream or oil and or other liquid styling tools
- Client record card/file

PROCEDURE

"The client consultation is an important part of your professional service. Be sure to complete this step prior to each client service you provide. Your successful retail sales and customer satisfaction rates depend upon it!"

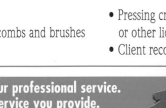

1. Drape the client in preparation for the service.
2. Thoroughly brush the client's hair to remove knots, tangles and hairspray.
3. Cleanse and condition the hair according to the client's needs. Rinse thoroughly and towel dry.
4. Comb the hair to detangle. Pressing cream or oil may be applied at this time, or once hair is dried. Using an excessive amount of oil may cause smoke or burning when contacted with heat.
5. Airform the hair, or place the client under a hood dryer.
6. Perform the style as shown.
7. Follow standard clean-up procedures.
8. Document the client record card/file.

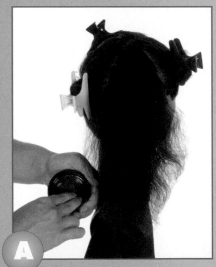

A

Section the hair into quadrants by parting from center front to nape and from ear to ear. Determine the technique to be applied. A soft press removes half of the hair's curl; a hard press will completely straighten the strand.

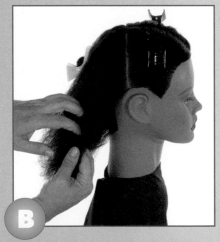

B

Work pressing cream through the first section in the back of the head. Adjust the heat and pressure used based on the hair's texture. Gray or lightened hair may discolor when pressed with too much heat.
Caution: For safety, always temperature test the pressing comb prior to use on the client's hair (see Chapter 2).

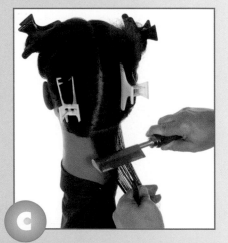

C

Taking a 1/4 inch (0.6 cm) parting, run the pressing comb along the surface of the hair to warm the subsection. Do not use high heat when pressing the fragile, short hair at the nape or temple areas. Breakage may occur with improper or too frequent pressing.

8

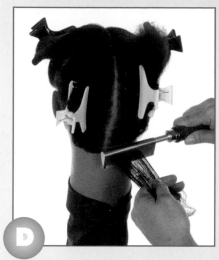

D Insert the pressing comb as close as possible to the base of the strand without touching the scalp. An all purpose comb may be placed between the scalp and the pressing comb to help avoid contact with the scalp.

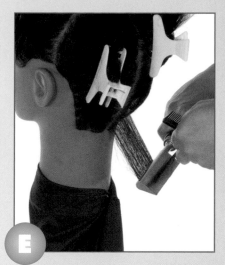

E Turn the teeth of the comb toward your body, and draw the comb out along the length of the strand. The back of the comb does the actual straightening.

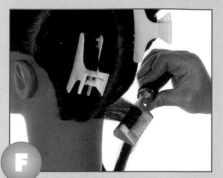

F Reinsert the pressing comb underneath each subsection, straightening down the length of the hair strand on both sides. In the soft press technique, the heated comb is used once on each side of the hair. The hard press is requires applying heat to both sides twice. A double press may be used for strong or resistant curl patterns; pass a hot curling iron over each section to pre-warm the strands and follow with a hard press.

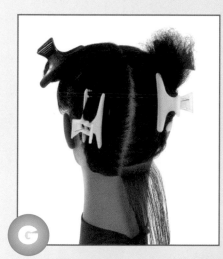

G Work from bottom to top in each section, pressing the hair until each subsection has been straightened. A touch-up treatment between shampoos is performed on new growth only.

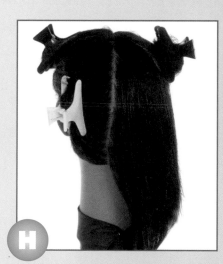

H The completed thermal press section. Continue pressing around the head until each section has been straightened. Burnt hair strands cannot be conditioned and must be trimmed.

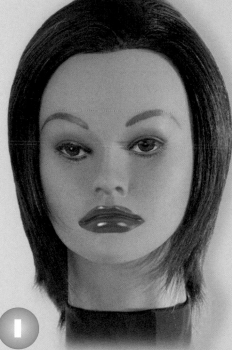

I A Marcel iron and finishing spray may also be used on the completed thermal press style, which lasts until the next shampoo.

EVALUATION

GRADE

STUDENT'S NAME

ID#

8

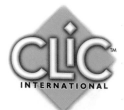

Crimping Wave

OBJECTIVE

To place an angular wave pattern into the hair using a crimping iron.

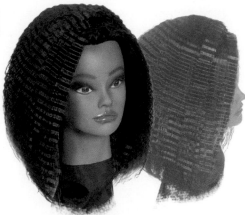

Crimping Wave

TOOLS & MATERIALS

- Neck strip and cape/smock
- Towels
- Clips

- Liquid styling tools
- Cleansing and conditioning products
- Styling combs and brushes

- Airformer and flat/crimping iron
- Client record card/file

PROCEDURE

"The client consultation is an important part of your professional service. Be sure to complete this step prior to each client service you provide. Your successful retail sales and customer satisfaction rates depend upon it!"

1. Drape the client in preparation for the service.
2. Thoroughly brush the client's hair to remove knots, tangles and hairspray.
3. Cleanse and condition the hair according to the client's needs. Rinse thoroughly and towel dry.
4. Comb the hair to detangle. Apply an appropriate liquid styling tool and airform the hair.
5. The hair may also be flat ironed after airforming to ensure it is completely smooth.
6. Perform the style as shown.
7. Follow standard clean-up procedures.
8. Document the client record card/file.

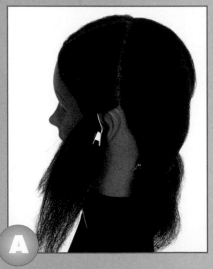

A The hair is divided into four sections or according to style pattern.

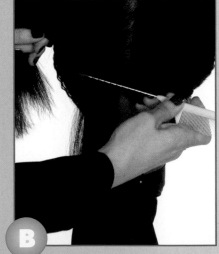

B Starting at the bottom of the section and take a 1/4 inch (0.6 cm) parting.

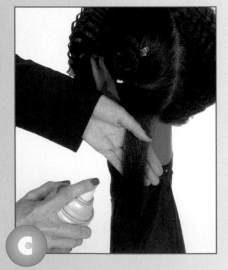

C Lightly apply finishing spray to the subsection in order to add better control to soft hair and increase definition of the wave pattern.

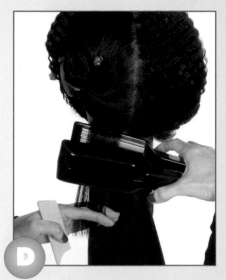

D

Place the crimping iron as close to the scalp as possible without touching the scalp. Close the iron and hold for approximately 10 seconds, or until heat thoroughly penetrates the strand.

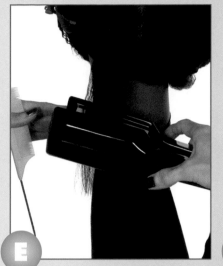

E

Working down the strand, place the iron next to the previously crimped hair.

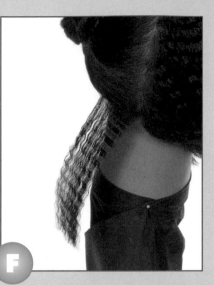

F

Continue until the ends of the strand are reached.

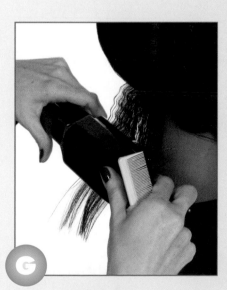

G

Move up the section of hair, continuing to take 1/4 inch (0.6 cm) subsections.

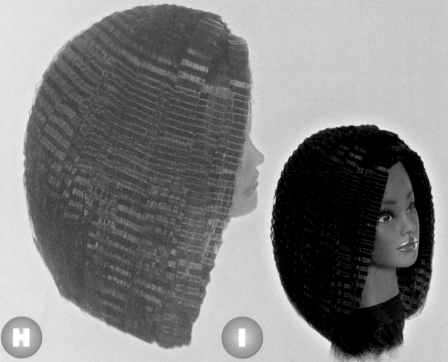

H

This pattern is followed until the entire hairdesign is complete.

I

An oil sheen may be lightly applied to the completed style.

EVALUATION

GRADE

STUDENT'S NAME

ID#

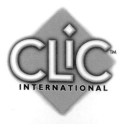

COMPLEX LAB PROJECT

Asymmetrical Finger Wave

OBJECTIVE

To create an asymmetrical finger wave, with the distribution of weight heavier on one side of the design and finished with the application of pin curls.

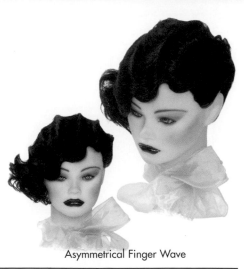

Asymmetrical Finger Wave

TOOLS & MATERIALS

- Neck strip and cape/smock
- Towels
- Single prong clips
- Hairnet
- Liquid styling tools
- Cleansing and conditioning products
- Styling combs and brushes
- Sectioning clamps or clips
- Hood dryer
- Client record card/file

PROCEDURE

"The client consultation is an important part of your professional service. Be sure to complete this step prior to each client service you provide. Your successful retail sales and customer satisfaction rates depend upon it!"

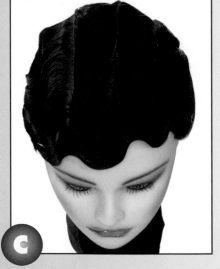

1. Drape the client in preparation for the service.
2. Thoroughly brush the client's hair to remove knots, tangles and hairspray.
3. Cleanse and condition the hair according to the client's needs. Rinse thoroughly and towel dry.
4. Comb the hair to detangle. Apply gel or another appropriate liquid styling tool.
5. Perform the finger wave as shown.
6. Follow standard clean-up procedures.
7. Document the client record card/file.

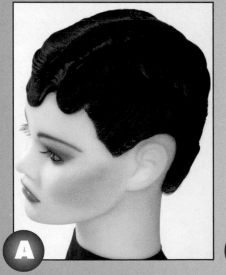

A

Start by combing all hair to one side of the head. Mold a "C" shape along the perimeter on the left side.

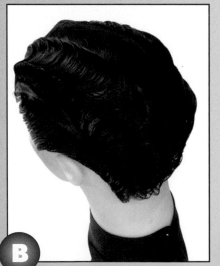

B

Form the first ridge above the ear at the open end of the oblong. Follow the five step method for forming the ridge of a finger wave outlined earlier in this chapter.

C

Each ridge and hollow must run parallel and be evenly spaced and of equal size. Use two fingers as a measurement guide to determine the width of the wave. Work across the top of the head to the other side.

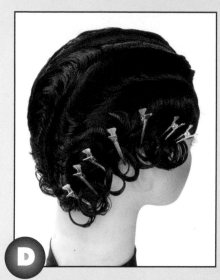

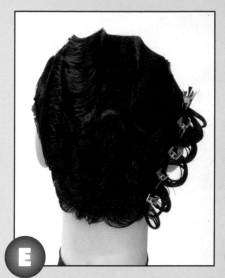

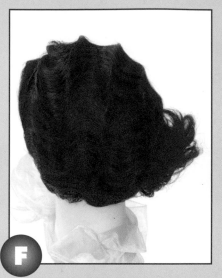

D Counter-clockwise pin curls may be placed along the perimeter of the style's heavier side. Pin curls must be a consistent size and shape.

E Secure the finished wave with a hairnet, and place the client under a hood dryer.

F When thoroughly dried, brush through the hair to relax the style and create a softer finish.

G Check for form and balance on the lighter side.

H Dry mold the asymmetrical design into the original wave pattern established before applying a finishing spray to set the style.

8

EVALUATION

GRADE

STUDENT'S NAME

ID#

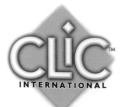
Push Wave

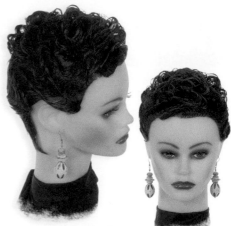

Push Wave

OBJECTIVE

To perform another hair waving variation, using two combs instead of fingers to lift the wave up from the head and create a three dimensional art form with length, depth, and width.

TOOLS & MATERIALS

- Neck strip and cape/smock
- Cleansing and conditioning products
- Clips
- Client record card/file
- Towels
- Styling combs and brushes
- Hood dryer
- Liquid styling tools

PROCEDURE

"The client consultation is an important part of your professional service. Be sure to complete this step prior to each client service you provide. Your successful retail sales and customer satisfaction rates depend upon it!"

1. Drape the client in preparation for the service.
2. Thoroughly brush the client's hair to remove knots, tangles and hairspray.
3. Cleanse and condition the hair according to the client's needs. Rinse thoroughly and towel dry.
4. Comb the hair to detangle. Apply gel or another appropriate liquid styling tool.
5. Perform the style as shown.
6. Follow standard clean-up procedures.
7. Document the client record card/file.

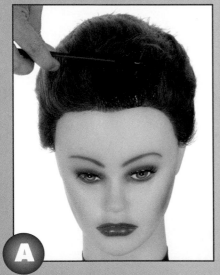

A Comb the hair smoothly along the front hairline, with the top and sides moving toward the back of the head.

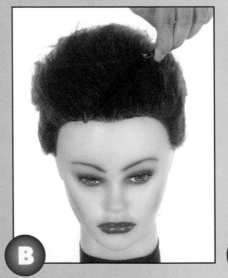

B Use a tail comb to lift the front hairline to the preferred height.

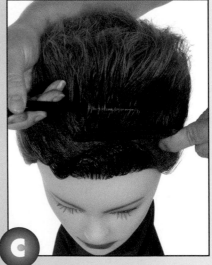

C Place another comb behind the first comb. Hold the hair between the two combs to force the ridge of a wave into the hair.

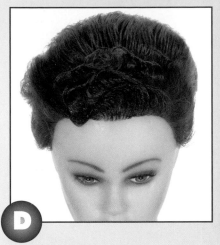

D Move back to the next area, and repeat this pattern until the desired amount of hair is completely lifted and pushed or scrunched into waves. If the hair is short, this procedure may be performed over the entire head. If the hair is long, push waves are created only from the front hairline to the crown area, and the back is finished with another technique.

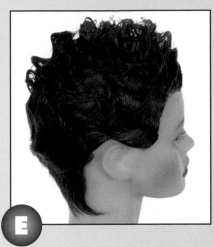

E Place the client under a hood dryer until the hair is partially dry.

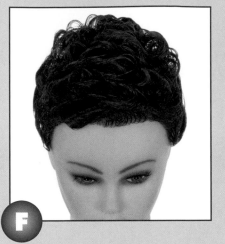

F Remove the client from the dryer, and mist the style with oil sheen and finishing spray. Return the client to the hood dryer, and allow the hair to dry completely.

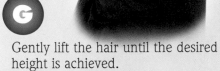

G Gently lift the hair until the desired height is achieved.

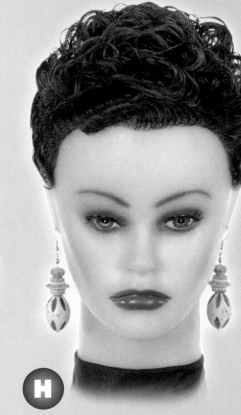

H Arrange the push wave style in its final form. Spray the hairdesign with an oil sheen to add luster, and apply finishing spray for support.

EVALUATION

GRADE

STUDENT'S NAME

ID#

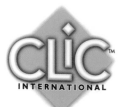
Undulating Wave

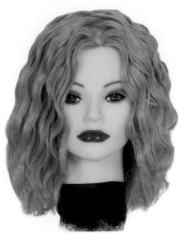

Undulating Wave

OBJECTIVE

To create a wave pattern in hair that has been air-formed to a straight smooth texture. The use of a thermal iron will produce the finished elegant appearance of soft, flowing waves.

TOOLS & MATERIALS

- Neck strip and cape/smock
- Clips
- Airformer
- Client record card/file
- Cleansing and conditioning products
- Flat/thermal/waver iron
- Styling combs and brushes
- Liquid styling tools

PROCEDURE

"The client consultation is an important part of your professional service. Be sure to complete this step prior to each client service you provide. Your successful retail sales and customer satisfaction rates depend upon it!"

1. Drape the client in preparation for the service.
2. Thoroughly brush the client's hair to remove knots, tangles and hairspray.
3. Cleanse and condition on the hair according to the client's needs. Rinse thoroughly and towel dry.
4. Comb the hair to detangle. Apply an appropriate liquid styling tool and airform the hair.
5. The hair may also be flat ironed after airforming to ensure complete smoothness.
6. Perform the style as shown.
7. Follow standard clean-up procedures.
8. Document the client record card/file.

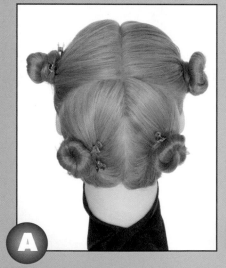

A The hair is divided into four sections, or according to the style pattern established in the design plan.

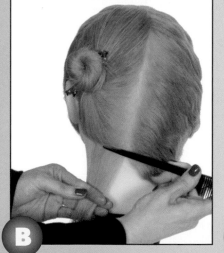

B Starting at the bottom of the section make a 1/4 inch (0.6 cm) parting.

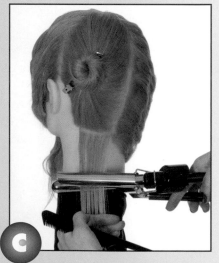

C Place a thermal iron on the subsection of hair, and glide down the strand to the ends to pre-warm the hair.

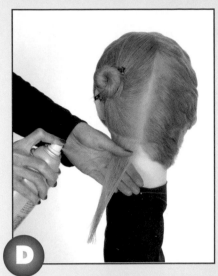

D

Lightly apply finishing spray to the subsection in order to increase definition of the wave pattern and add better control to soft hair.

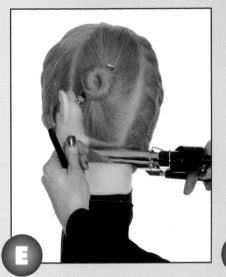

E

Place the shell of the iron on top of the subsection. Pull the ends of the hair up, allowing the shell to rest briefly on the hair, approximately five seconds.
Caution:
To prevent crimping, the shell must not rest too tightly on the hair.

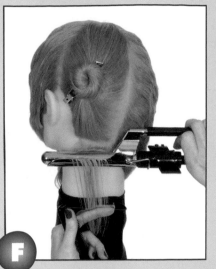

F

Place the iron next to the previous movement with the rod on top of the subsection. Pull the ends of the hair down, and allow the rod to rest on the hair for approximately five seconds, or until the heat causes the hair to take the form of the iron.

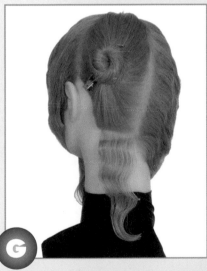

G

Continue to work down the strand in the same manner until the ends are reached. Move up the section following this pattern.

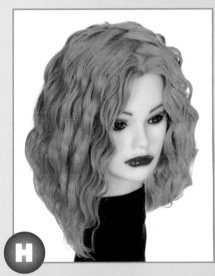

H

Follow the same steps for each section until the pattern is achieved throughout the head.

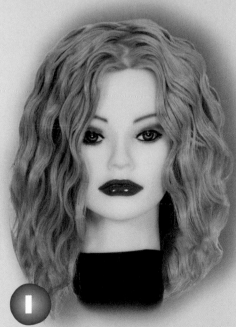

I

A finishing spray may be used on the completed style for better hold.

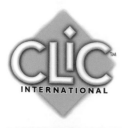

Cornrows

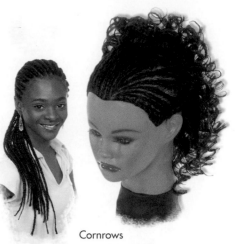

Cornrows

OBJECTIVE

To place individual cornrow braids in any length hair for a design partially or completely covering the head form.

TOOLS & MATERIALS

- Neck strip and cape/smock
- Clips and bobbie pins
- Airformer
- Small elastic bands
- Client record card/file
- Cleansing and conditioning products
- Towels
- Flat/waving/curling iron
- Styling combs and brushes
- Liquid styling tools

PROCEDURE

"The client consultation is an important part of your professional service. Be sure to complete this step prior to each client service you provide. Your successful retail sales and customer satisfaction rates depend upon it!"

RETAIL • RE-BOOK • REFERRAL

1. Drape the client in preparation for the service.
2. Thoroughly brush the client's hair to remove knots, tangles and hairspray.
3. Cleanse and condition the hair according to the client's needs. Rinse thoroughly and towel dry.
4. Comb the hair to detangle. Apply an appropriate liquid styling tool. This procedure may be performed on damp hair or on airformed hair that has been smoothed with a chemical relaxer, flat iron or pressing comb.
5. Perform the style as shown.
6. Follow standard clean-up procedures.
7. Document the client record card/file.

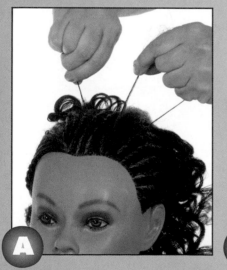

A Divide the hair according to the desired design plan (partial or whole head). Start at the front hairline. Separate a 1/4 inch (0.6 cm) subsection into three individual strands.

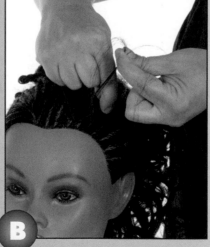

B An under braid technique is used, keeping the hair very close to the head. Cross the outside strand from either side under the center strand.

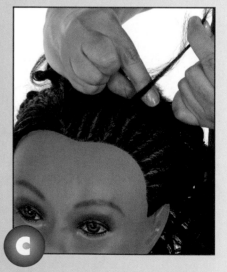

C Continue to under braid into cornrows while moving down the subsection of hair.

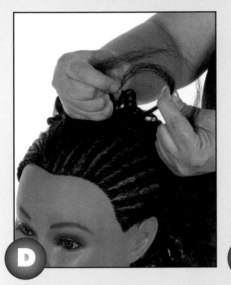

D Keep fingers close to the scalp to maintain a low elevation. Apply firm tension on the hair, but not too tight to prevent scalp redness or hot spots.

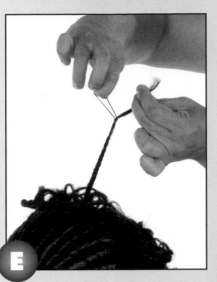

E Continue to cornrow down the strand to the hair ends. Secure each braid at the end with a small elastic band.

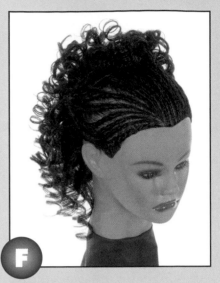

F The braided ends can be arranged and secured at the scalp. Finish the hair remaining as desired (curling iron, flat iron, etc.).

Variation

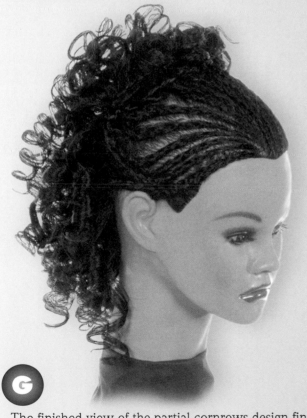

G The finished view of the partial cornrows design finished with spiral curls. Oil sheen may be lightly applied to the hair.

H **Full head cornrows**
Under braid the entire strand close to the head form, and secure the ends of each strand in the style with a small elastic band.

EVALUATION

GRADE

STUDENT'S NAME

ID#

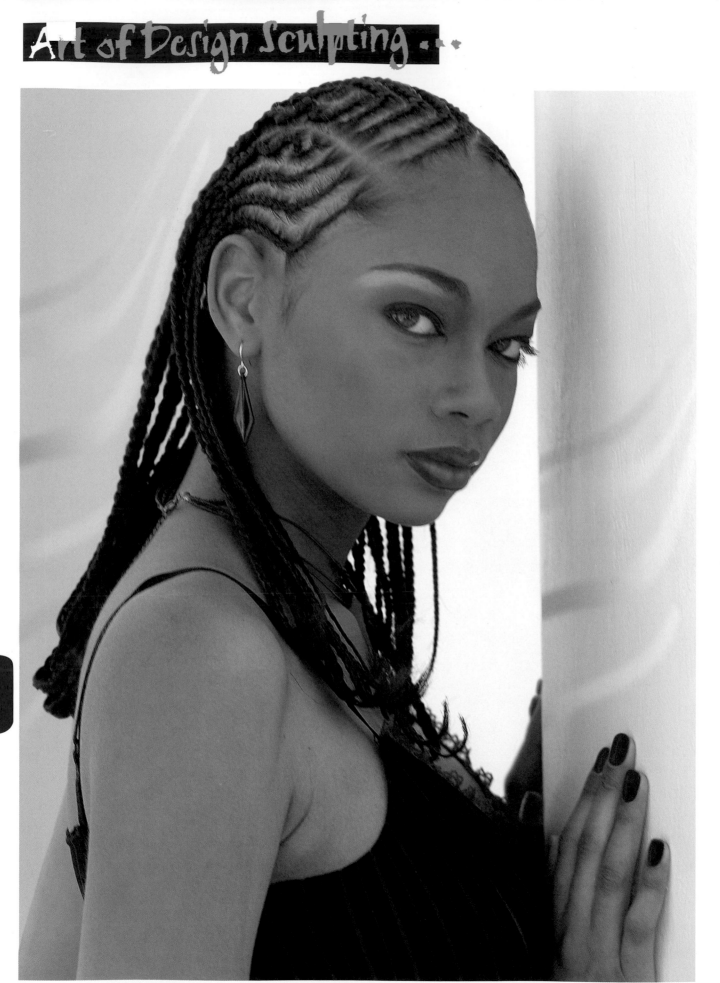

8

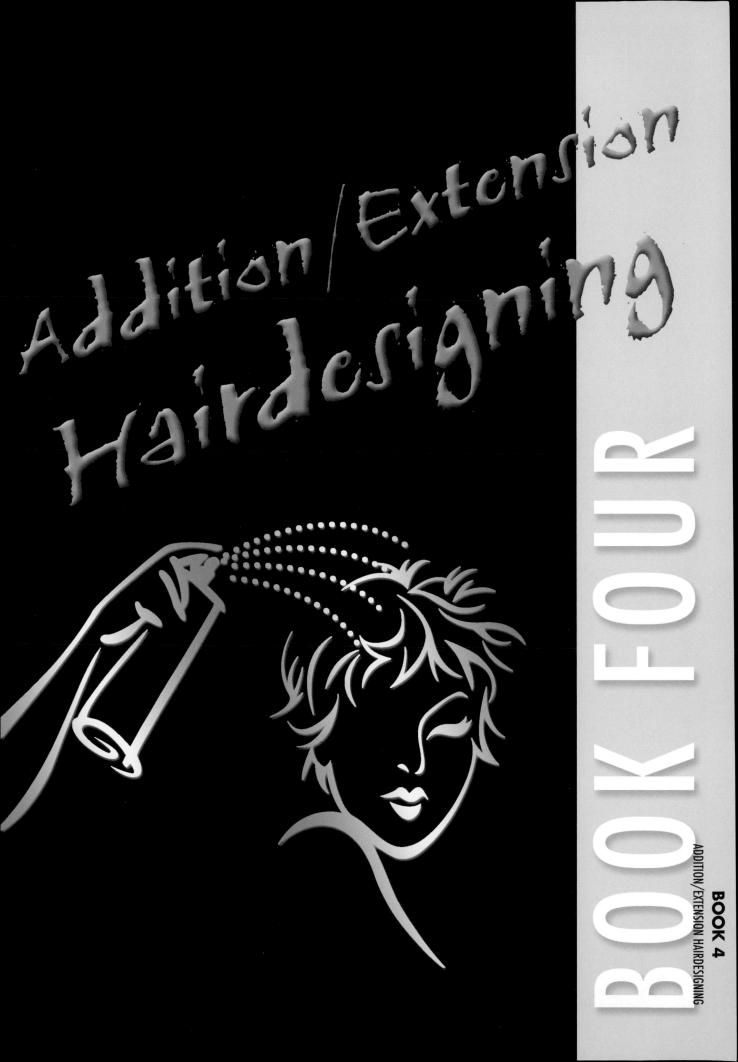

Addition/Extension Hairdesigning

BOOK FOUR

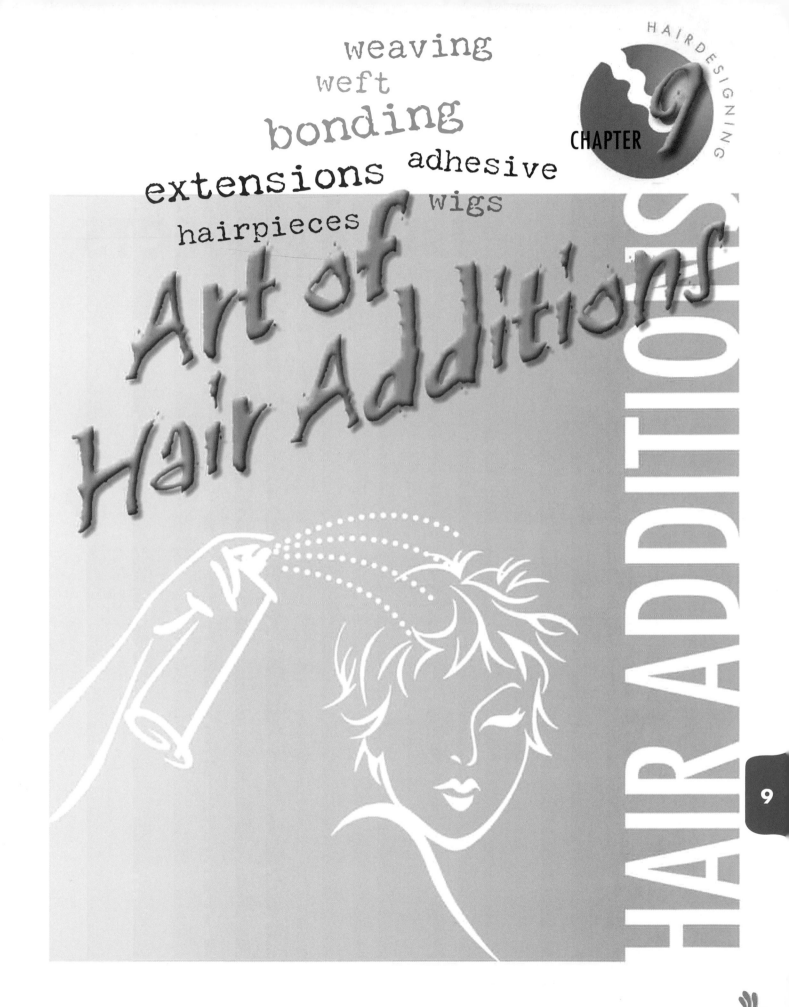

weaving
weft
bonding
extensions   adhesive
hairpieces   wigs

Art of
Hair Additions

Hair Additions
LAB PROJECTS

Simple

Intermediate

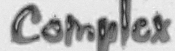

Complex

Extra Credit Lab Projects

1

2

9

Hair additions services provide the client with the appearance of any hair texture, length or color he/she desires. A good illusionist performs all kinds of tricks the eye can see but not believe. However, there is no magic secret involved; it is about simply knowing how the illusion is achieved. With the proper training and practice, hairdesigners who study and practice this art of illusion may provide one of the most in demand, lucrative services in the beauty industry.

The first **secret** is that there are many ways to accomplish what the client needs and wants. The choices are broad when selecting both the tool used and the service. Although descriptions for tools used with hair additions services were covered in Chapter 2, this knowledge will now be incorporated into choosing the **proper tool**, **service** and **application technique** to fit the client's demands.

As with all services, the **consultation** is the key to a successful service. Clients come to you as a knowledgeable professional for help with their hair problems. Make a client in need of hair additions services more **comfortable** by keeping a separate room available for consultations and application. Know what the client wishes to gain from his/her hair additions service.

9

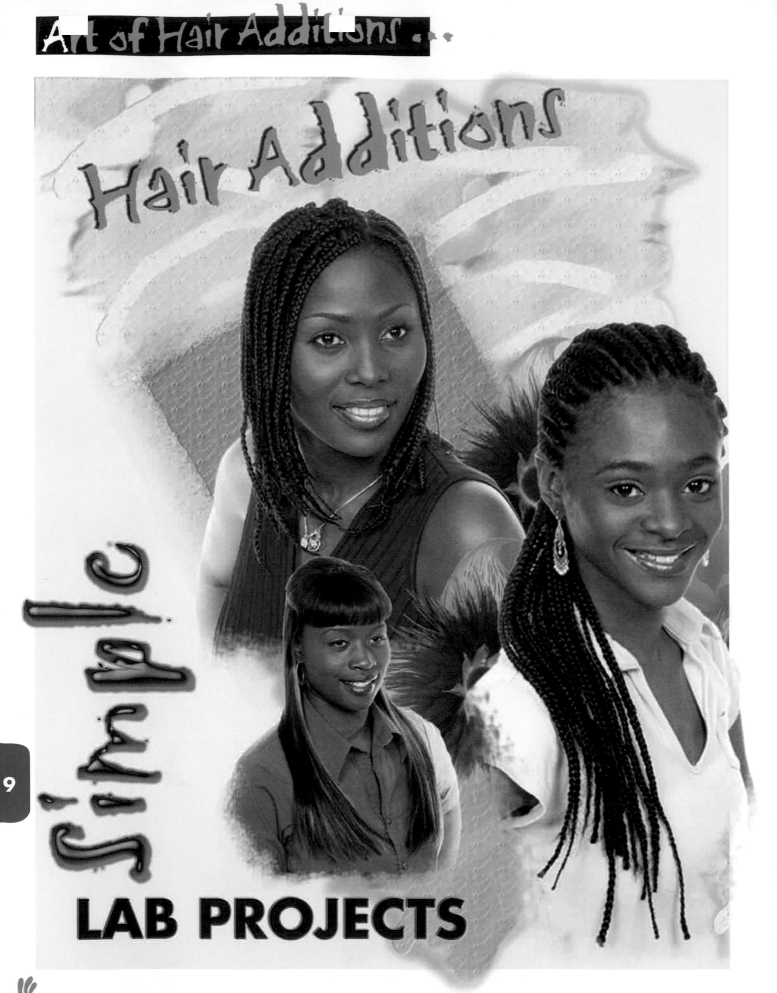

Hair Additions

Simple

LAB PROJECTS

9

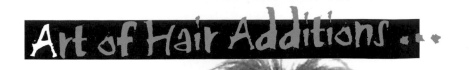
Intermediate
LAB PROJECTS

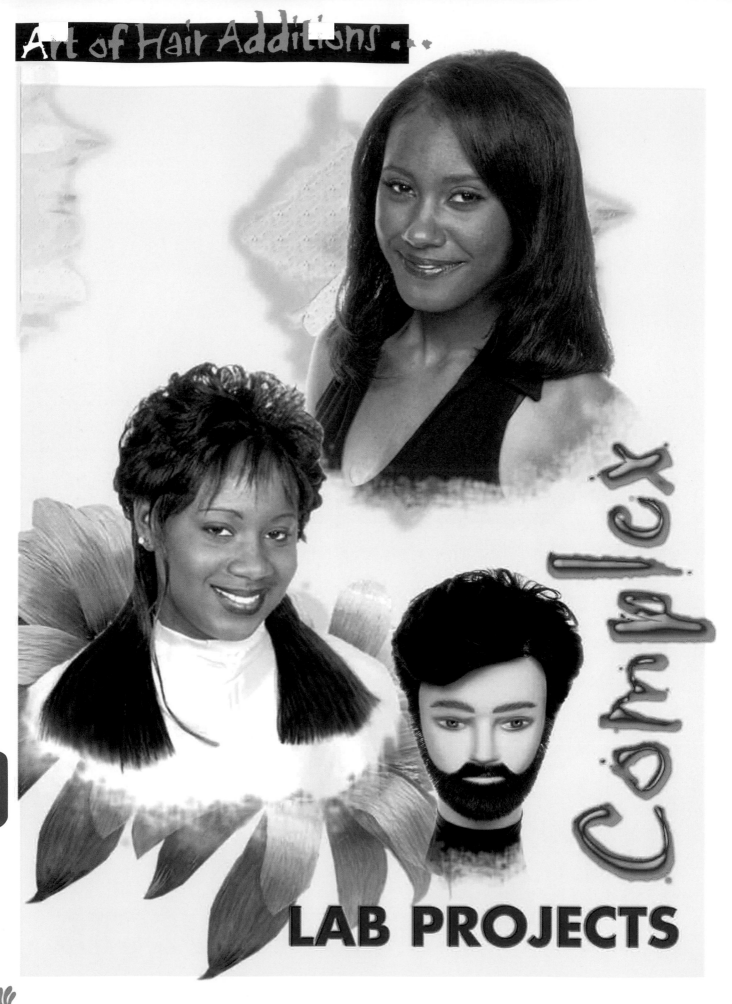

Complex

LAB PROJECTS

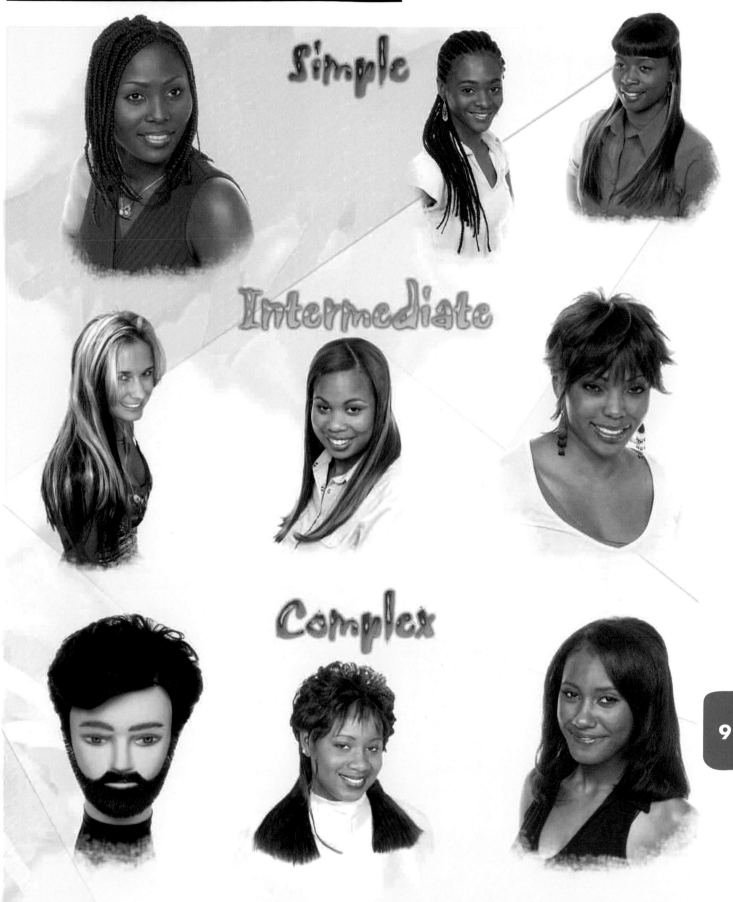

Simple

Intermediate

Complex

Reasons clients seek hair additions services:

To add length –
Hair additions provide a valuable service for clients who may be unable to grow their hair to the length desired, or are unwilling to wait for additional length to grow before changing their style.

To replace hair that has been lost –
The variety of hair additions services available, along with the versatility of application techniques, enables the hairdesigner specializing in these services to offer a customized look to a client who requires partial to full coverage of missing hair. Hair additions services help to improve a client's self-image in times of great psychological stress.

To add volume –
Clients with naturally fine or thinning hair due to either damage or medical reasons will benefit from immediate improvement in the appearance of increased hair texture and healthy-looking condition a hair addition service provides.

To change appearance –
Fashionable clients often change hairdesigns at a whim, while others will choose hair additions services to wear elaborate styles for special occasions.

Before

After

There are three categories of hair additions services:

1 Extensions –
Hair or fiber is placed into the client's own hair, using the client's hair to hold the addition on the head. The addition may be purchased as tracks of hair or fiber sewn into a weft or individual strands attached with adhesive or clips.

2 Hairpieces –
Hair or fiber is attached to a "base" and attached to the client's head or hair, allowing partial coverage while incorporating at least some of the client's own hair into the design. Falls, switches, and wiglets in this category are designed to be added and removed by the client.

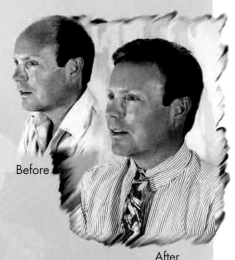

Before

After

3 Wigs –
The "base" allows full coverage of the client's head and hair. This service is designed to replace missing hair and/or be a fashion item for religious or social reasons. Special styles with net bases allow "integration" of the client's own hair with the wig hair or fiber. A hairpiece for men is referred to as a "unit," toupee or non-medical hair replacement system. For medical insurance purposes, a wig is also known as a cranial prosthesis.

Before

After

Art of Hair Additions...

The three types of hair or fibers to consider are:

1 Synthetic –
Best used for off scalp application techniques, synthetic (nylon, acetate, dynel, kanekalon, modacrylic and polyester) fibers require minimal care to maintain and are relatively inexpensive. Synthetic fibers are designed to stay and look the way they were purchased and will not accept a permanent wave or color change. They are maintained using only water-soluble based products and are air-dried, since synthetic material may melt with the application of heat styling tools.

2 Animal –
This source from goat or rabbit (angora), horse, yak (ox), camel, boar, or sheep hair may be blended with other types of hair additions or fibers. A type of animal hair fiber called "yaki" may be made from any combination of animal hair, and is a comparatively inexpensive alternative to human hair, with similar properties.

3 100% Human –
The preferred and most natural source, which can be chemically serviced and styled the same as the client's own hair. Hair is often harvested from China (most popular and least expensive), India (most readily available source), Italy and Russia (thinner hair diameter). A special "Remy" processing technique tags and aligns the cuticle from each hair in one direction, allowing for stronger color hold and less matting of this more expensive type of human hair.

It is extremely important to know the **material** a hair addition is made from, since it will affect the method of styling and care it is given. To identify the type of hair from unknown sources, pull (very carefully) a few strands from the test sample and hold them to a flame for a **burn test**. **Human hair** singes and smells similar to sulfur. It will burn completely, leaving a residue like white ashes. **Synthetic fiber** melts and smells like burnt plastic, curling up and forming small plastics beads at the ends that feel hard between the fingers and thumb.

Select the correct hair or fiber for each hair addition service based on the look desired, whether the client wants to alter the appearance of the hair addition, and the wear and maintenance involved with the hair or fiber selected. Choose the curl pattern and color to either **blend** into or **contrast** with the client's natural hair. Cover service and hair or fiber costs, and gain client commitment on the in-salon follow-up involved and maintenance time required at home. Sell **additional services** and products to help with maintenance of hair additions.

RETAIL · RE-BOOK · REFERRAL

9

Chapter 9 • ART OF HAIR ADDITIONS 375

Health and safety are top priority!

Check the condition of the scalp for irritations such as abrasions and "hot" spots, and condition the scalp, if necessary. Clients with an allergy to latex may be sensitive to bonding adhesive or hair tape with latex as a base. If a **predisposition test** shows the client has an allergy to the adhesive, an alternative attachment method such as the individual braiding or latch hook technique should be used.

Analyze the client's hair growth patterns. Placing hair additions against the natural growth pattern may be uncomfortable for the client and cause breakage in fragile or finely-textured hair. When braiding, do not pull hair too tightly to avoid causing **traction alopecia** (hair loss due to repetitive pulling of hair along tracks). Any hair addition attached to a cornrow base that is uncomfortably tight should be removed immediately.

When attaching a hair addition, base the size of the subsection of the client's hair on the weight of the hair addition. If the hair addition is too heavy for the subsection it is attached to, gravity will naturally **pull the hair out**. Remember, hair that has had chemical services is in a weakened state, and can therefore support less weight.

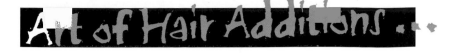

A good balance between hair extension weight and the size of the subsection it is attached to has actually been shown to **increase blood circulation** to the area and potentially stimulate hair growth. However, the base where the hair addition is attached will naturally weaken as the client's natural hair grows out, placing more stress and weight on the hair and scalp. It is for this reason a client must have extensions serviced on a regular basis. This involves removing the extensions, cleansing and conditioning the hair and scalp, and repositioning or replacing the extensions closer to the scalp area to adjust for hair growth. See the procedures in this chapter for **maintenance and removal** of hair additions services.

In addition to standard notations of hair color, wave pattern and hair conditions on the client record card, note the placement location of the hair additions, the type of hair additions used and the method of attachment. Vary the placement of attachments with each maintenance visit to avoid placing stress on the hair and scalp in the same location.

If there is any doubt about performing a service, have the client sign a release form or reschedule the appointment until hair and scalp are in the condition necessary to ensure the success of the service.

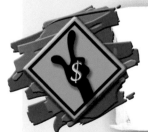

Help service the needs of your clients by providing appropriate retail styling tools and professional hair care products for home maintenance that are both safe and effective.

EXTRA CREDIT LAB PROJECT

OBJECTIVE:
To provide the client with home care instructions on how to maintain a hair additions design.

TOOLS & MATERIALS:
Cleansing and conditioning products
Liquid styling tools (no oil base)
Airformer and curling/flat iron
Styling combs and brushes
Towels
Clips

PROCEDURE:

1. Know what source your hair addition is made from (human or synthetic), and follow manufacturer's care, styling, and maintenance product recommendations.

2. Separate braided hair extensions, if any, from the natural hair before brushing gently with a wire wig (pin) brush. Hold the hair additions firmly in one hand, and work from ends to scalp.

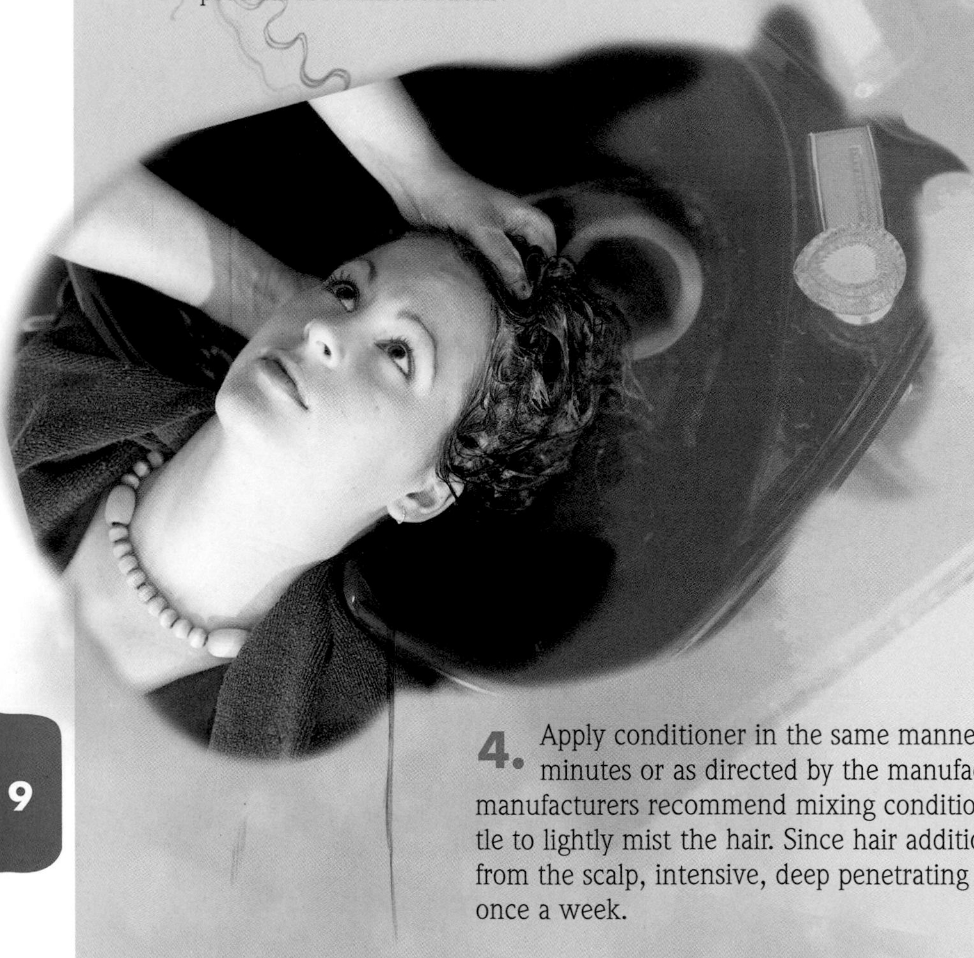

3. Wet the hair and scalp. Spread shampoo in palms first to generate lather, and then work into hair from the scalp area down toward the ends. Avoid circular motions, which will cause hair to tangle. The scalp requires the most attention. Rinse and repeat the shampoo, if necessary. Squeeze out excess water. Wigs should be turned inside out to clean, and care should be taken to avoid prolonged immersion in water, which may swell, damage or loosen the hair or fiber from its base.

4. Apply conditioner in the same manner as the shampoo. Leave in for 3 to 5 minutes or as directed by the manufacturer's instructions; some wig manufacturers recommend mixing conditioner with water and using a spray bottle to lightly mist the hair. Since hair additions do not contain the natural oils from the scalp, intensive, deep penetrating conditioners should be used once a week.

5. Rinse and pat hair dry with a towel. Be careful not to rub the hair with the towel to avoid matting or tangling of the hair addition.

6. A leave-in detangling conditioner may be liberally applied. Use your fingers to work the conditioner through the hair.

7. When styling the hair with a thermal iron or applying pomade, avoid contact with any adhesive if used to secure the hair addition. Heat appliances or styling tools containing heavy oils may soften the adhesive and loosen the human hair addition. Synthetic blends should be wet-styled with rollers and allowed to air dry. Wigs and hairpieces may be dried and stored on a wig block to maintain their shape. Use only low-alcohol spray on wigs and hairpieces. Braided hair may require a light oil spray, since acid-or water-based sprays may revert hair previously straightened with a pressing comb or chemical relaxer back to its natural curl.

8. Do not go to bed with wet hair. A hair net or scarf will help keep the style in place. Sleeping on a satin pillow case will also minimize friction. Long hair extensions may be braided before sleeping to prevent tangling.

9. Prolonged exposure to heat or water (hot tub, swimming, sauna, etc.) may swell the hair additions and cause matting or tangling. Cleanse and condition immediately after these activities. Never allow the hair to dry with tangles in it.

10. Hair additions require professional maintenance about as often as you would get a haircut; no longer than 6 to 8 weeks. Due to the growth of your natural hair at the scalp and normal shedding, the hair will begin to weigh down or become entangled in the extension if the hair addition is not serviced regularly to adjust for new growth. With proper care and professional maintenance adjustments, hair additions can be worn indefinitely.

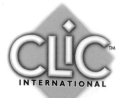

Boxed Braid Hair Additions

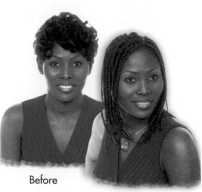

Before

After

OBJECTIVE

To create a three-strand under braid (off the scalp) using synthetic fiber or human hair additions to increase length in the finished design.

TOOLS & MATERIALS

- Cleansing and conditioning products
- Neck strips and cape/smock
- Liquid styling tools
- Airformer/hood dryer
- Client record card/file
- Towels
- Clips
- Styling combs and brushes
- Mineral oil
- Water bottle
- Ornamentation
- Synthetic or human hair fiber
- Color swatch ring
- Braid sealer
- Small elastic bands

PROCEDURE

"The client consultation is an important part of your professional service. Be sure to complete this step prior to each client service you provide. Your successful retail sales and customer satisfaction rates depend upon it!"

RETAIL RE-BOOK REFERRAL

1. Drape the client in preparation for the service.
2. Thoroughly brush the client's hair to remove knots, tangles and hairspray.
3. Cleanse and condition the hair and scalp according to the client's needs. Rinse thoroughly and towel dry.
4. Comb the hair to detangle. Apply an appropriate liquid styling tool to the entire head. Mineral oil may be applied to the scalp area to act as a lubricant for dry scalp.
5. Airform the hair or place the client under a hood dryer.
6. Perform the style as shown.
7. Suggest appropriate retail tools for the client's at-home hairdesign maintenance.
8. Follow standard clean-up procedures.
9. Document the client record card/file.

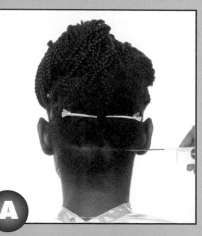

A Section the hair according to style pattern. Start at the lower nape with a 1/4 to 1/2 inch (0.6 - 1.3 cm) horizontal subsection. Use a color swatch ring to determine the closest match to the client's natural hair color, although more than one color may be used to add dimension to the style.

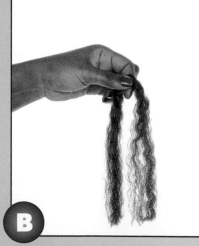

B Prepare the synthetic or human hair addition. To eliminate tangles, spray the hair addition with water or oil sheen and use a wig brush as necessary. Trim the length according to the finished design plan.

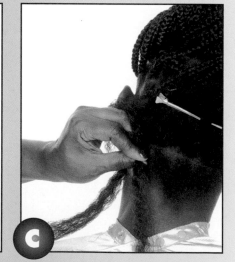

C Using a 1/4 or 1/2 inch (0.6 - 1.3 cm) square subsection, separate the hair addition into three strands, and place it at the scalp next to the client's natural hair.

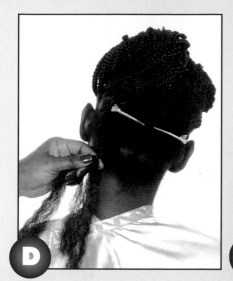

D

Combine the center strand of the hair addition with the natural hair and begin an under braid (off the scalp) technique.

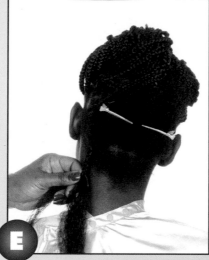

E

Continue under braiding to the bottom of the strand. Use sufficient tension to keep the hair addition entwined with the natural hair.

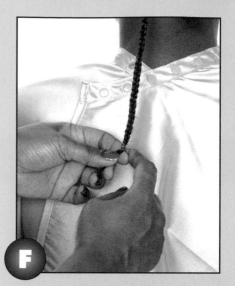

F

Secure the hair ends with a small elastic band or a braid sealer.

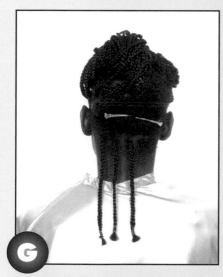

G

Apply subsequent hair additions in the same manner as listed above. Keep the bricklayer partings clean, and the hair centered within each square subsection.

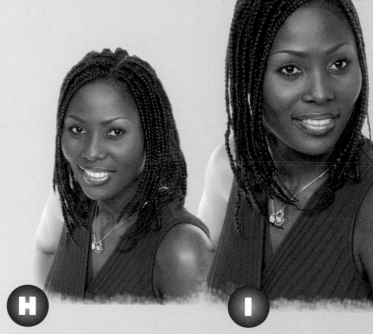

H

Gradually reduce the size of the squares to approximately 1/4 inch (0.6 cm) toward the top of the head for a better appearance.

I

Ornamentation may be added to the finished boxed braid hair additions style.

EVALUATION

GRADE   STUDENT'S NAME   ID#

9

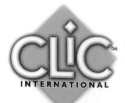

Cornrow with Hair Additions

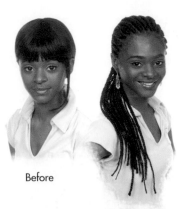

Before

After

OBJECTIVE

To incorporate hair or fiber additions into a three-strand cornrow under braid (on the scalp) to provide more fullness in the finished design.

TOOLS & MATERIALS

- Cleansing and conditioning products
- Neck strips and cape/smock
- Liquid styling tools

- Airformer/hood dryer
- Client record card/file
- Towels

- Clips
- Styling combs and brushes
- Mineral oil
- Water bottle
- Ornamentation

- Synthetic or human hair fiber
- Color swatch ring
- Braid sealer
- Small elastic bands

PROCEDURE

"The client consultation is an important part of your professional service. Be sure to complete this step prior to each client service you provide. Your successful retail sales and customer satisfaction rates depend upon it!"

RETAIL RE-BOOK REFERRAL

1. Drape the client in preparation for the service.
2. Thoroughly brush the client's hair to remove knots, tangles and hairspray.
3. Cleanse and condition the hair and scalp according to the client's needs. Rinse thoroughly and towel dry.
4. Comb the hair to detangle. Apply an appropriate liquid styling tool to the entire head. Mineral oil may be applied to the scalp area to act as a lubricant for dry scalp.
5. Airform the hair or place the client under a hood dryer.
6. Perform the style as shown.
7. Suggest appropriate retail tools for the client's at-home hairdesign maintenance.
8. Follow standard clean-up procedures.
9. Document the client record card/file.

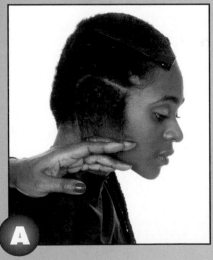

A Section the hair according to style pattern. Start at the hairline in the lower front side. Take a 1/4 to 1/2 inch (0.6 - 1.3 cm) horizontal subsection that conforms to the head curve.

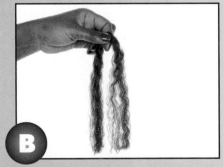

B Prepare the synthetic or human hair addition. Use a color swatch ring to determine the closest match to the client's natural hair color, although more than one color may be used to add dimension to the style. To eliminate tangles, spray the hair extension with water or oil sheen and use a wig brush as necessary. Trim the length according to the finished design plan.

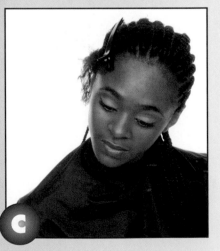

C The hair above the working subsection is clipped out of the way to maintain clean partings and keep stray hair from becoming entangled in another track.

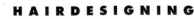

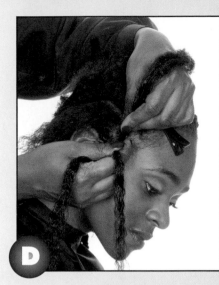

D Using a 1/4 or 1/2 inch (0.6 - 1.3 cm) square subsection, separate the hair addition into three strands and place it at the scalp next to the client's natural hair.

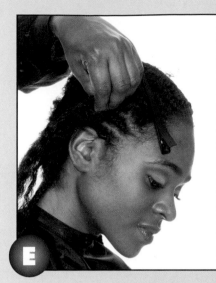

E Combine the center strand of the hair addition with the natural hair and begin a three-strand under braid (on the scalp) cornrow technique. Pick up and add the natural hair at the scalp into the braid along with the hair addition or fiber.

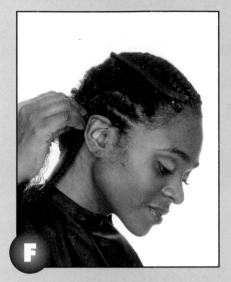

F Keep fingers close to the scalp while creating cornrows. Maintain even tension while braiding the hair to keep the hair addition entwined with the natural hair.

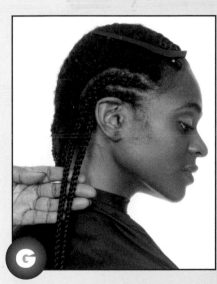

G Add a consistent amount of natural hair into the braid.

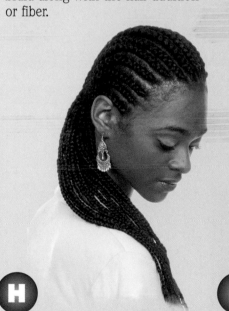

H The finished braid may be sealed with heat if synthetic fiber has been used. Natural fiber hair additions may be finished with an elastic band.

I Finished view of the cornrowed hair additions design.

9

EVALUATION

GRADE   STUDENT'S NAME   ID#

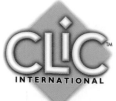

Weft Bonding with Cold Adhesive

OBJECTIVE

Utilize a cold adhesive to quickly bond a weft hair addition to the client's natural hair.

Before

After

TOOLS & MATERIALS

- Cleansing and conditioning products
- Neck strips and cape/smock
- Towels
- Scissors
- Clips
- Cold adhesive
- Airformer/hood dryer
- Flat iron
- Hair wefts (synthetic or human)
- Color swatch ring
- Styling combs and brushes
- Liquid styling tools (no oil base)
- Client record card/file

PROCEDURE

"The client consultation is an important part of your professional service. Be sure to complete this step prior to each client service you provide. Your successful retail sales and customer satisfaction rates depend upon it!"

RETAIL · RE-BOOK · REFERRAL

1. Drape the client in preparation for the service.
2. Thoroughly brush the client's hair to remove knots, tangles and hairspray.
3. Cleanse and condition the hair and scalp according to the client's needs. Rinse thoroughly and towel dry.
4. Comb the hair to detangle. Apply a non-oil based liquid styling tool to the entire head.
5. Airform the hair or place the client under a hood dryer. Use a flat iron to smooth the hair if it is curly in texture.
6. Perform the style as shown.
7. Suggest appropriate retail tools for the client's at-home hairdesign maintenance.
8. Follow standard clean-up procedures.
9. Document the client record card/file.

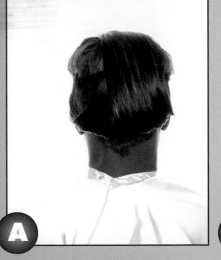

A

Section the hair according to style pattern. Start at the lower nape with a 1/4 to 1/2 inch (0.6 - 1.3 cm) horizontal subsection.

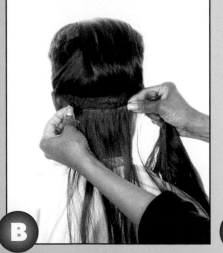

B

Prepare the synthetic or human hair weft. Use a color swatch ring to determine the best match to the client's natural hair color, although more than one color may be used to add dimension to the style.

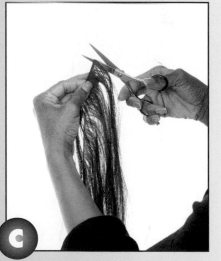

C

Cut the weft to match the length of the parting.

9

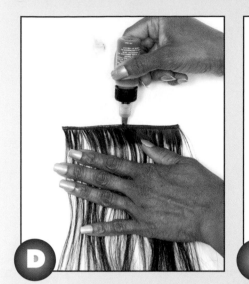

D Apply a thin line of cold adhesive to the back seam of the hair weft.

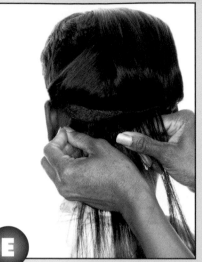

E Match the weft up to the part line.

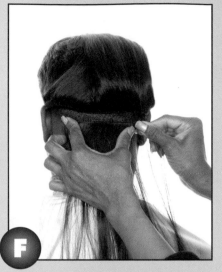

F Press the seam of the weft along the parting. Hold the weft in place approximately ten seconds for the adhesive to set. An airformer may be used to speed drying time.

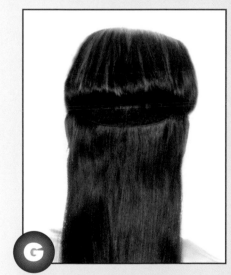

G Secure the weft along the line of the parting. Press an absorbent towel against areas with an excessive amount of adhesive to blot up the excess.

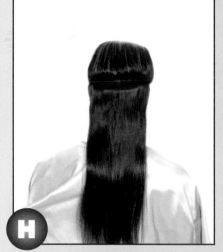

H Follow the same procedure while continuing up the head form to complete the style.

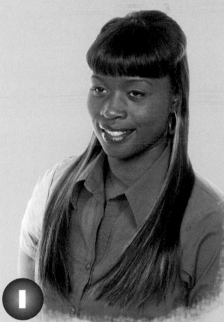

I A light oil-free finishing spray may be added to support the cold weft attachment style.

9

EVALUATION

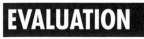

GRADE   STUDENT'S NAME   ID#

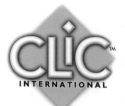
INTERMEDIATE LAB PROJECT

Clip-In Extensions

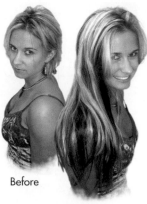

Before

After

OBJECTIVE

Create an inexpensive, fun, temporary design using clip-in hair extensions.

TOOLS & MATERIALS

- Cleansing and conditioning products
- Neck strip and cape/smock
- Styling combs and brushes
- Client record card/file
- Clips
- Towels
- Scissors
- Airformer/hood dryer
- Clip-in weft (synthetic or human)
- Color swatch ring
- Liquid styling tools
- Curling or flat iron

PROCEDURE

"The client consultation is an important part of your professional service. Be sure to complete this step prior to each client service you provide. Your successful retail sales and customer satisfaction rates depend upon it!"

RETAIL • RE-BOOK • REFERRAL

1. Drape the client in preparation for the service.
2. Thoroughly brush the client's hair to remove knots, tangles and hairspray.
3. Cleanse and condition the hair and scalp according to the client's needs. Rinse thoroughly and towel dry.
4. Comb the hair to detangle. Apply an appropriate liquid styling tool.
5. Airform the hair or place the client under a hood dryer. Use a flat iron to smooth the hair if it is curly in texture.
6. Perform the style as shown.
7. Suggest appropriate retail tools for the client's at-home hairdesign maintenance.
8. Follow standard clean-up procedures.
9. Document the client record card/file.

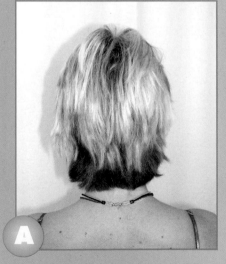

A Begin in the nape area at the back of the head. Work along 1/4 to 1/2 inch (0.6 - 1.3 cm) partings.

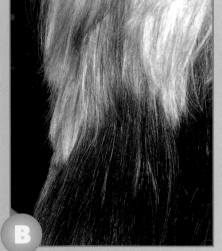

B Use a color swatch ring to determine the best match to the client's natural hair color, although more than one color may be used to add dimension to the style.

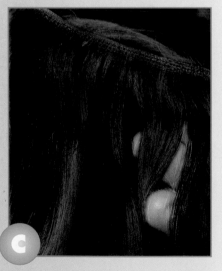

C Place a clip-in hair weft that closely matches the client's hair color along the parting. Attach the clip to the hair in the scalp area.

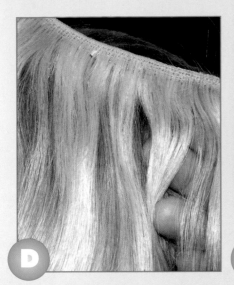

D If desired, place a different color weft along the next parting, allowing the clip to attach securely to the hair at the scalp.

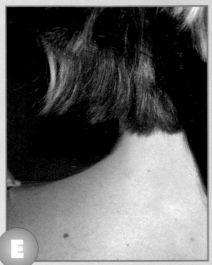

E Various lengths created by adding the clip-in wefts are shown here. Alternate weft colors for placement along every other parting.

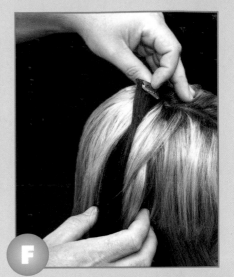

F Continue placing clip-in wefts while moving up the head form.

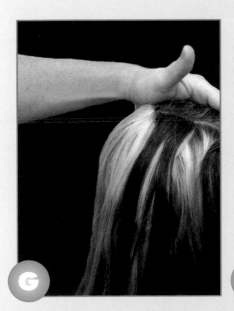

G A row of clip-in wefts being placed along a parting.

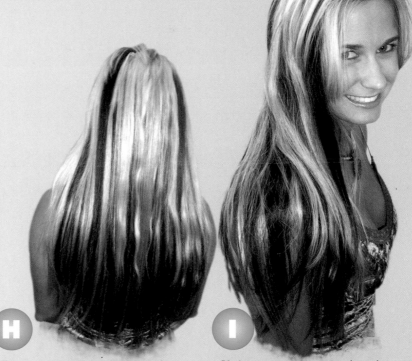

H The completed back view of clip-in hair extensions. Cut if desired, taking note of the additional length.

I If the extensions are placed carefully along the perimeter hairline, the client should be able to wear the hair either up or down in any style without detection.

9

EVALUATION

_____

_____

GRADE _____   STUDENT'S NAME _____   ID# _____

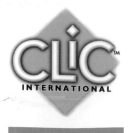

Hair Weaving

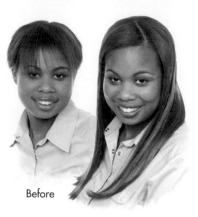

OBJECTIVE

This procedure will provide added thickness and length to the finished design by braiding the natural hair and sewing the hair additions into the braided hair.

Before

After

TOOLS & MATERIALS

- Cleansing and conditioning products
- Neck strips and cape/smock
- Styling combs and brushes

- Airformer/hood dryer
- Client record card/file
- Clips

- Towels
- Liquid styling tools
- Mineral oil
- Flat iron

- Curved needle
- Thread
- Hair wefts (synthetic or human)
- Color swatch ring
- Scissors

PROCEDURE

"The client consultation is an important part of your professional service. Be sure to complete this step prior to each client service you provide. Your successful retail sales and customer satisfaction rates depend upon it!"

RETAIL RE-BOOK REFERRAL

1. Drape the client in preparation for the service.
2. Thoroughly brush the client's hair to remove knots, tangles and hairspray.
3. Cleanse and condition the hair and scalp according to the client's needs. Rinse thoroughly and towel dry.
4. Comb the hair to detangle. Apply an appropriate styling product.
5. Airform the hair or place the client under a hood dryer. Use a flat iron to smooth the hair if it is curly in texture.
6. Perform the style as shown.
7. Suggest appropriate retail tools for the client's at-home hairdesign maintenance.
8. Follow standard clean-up procedures.
9. Document the client record card/file.

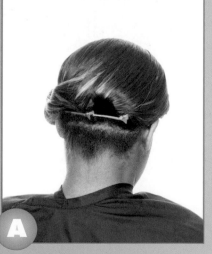

A Section the hair according to style pattern. Begin at the nape, excluding the hairline, with a 1/4 to 1/2 inch (0.6 - 1.3 cm) horizontal subsection.

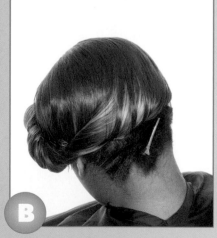

B Prepare the synthetic or human hair weft. Use a color swatch ring to determine the best match to the client's natural hair color, although more than one color may be used to add dimension to the style.

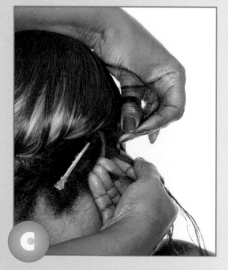

C Divide the hair at the scalp into three subsections. Separate the hair addition into three strands and join it with the natural hair at the scalp.

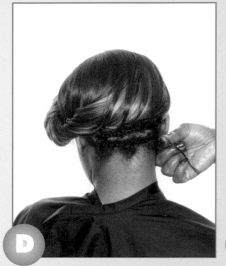

D

Complete a horizontal under braid technique, making sure the ends are secured within the cornrow (needle and thread may be used).

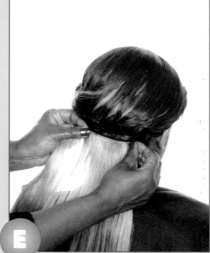

E

Size the length of the weft according to the length of parting.

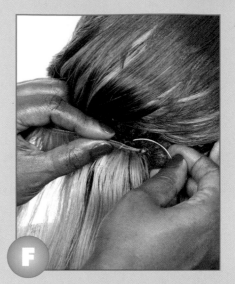

F

Place the weft along the cornrow and secure the weft with thread and curved needle, pulling through the cornrow and the seam of the weft, working along the parting.

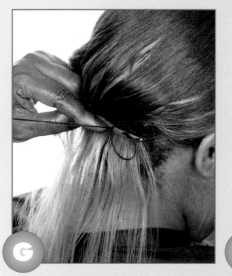

G

Use a slip knot to secure the end of the weft to the cornrow. To form a slip knot, make a loop, then push another loop through it. Tighten gently and slide the knot up to the base.

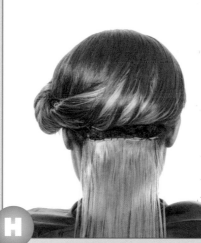

H

Attach another weft to the next cornrowed base at the scalp. Continue in this manner to complete the hairdesign pattern.

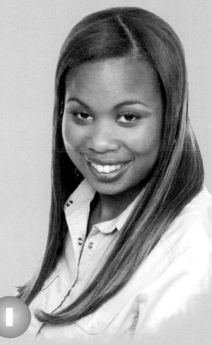

I

The completed weave is a natural "extension" of the client's own hair.

9

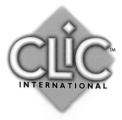

CLIC INTERNATIONAL

Wig Application

OBJECTIVE

To effectively measure and fit a client with a full coverage natural human hair or synthetic wig for cosmetic or fashion purposes.

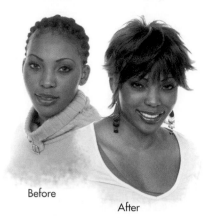

Before

After

TOOLS & MATERIALS

- Cleansing and conditioning products
- Neck strips and cape/smock
- Clips
- Towels
- Client record card/file
- Styling combs and brushes
- Airformer/hood dryer
- Liquid styling tools
- Rollers or thermal irons
- Wig (synthetic or human)
- Color swatch ring
- Measuring tape
- Scissors
- Weave or mesh cap

PROCEDURE

"The client consultation is an important part of your professional service. Be sure to complete this step prior to each client service you provide. Your successful retail sales and customer satisfaction rates depend upon it!"

RETAIL RE-BOOK REFERRAL

1. Drape the client in preparation for the service.
2. Thoroughly brush the client's hair to remove knots, tangles and hairspray.
3. Cleanse and condition the hair and scalp according to the client's needs. Rinse thoroughly and towel dry.
4. Comb the hair to detangle. Apply an appropriate liquid styling tool.
5. Airform the hair or place the client under a hood dryer.
6. Perform the style as shown.
7. Suggest appropriate retail tools for the client's at-home hairdesign maintenance.
8. Follow standard clean-up procedures.
9. Document the Client Record Card/File.

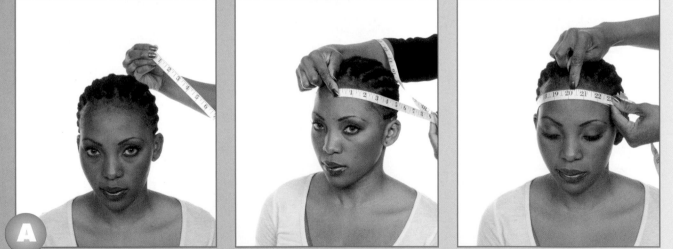

A

Getting the correct fit for the client's head size is perhaps the most important step in keeping a wig securely attached. This information is vital in selecting a good-fitting wig or ordering one to be custom made. Measure the circumference of the client's head. Place a tape measure at the center of the forehead at the hairline. The tape should go above the ears, below the occipital and back to the front hairline, working around the perimeter of the head form.

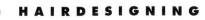

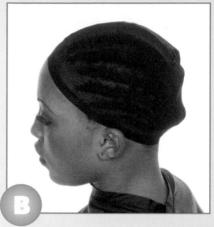

B Brush the client's own hair back, pinning long hair up and away from the hairline around the hairline's entire perimeter. Apply a breathable nylon wig cap over the entire head above the ears to hold existing hair in place and keep the wig comfortable and snug.

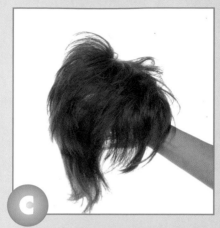

C Hold the wig in the palm of the hand, and shake gently to separate the strands. Identify the front and back of the wig by locating the label in the back of the wig's underside. Adjust the front edge to line up with the client's front hairline.

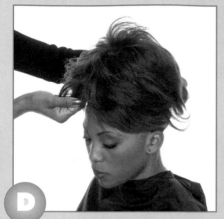

D Hold the wig from the front over the front hairline and position it over the entire head, slipping it on from front hairline to nape. The wig should feel secure, but not too tight. Most wigs come with adjustable hooks, elastic straps or Velcro® to be altered at the crown or back to a smaller size, but they cannot be made larger. Two wig tabs usually present in the manufacturer's design should be set in front of the client's ears. Pull the ears out from under the wig hair, just as they would be in a natural hairline.

Variation

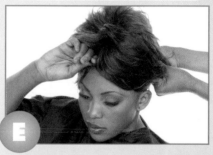

E Allow the client to hold the front of the wig at the hairline while it is pulled over the head and secured into position. Check to make sure the wig starts at the client's natural hairline or estimate its proximity on hair loss clients. The wig may have combs sewn into the cap or contain a tape tab along the edges to adhere it to areas with partial hair loss. Wigs with special bases designed to be bonded to the head with adhesive for complete or permanent hair loss must be removed periodically to care for the scalp.

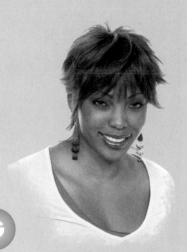

F The wig may be cut and styled either on or off the client's head. A wig comes from the manufacturer with extra hair or fiber so it can be trimmed or texturized as desired. Fine tune the hairdesign to complement the client's features. Natural styles include a fringe or wisps to obscure the hairline of the wig.

G The finished design shows no indication of a wig in place. Many clients keep at least one extra wig to use while one is being serviced or to use as an alternate hairstyle.

EVALUATION

GRADE

STUDENT'S NAME

ID#

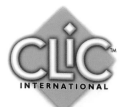

COMPLEX LAB PROJECT

Hairpiece for Balding Male

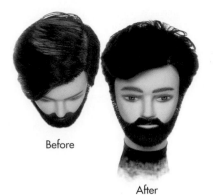

Before

After

OBJECTIVE To provide proper coverage of the balding area(s) for cosmetic purposes.

TOOLS & MATERIALS

- Cleansing and conditioning products
- Neck strips and cape/smock
- Styling combs and brushes
- Client record card/file
- Towels
- Transparent adhesive tape
- Transparent plastic wrap
- Permanent marker/grease pencil
- Hairpiece (synthetic or human)
- Airformer/hood dryer
- Color swatch ring
- Liquid styling tools
- Hairpiece tape
- Scissors
- Clips

PROCEDURE

"The client consultation is an important part of your professional service. Be sure to complete this step prior to each client service you provide. Your successful retail sales and customer satisfaction rates depend upon it!"

RETAIL RE-BOOK REFERRAL

1. Drape the client in preparation for the service.
2. Thoroughly brush the client's hair to remove knots, tangles and hairspray.
3. Cleanse and condition the hair and scalp according to the client's needs. Rinse thoroughly and towel dry.
4. Comb the hair to detangle. Apply an appropriate liquid styling tool.
5. Airform the hair or place the client under a hood dryer.
6. Perform the style as shown.
7. Suggest appropriate retail tools for the client's at-home hairdesign maintenance.
8. Follow standard clean-up procedures.
9. Document the Client Record Card/File.

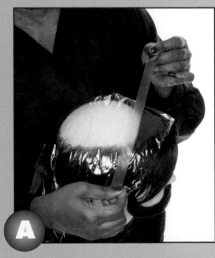

A Apply plastic film wrap to the balding area, and place tape horizontally and vertically across the entire surface of the plastic wrap.

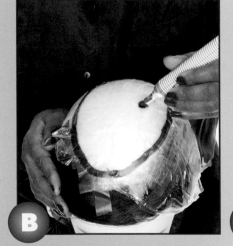

B Using a standard permanent marker or grease pencil, outline the circumference of the area with male pattern baldness. **Important:** Make sure the plastic wrap being used to make a template remains securely conformed to the head curve.

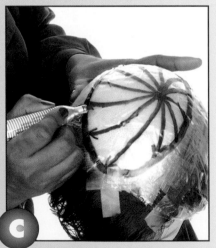

C Mark the placement and direction of hair movement. Note any cowlicks, whorls, wave patterns or other changes in the hair's directional flow.

9

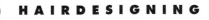

HAIRDESIGNING

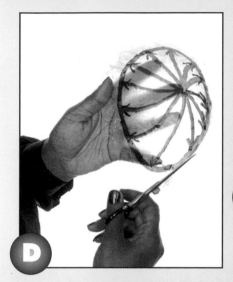

D Cut the plastic along the marked circumference. This becomes the template to be used by the hair-piece manufacturer.

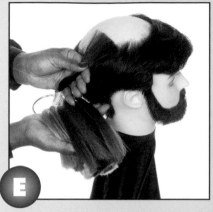

E Use a color swatch ring to determine the closest match to the client's natural hair color, although more than one color may be used to add dimension to the style. Include this information or a sample of the client's hair color and texture along with the custom template design made of the client's head, and submit a purchase order request to the manufacturer.

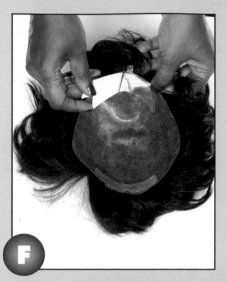

F When the hairpiece has been completed by the manufacturer and returned, tape is placed along the circumference on the inside of the hairpiece.

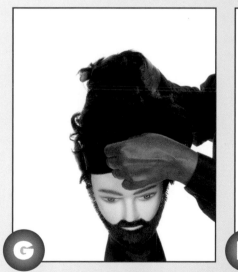

G Place the custom hairpiece at the front of the balding area and press to secure the adhesive tape to the scalp.

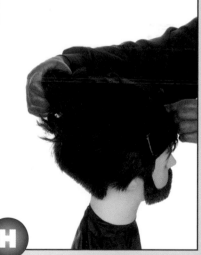

H Position the hairpiece over the top of the bald area. Cut to blend the hairpiece into the adjacent hair and finish according to the desired style.

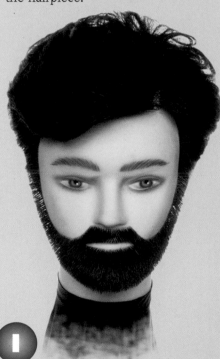

I There should be no indication of the absence of hair in the completed male hairpiece design.

EVALUATION

GRADE   STUDENT'S NAME   ID#

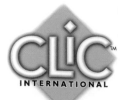

COMPLEX LAB PROJECT

Strand Bonding with Hot Adhesive

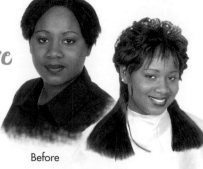

Before

After

OBJECTIVE

To perform strand bonding of hair additions with a hot adhesive. This method produces a thicker feel to the hair.

TOOLS & MATERIALS

- Cleansing and conditioning products
- Neck strip and cape/smock
- Towels
- Airformer/hood dryer
- Clips
- Flat/curling iron
- Styling combs and brushes
- Liquid styling tools (no oil base)
- Bulk synthetic/human hair or weft
- Thermal molding adhesive colors
- Color swatch ring
- Applicator gun
- Placement disks
- Client record card/file
- Scissors

PROCEDURE

"The client consultation is an important part of your professional service. Be sure to complete this step prior to each client service you provide. Your successful retail sales and customer satisfaction rates depend upon it!"

RETAIL • RE-BOOK • REFERRAL

1. Drape the client in preparation for the service.
2. Thoroughly brush the client's hair to remove knots, tangles and hairspray.
3. Cleanse and condition the hair and scalp according to the client's needs. Rinse thoroughly and towel dry.
4. Comb the hair to detangle. Apply an appropriate (no oil base) liquid styling tool.
5. Airform the hair or place the client under a hood dryer. Use a flat iron to smooth the hair if it is curly in texture.
6. Perform the style as shown.
7. Suggest appropriate retail tools for the client's at-home hairdesign maintenance.
8. Follow standard clean-up procedures.
9. Document the client record card/file.

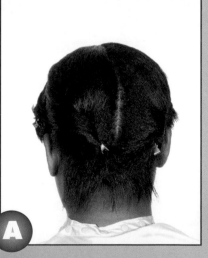

A

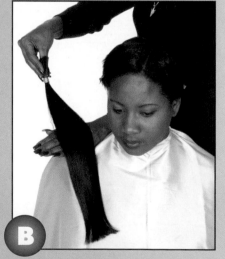

B

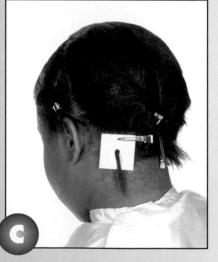

C

Section hair according to desired style. Take a 1/8 to 1/4 inch (0.3 - 0.6 cm) parting along the hairline at the lower nape.
Caution: Leave the hairline untouched if it is too fine or broken and use the next parting of hair.

Use a color swatch ring to determine the best match to the client's natural hair color, although more than one color may be used to add dimension to the style. Twist the bulk hair or fiber together and cut to clean up the ends.

Place the client's hair through the hole in the placement disk, allowing the hair to hang in the natural growth direction.

9

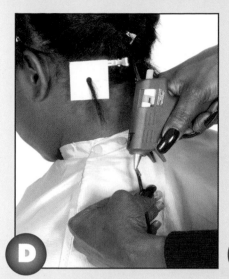

D

Choose the amount of bulk hair or fiber to be used according to the density of the hair desired. Place the applicator gun nozzle 1/8 inch (0.3 cm) below the ends of the hair extension. Push gently to dispense a small bead of adhesive.

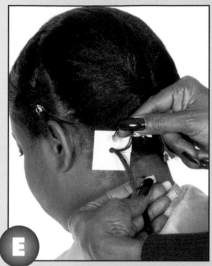

E

Place the hair addition underneath the natural hair strand, allowing it to blend into one strand of hair.

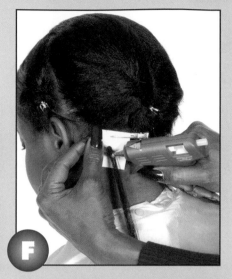

F

Place an additional bead of adhesive on top at the point where the natural hair and bulk hair or fiber blends to form a seal.

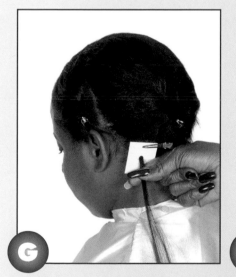

G

Press down on the adhesive area to ensure an extended seal.

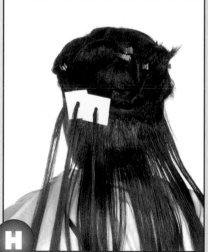

H

Use a staggered bricklayer pattern to prevent splits within the design and to create more hair density. Continue application until the strand bonding method is complete.

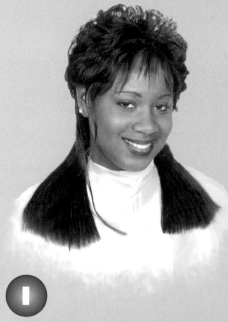

I

Add variety to the finished strand bonded hair extensions design by adding a strategically placed fashion accent color.

9

EVALUATION

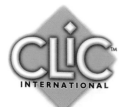

Latch Hook Braids

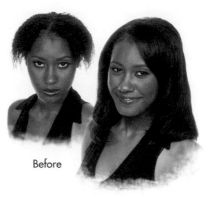

Before

After

OBJECTIVE

To provide an alternative method of producing longer lengths of hair by securing hair additions with the latch hook braiding technique.

TOOLS & MATERIALS

- Cleansing and conditioning products
- Neck strips and cape/smock
- Towels

- Styling combs and brushes
- Liquid styling tools
- Thread

- Latch hook tool
- Clips
- Flat/curling iron
- Airformer/hood dryer

- Mineral oil
- Color swatch ring
- Synthetic/human hair extensions
- Client record card/file
- Scissors

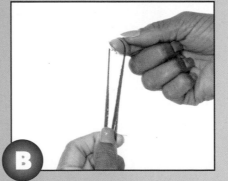

PROCEDURE

"The client consultation is an important part of your professional service. Be sure to complete this step prior to each client service you provide. Your successful retail sales and customer satisfaction rates depend upon it!"

1. Drape the client in preparation for the service.
2. Thoroughly brush the client's hair to remove knots, tangles and hairspray.
3. Cleanse and condition the hair according to the client's needs. Rinse thoroughly and towel dry. Apply a liquid styling tool. Comb the hair to detangle.
4. Airform the hair if desired (braiding the hair while damp may make it easier to braid).
5. The hair may be flat ironed if the hair is of a curly texture.
6. Perform the style as shown.
7. Suggest appropriate retail tools for the client's at-home hairdesign maintenance.
8. Follow standard clean-up procedures.
9. Document the client record card/file.

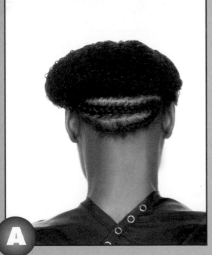

A Section the hair according to style pattern. Complete an under braid technique at the hairline. Secure the ends of the braid with thread.

B Prepare the synthetic or human hair extensions. Use a color swatch ring to determine the closest match to the client's natural hair color, although more than one color may be used to add dimension to the style. To eliminate tangles, spray the extensions with water or oil sheen and use a wig brush as necessary. Trim the length according to the finished design plan.

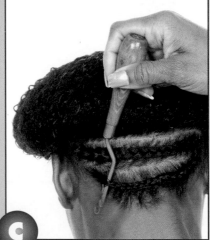

C Insert the latch hook under the cornrows at the beginning of the track.

9

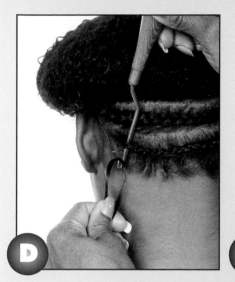

D Form a loop with the hair extension and place the loop onto the hook.

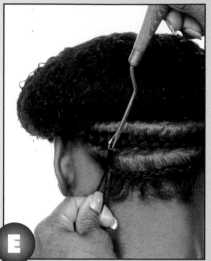

E Pull the hook containing the hair extension loop carefully through the cornrowed base on an angle to avoid scratching the scalp.

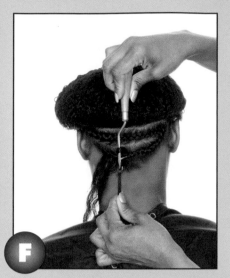

F Reinsert the latch hook tool beneath the next cornrowed track section, and place the ends of the next hair extension loop onto the latch hook.

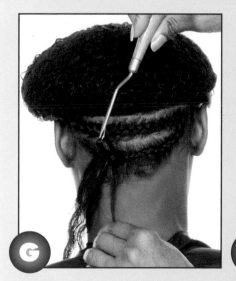

G Pull the ends of the hair extension through the top of the cornrow.

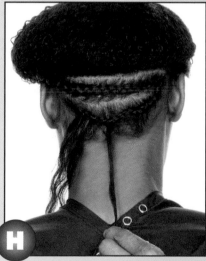

H Pull each hair extension down toward the nape to secure the hair within the cornrow.

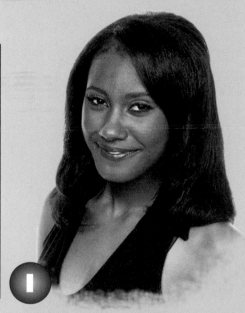

I A view of the completed latch hook extensions hairdesign. A light finishing spray may be used to support the style.

EVALUATION

GRADE STUDENT'S NAME ID#

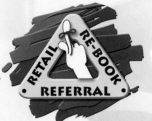

"The client consultation is an important part of your professional service. Be sure to complete this step prior to each client service you provide. Your successful retail sales and customer satisfaction rates depend upon it!"

OBJECTIVE:

OBJECTIVE:

To remove hair additions services safely and effectively without stress on the client's natural hair or scalp.

TOOLS:

TOOLS & MATERIALS:

Cleansing and conditioning products
Neck strips and cape/smock
Styling combs and brushes
Curling and/or flat iron
Adhesive solvent (oil)
Airformer/hood dryer
Client record card/file
Liquid styling tools
Applicator gun
Clips
Towels

PROCEDURE:

1. Drape the client in preparation for the service.

2. Gently brush the hair, starting from the ends and working toward the scalp.

3. Cleanse and condition the hair and scalp according to the client's needs. Rinse and pat the hair to towel dry without rubbing.

4. Place the client under a hood dryer set on low or medium heat to remove excess moisture from the hair without irritating the scalp.

5. Separate the hair into sections according to the order to be worked on for hair additions removal.

 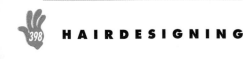

6. For removal of single bonded strands: Apply one or two drops of oil directly to the adhesive connection, then place the heated applicator gun directly on top of the adhesive to help soften the adhesive and free the extension from the natural hair. Some manufacturers recommend cracking the adhesive seal with needle nose pliers in conjunction with the application of oil or another solvent.

7. For removal of multiple bonded strands: Use the manufacturer's recommended adhesive solvent or oil directly on the adhesive connection of each strand. Place the heated barrel of a curling or flat iron directly on top of the adhesive until it softens the adhesive bonding agent through to the point of contact with the natural hair. Extensions which are sewn into place are removed by carefully cutting only the thread and gently releasing the client's hair. Extensions may also be removed by simply cutting them off if they are to be reapplied immediately or the hair has matted together.

8. For wig and hairpiece removal: Wigs and hairpieces that are fastened by temporary means such as attached combs or straps should be carefully lifted off of the client's head a section at a time, gently detaching any contact points to avoid tangling with the cap or hair underneath. Semi-permanent attachment methods, such as tape or bonding adhesive may require the placement of a spray or drip adhesive solvent between the scalp and the bonded attachment point to make it easier to soften and release the prosthesis and peel it away from the scalp like a large bandage.

9. The hair addition should separate from the natural hair easily. No tugging or pulling on hair is necessary. Hair should be totally free of adhesive. If not, add a few drops of oil and reapply heat to soften the adhesive. Use a towel to wipe the hair clean while it is still warm, since the adhesive will begin to harden again as the hair cools.

10. When all hair additions have been removed, shampoo the hair using a deep cleansing product to eliminate residue.

11. Apply an intensive conditioner to the hair and scalp, following directions as recommended by the manufacturer.

12. Rinse thoroughly and style the client's hair as desired, or begin a new application.

13. Suggest appropriate retail tools for the client's at-home hairdesign maintenance.

14. Follow standard clean-up procedures.

15. Document the client record card/file.

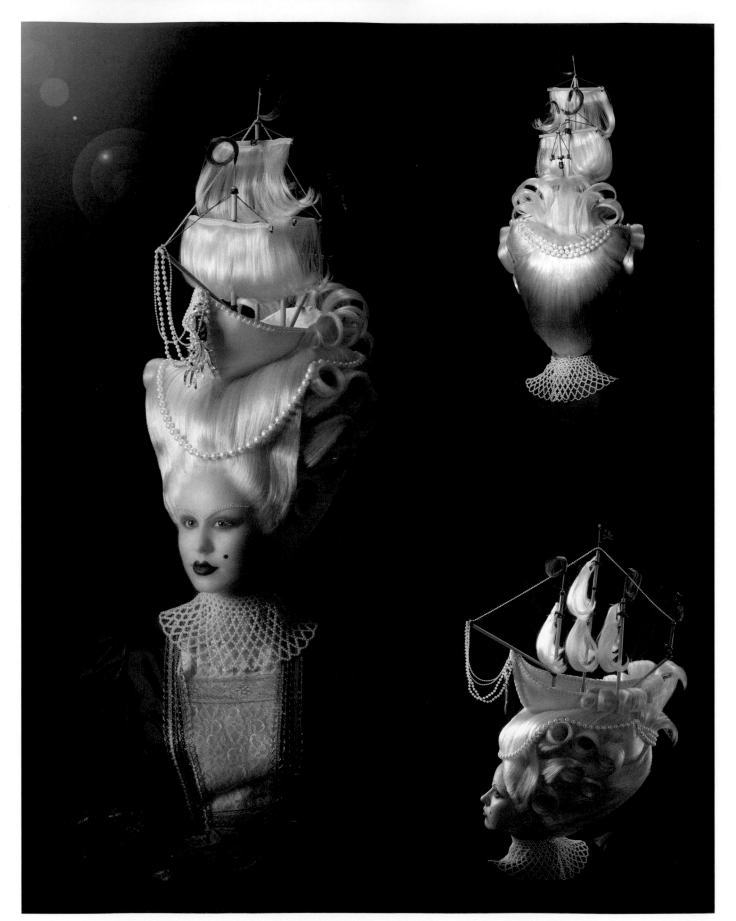

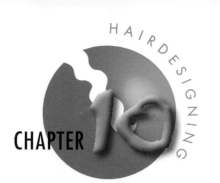

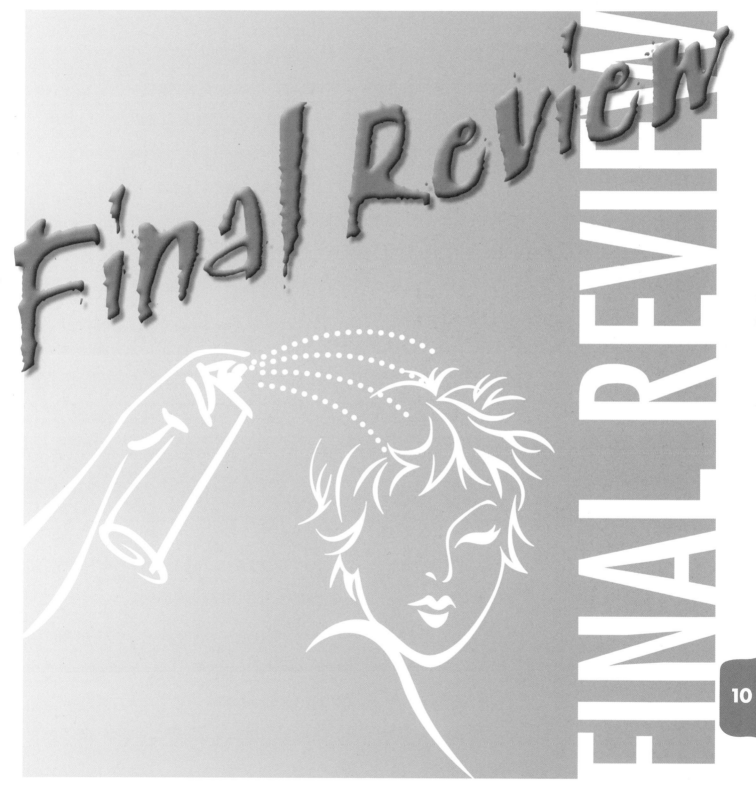

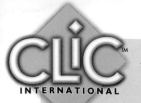
MATCHING

A.	Acceleration
B.	Artistry
C.	Brushing
D.	Coarse
E.	Composition
F.	Contrast
G.	Density
H.	Design Comb
I.	Direction
J.	Electric Iron
K.	Interlocked
L.	Lines
M.	Mannequin
N.	Ovaloid
O.	Ridge
P.	Synthetic
Q.	Triangle
R.	Value
S.	Volume
T.	Whorl

_____ 1. The raised section of a wave.

_____ 2. The arrangement of components to create a finished hairstyle.

_____ 3. Imaginative skill or ability in arrangement or execution.

_____ 4. The most perfect shape in hairdesign, with a naturally strong base.

_____ 5. Three-dimensional head forms used to perfect hairdesign skills.

_____ 6. The rate in which line, movement, wave or curl increases.

_____ 7. A circular pattern of follicles found at the crown or hairline.

_____ 8. Stimulates blood flow to the scalp and nourishes the hair.

_____ 9. Temporarily curls, waves, straightens and shines hair of any texture.

_____ 10. Used to sketch and distribute a two-dimensional design into the hair or comb finished hairdesigns.

_____ 11. The amount of follicles and hair per square inch.

_____ 12. The amount of light or darkness in the tone of a color.

_____ 13. Occurs when two or more opposing colors are placed close to each other within a hairdesign.

_____ 14. Hair that tends to have a thicker texture and larger diameter.

_____ 15. Placement creating fullness or lift in the hairdesign.

_____ 16. Created by shifting points in a straight or curved direction.

_____ 17. This shape placed in alternating directions creates a finger wave.

_____ 18. A type of hair additions fiber that should NOT be styled with heat.

_____ 19. Created by joining straight or curved lines within a hairdesign.

_____ 20. Lacing technique that joins hair from one section into the next.

10

STUDENT'S NAME   DATE   GRADE

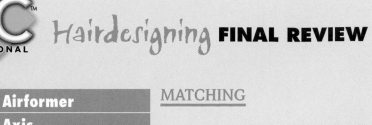
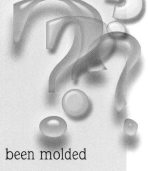

A.	**Airformer**
B.	**Axis**
C.	**Compact**
D.	**Concave**
E.	**Conical**
F.	**Curl**
G.	**Decelerated**
H.	**Double Prong Clips**
I.	**Eyes**
J.	**Fixative**
K.	**Keratin**
L.	**Mannequin Stand**
M.	**Natural Part**
N.	**On Base**
O.	**Oval**
P.	**Pressing Comb**
Q.	**Subsections**
R.	**Vertical**
S.	**Wet**
T.	**Zigzag**

<u>MATCHING</u>

_____ 1. A circle at the ends of the hair.

_____ 2. The type of memory achieved when hair has been molded into a specific design.

_____ 3. Dries hair by reforming hydrogen bonds, broken while the hair was being shampooed.

_____ 4. A paper neck strip may be used to temperature test this tool.

_____ 5. Used to secure roller and pin curl settings.

_____ 6. Holds a model head form while stylists practice or demonstrate hairdesigning.

_____ 7. A styling tool used for maximum hold and control.

_____ 8. This face shape has an ideally balanced vertical and horizontal proportion for hairdesigning.

_____ 9. A visible line on the scalp with growth patterns of the hair falling on either side.

_____ 10. Type of parting that creates drama and interest.

_____ 11. Most expressive facial feature, and often the focal point of the overall hairdesign.

_____ 12. Protein from which the hair is formed.

_____ 13. The tempo of straight hair.

_____ 14. Lines that create the illusion of length or height.

_____ 15. Created by dividing sections into smaller areas.

_____ 16. Placement creating maximum volume with no stem mobility.

_____ 17. Type of roller always fastened at the smaller end.

_____ 18. A base placement that creates closeness or indentation.

_____ 19. A fixed point of reference from which a body or geometric shape rotates.

_____ 20. Lacing technique that creates the most volume.

10

MULTIPLE CHOICE

1. Five chemical elements present in the hair are carbon, oxygen, hydrogen, nitrogen and:
   A. Sodium   B. Sulfur   C. Calcium   D. Keratin

2. The three layers of the hair are called the cuticle, medulla, and:
   A. Cortex   B. Follicle   C. Papilla   D. Root

3. Five basic styling elements utilized in hairdesigning are space, color, texture, line and:
   A. Balance   B. Proportion   C. Emphasis   D. Form

4. This factor, plus the diameter of the small end of a conical roller, determines the size of a circle shaping.
   A. Hair density   B. Color   C. Length   D. Shape

5. The five straight geometric shapes are triangle, kite, rectangle, square and:
   A. Circle   B. Diamond   C. Ovaloid   D. Line

6. When creating a design with indentation (concave) movement, the ends turn:
   A. Down   B. Sideways   C. Up   D. Under

7. Which pin curl stem placement creates maximum movement with the least amount of curl?
   A. Full stem   B. No stem   C. Half stem   D. Off base

8. When airforming, a stylist's elbows are extended outward with the air flow directed:
   A. Forward   B. Inward   C. Outward   D. Upward

9. What factor does NOT help determine the amount of curl produced in a hairdesign?
   A. Heredity   B. Hair length   C. Tool diameter   D. Wrap technique

10. What is achieved by relaxing the dry form with a brush?
    A. Shaping   B. Sculpting   C. Scaling   D. Directional memory

11. The four senses stylists use in hairdesigning are sight, hearing, touch and:
    A. Intuitive   B. Smell   C. Taste   D. Common

12. A hairdesign that coordinates well with a client's dramatic fashion personality.
    A. Elegant   B. Soft curls   C. Uncomplicated   D. Angular

13. The three parts of a pin curl are the base, stem, and:
    A. Curl   B. Parting   C. Scale   D. Clip

14. Mesomorph, Endomorph, and Ectomorph are the three major body:
    A. Tissues   B. Functions   C. Types   D. Parts

15. The facial shape with a narrow forehead and jaw.
    A. Diamond   B. Circle   C. Oblong   D. Pear

16. The three French lacing techniques are compact, interlocked and:
    A. Cushioning   B. Directional   C. Backcombing   D. Applied

17. The three curvature shapes are circle, oval, and:
    A. Oblong   B. Ovaloid   C. Pear   D. Inverted triangle

18. Three scientific influences that control the physical properties of hair are energy, tempo and:
    A. Mass   B. Balance   C. Rotation   D. Force

19. Motion is the action of movement, direction or:
    A. Energy   B. Force   C. Speed   D. Distance

20. The second stage in the chronological order of a hairdesign, where the hair is proportioned into distinct areas.
    A. Sculpt   B. Set   C. Sketch   D. Scale

10

STUDENT'S NAME   DATE   GRADE

A.	Allergy
B.	Asymmetry
C.	Balance
D.	Concentration
E.	Cortex
F.	Curved
G.	Cuticle
H.	Elevation
I.	Emphasis
J.	Follicle
K.	Force
L.	Full Over-directed
M.	Hair Root
N.	Half Over-directed
O.	Hollow
P.	Ornamentation
Q.	Papilla
R.	Part
S.	Rectangle
T.	Sections

MATCHING

_____ 1. Used as an element within a hairdesign to divide the head.

_____ 2. Portion of hair below the scalp.

_____ 3. Layer providing hair's elasticity and the pigment melanin.

_____ 4. A 10-degree placement, secured above the top parting.

_____ 5. Geometric shapes placed on various areas of the head.

_____ 6. Height or angle the hair is lifted off of the scalp.

_____ 7. Concave (indentation) ovaloid section directly under the ridge.

_____ 8. A facial shape that is longer than it is wide.

_____ 9. Receives the blood supply and stimulates hair growth.

_____ 10. Causes the immune system to overreact to a normally harmless substance.

_____ 11. Lines that create movement and waves.

_____ 12. Overall thickness of hair, determined by diameter, density and distribution.

_____ 13. Cavity that contains the hair root.

_____ 14. Visual comparison of weight used to offset or equalize proportion.

_____ 15. Protective hair layer, responsible for sheen and porosity.

_____ 16. Visual weights in hairdesign which are unequal and/or placed at different distances from the axis.

_____ 17. Also referred to as a focal point or the heart of interest.

_____ 18. A 30-degree angle above the base, secured on the top parting.

_____ 19. Decorative items in fashion and hairdesign used to attract the eye and create interest.

_____ 20. How far hair must travel and the momentum that it takes to get there.

10

STUDENT'S NAME   DATE   GRADE

MULTIPLE CHOICE

1. During the consultation with a client in a wheelchair, sit at:
    A. A mirror
    B. The reception Area
    C. Eye level
    D. A private room

2. Sensation experienced when light of varying wave lengths reaches the eye.
    A. Kinesthetic
    B. Visual
    C. Auditory
    D. Primitive

3. Hairdesigns with soft lines fit this fashion personality best.
    A. Classic
    B. Sporty
    C. Romantic
    D. Dramatic

4. A rounded body type with short limbs.
    A. Endomorph
    B. Ectomorph
    C. Mesomorph
    D. Androgynous

5. Lined pouches are used to store hot:
    A. Towels
    B. Solutions
    C. Photos
    D. Thermal equipment

6. Aqueous solution into which hair tools are submerged after each use.
    A. Wet sanitizer
    B. Developer
    C. Shampoo cap
    D. Smoothing lotion

7. At what angle is the hair held for an indentation half under-directed base placement?
    A. 30-degree
    B. 45-degree
    C. 90-degree
    D. 15-degree

8. Used to thank the client for a referral or remember a special event.
    A. Stylists
    B. Gift certificates
    C. Managers
    D. Client record cards

9. A three-dimensional design has length, width and:
    A. Depth
    B. Texture
    C. Color
    D. Space

10. Using correct body posture communicates confidence and helps prevent:
    A. Injury
    B. Errors
    C. Relaxation
    D. Interruption

11. Profile having a protruding chin and forehead, giving the impression of a receding nose.
    A. Converse
    B. Convex
    C. Concave
    D. Straight

12. Fine, medium, and coarse are descriptions of hair:
    A. Density
    B. Distribution
    C. Diameter
    D. Tempo

13. Type of part that should NOT be placed on a client with a prominent nose.
    A. Center
    B. Side
    C. Diagonal
    D. Curved

14. The primary function of a flat iron.
    A. Straighten
    B. Color
    C. Condition
    D. Crimp

15. Effect of a natural boar bristle round brush on the hair.
    A. Polishes
    B. Tangles
    C. Damages
    D. Straightens

16. Tool used to disperse airflow in multiple directions.
    A. Airformer
    B. Diffuser
    C. Concentrator
    D. Soft bonnet

17. Position hair is held in relation to the scalp to produce indentation.
    A. Away
    B. Angled
    C. Close
    D. Below

18. Angle used for a volume full under-directed base placement.
    A. 10-degree
    B. 90-degree
    C. 45-degree
    D. 30-degree

19. Redirecting the eye away from an undesirable area to a more pleasing one.
    A. Emphasis
    B. Diversion
    C. Illusion
    D. Movement

20. Describes curls formed against the direction that hands move on a timepiece.
    A. Clockwise
    B. Rotational
    C. Spiral
    D. Counter-clockwise

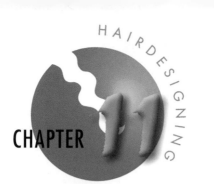

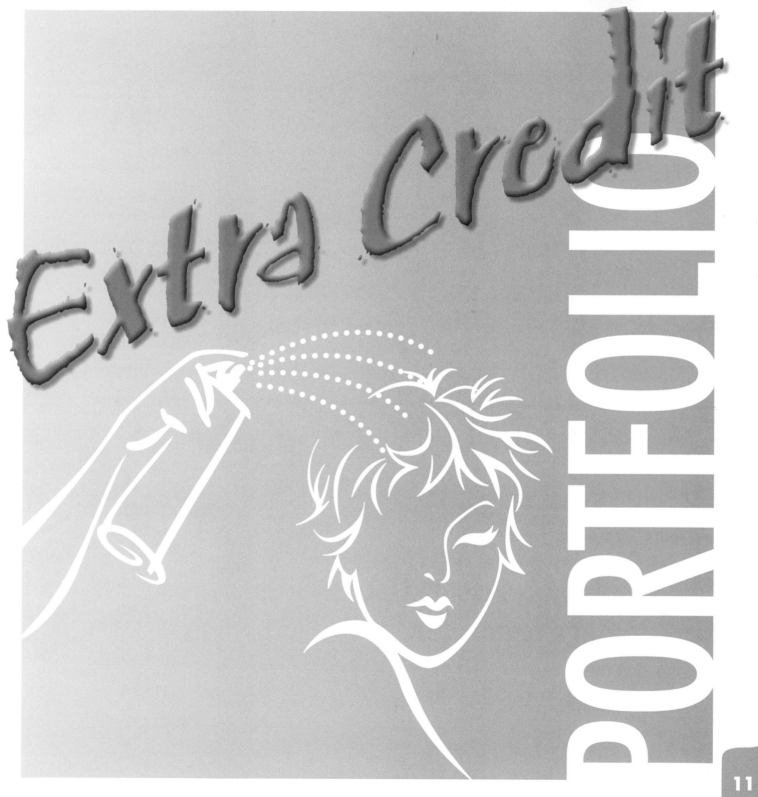

Extra Credit

PORTFOLIO

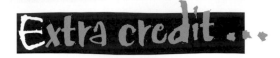

The following Extra Credit pages will help you create your own portfolio.

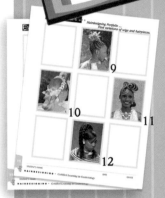

- Find pictures in magazines showing variations of the hairstyles pictured on the following pages.

- Attach your pictures in the open frames.

- Remove the pages and place in a 3-ring binder.

- Your first portfolio is ready to show the guests you service and should be updated as you learn more complex hairdesigns.

As you move from your student portfolio to a professional portfolio, you will showcase the hairdesigns you have created. Purchase a portfolio case with individual acetate sleeves and insert 8" x 10" photographs (color or black and white) of your hairdesigns.

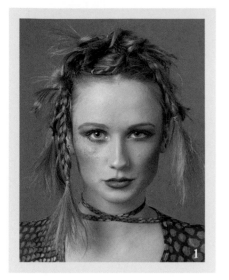

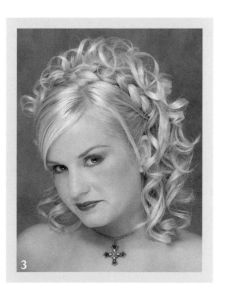

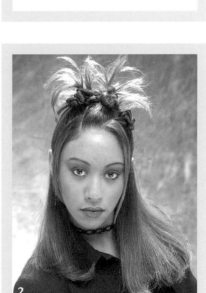

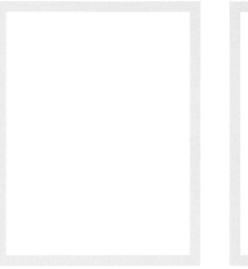

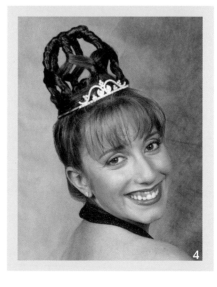

STUDENT'S NAME   DATE   GRADE

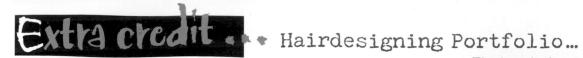
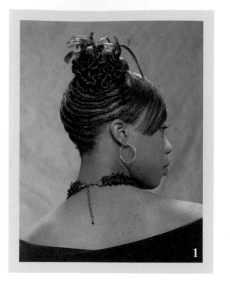

1

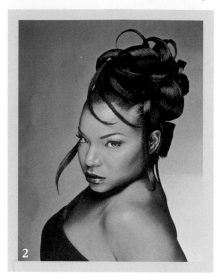

2

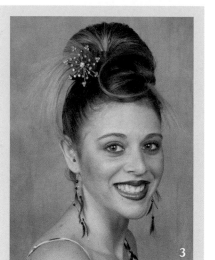

3

4

11

STUDENT'S NAME   DATE   GRADE

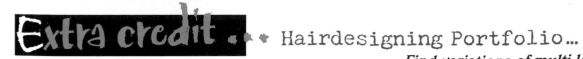
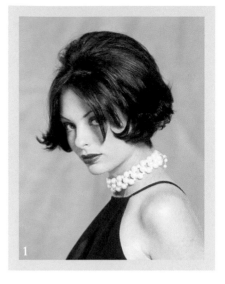

1

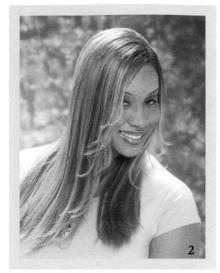

2

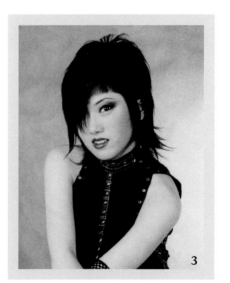

3

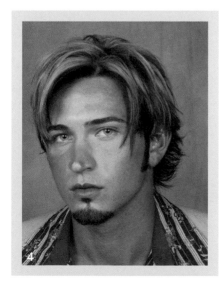

4

STUDENT'S NAME   DATE   GRADE

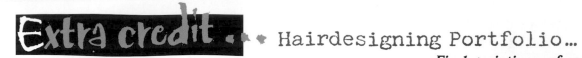
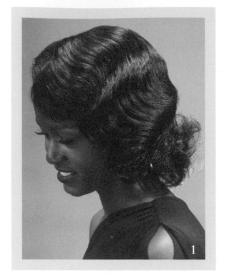

1

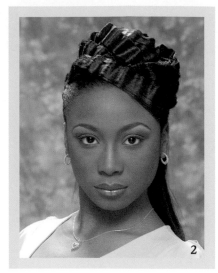

2

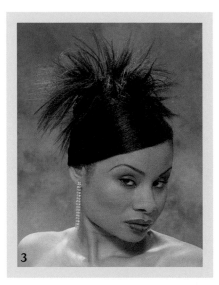

3

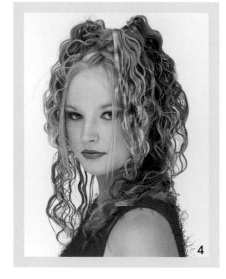

4

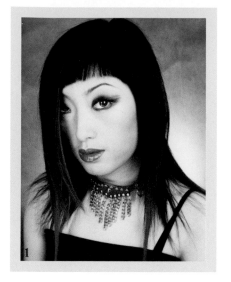

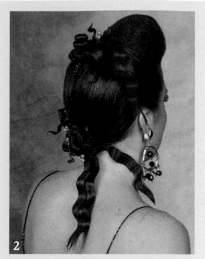

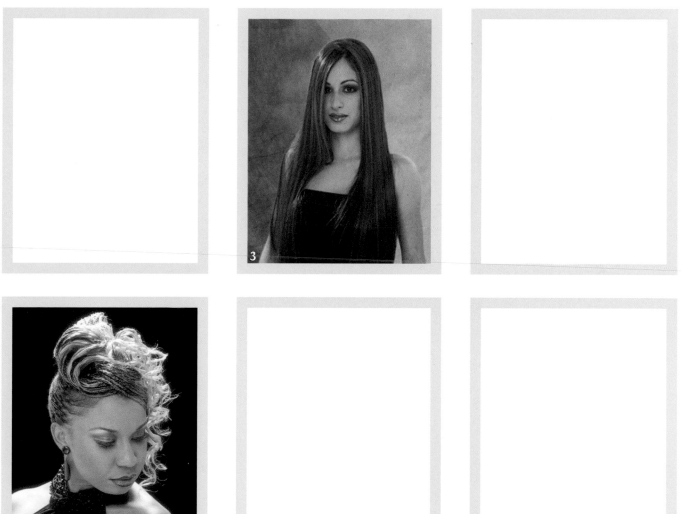

STUDENT'S NAME

DATE   GRADE

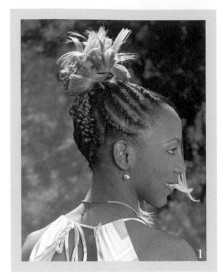

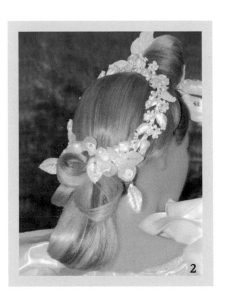

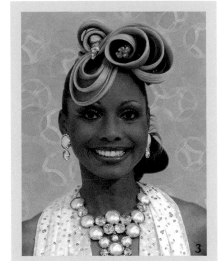

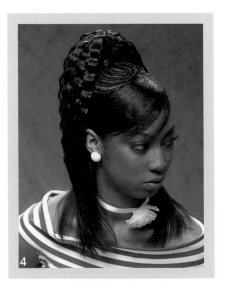

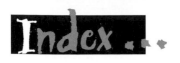

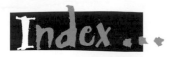

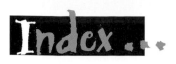

Index...

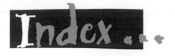

CLiC Classmates Sign In...

School _____   Class of _____

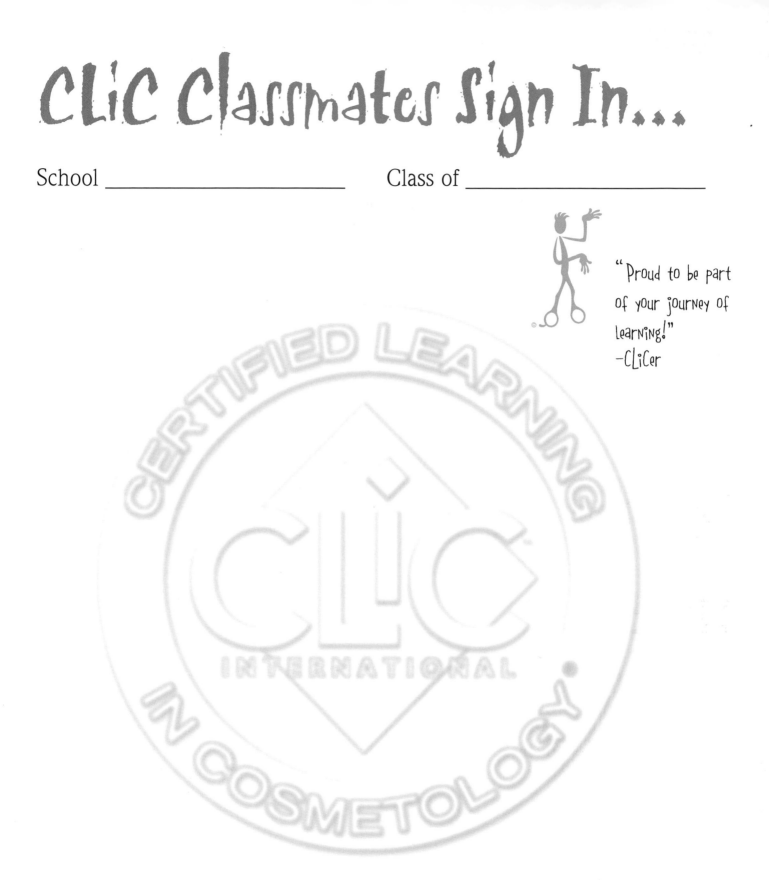

"Proud to be part of your journey of learning!"
—CLiCer

Thank you for joining our professional team of great hairdesigners!

 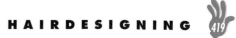

National certification makes the difference in career success...

CONGRATULATIONS!

Now that you have completed your journey through the **Hairdesigning** module, you are ready to take the Student Certification Exam. With a passing grade, you will receive official certification documenting that you have mastered the skills presented in the **Hairdesigning** module.

As you continue on your journey through each of the **CLiC** learning modules, you will receive a certificate for each module completed successfully. After completing all modules with passing grades, you will receive a **CLiC** masters certification award.

Best of success to you!

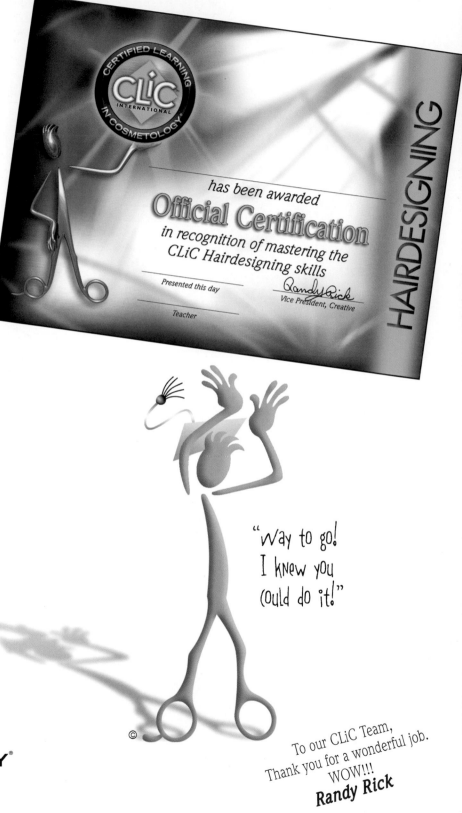

For more information call:
CLiC INTERNATIONAL®
1.800.207.5400
info@clicusa.com

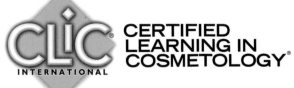

CLiC
INTERNATIONAL

**CERTIFIED
LEARNING IN
COSMETOLOGY**®

"Way to go!
I knew you
could do it!"

To our CLiC Team,
Thank you for a wonderful job.
WOW!!!
Randy Rick